Williams & Wilkins'

DENTAL HYGIENE
HANDBOOK

*This book is dedicated to my friends, colleagues, and staff
of the American Dental Hygienists' Association,
my teachers and mentors,
Phyllis Beemsterboer and Ulla Lemborn,
and my daughter, Beverly A. Cornell, R.D.H.,
who have given me the opportunities
and inspiration for all things possible.*

PREFACE

This book is intended for dental hygienists who have been in practice for several years. It is intended as a resource and reference guide to help the practitioner review processes and protocols as needed. The text considers the foundation knowledge attained through the dental hygiene education process and work experience and provides information relevant to that knowledge. The format is in the form of tables that facilitate reference to specific areas of care.

AUTHOR'S NOTE

The word "patient" is used in the text; I prefer the word "client" because I believe it better describes the relationship between the practitioner and the consumer of our services. It is a relationship that assumes both participants are working together toward a mutual goal of optimum oral health, not one of unequal individuals, one dominant and one passive. Reviewers and the publisher did not want the word substituted. I have acquiesced to their wishes.

ACKNOWLEDGMENTS

A sincere debt of gratitude is owed by this author and the dental hygiene profession to Esther M. Wilkins. Her extensive research, work, and continuous support of the profession is phenomenal. Esther is a "living treasure" to dental hygienists the world over—a role model and mentor to so many of us. Thank you.

To my husband, Richard, I thank you for all your support and encouragement and for putting up with the countless hours, days, and years spent, working into the "wee hours," for the profession. You are always there for me with patience and love.

To John L. Vicelja, D.D.S., and Vickie Sansom, we have shared so much through the years together and you have always been so supportive of all my endeavors. Thank you so much.

CONTENTS

INFECTION CONTROL RECOMMENDATIONS FOR THE DENTAL OFFICE AND THE DENTAL LABORATORY

Dental professionals are exposed to a wide variety of microorganisms in the blood and saliva of patients. These microorganisms may cause infectious diseases such as the common cold, pneumonia, tuberculosis, herpes, hepatitis B, and acquired immune deficiency syndrome (AIDS). The use of effective infection control procedures and universal precautions in the dental office and the dental laboratory will prevent cross contamination that could extend to dentists, dental office staff, dental technicians, and patients.

The American Dental Association has advocated the use of infection control procedures in the dental practice for many years.[1-4] As new information has become available, the Association has disseminated it to the profession and will continue to do so. Currently available Association publications that provide detailed information about infection control and treatment of patients with infectious diseases are: *Facts about AIDS for the Dental Team*,[5] *Monograph on Safety and Infection Control*,[6] *Infection Control in the Dental Environment*,[7] and now this report. The Association has also provided *The American Dental Association Regulatory Compliance Manual*,[8] and a videotape entitled *OSHA: What You Must Know*,[9] both designed to help dentists come into compliance with OSHA's Standards on Occupational Exposure to Bloodborne Pathogens and Hazard Communication.

This report is based on the recommendations of the Centers for Disease Control (CDC)[10-12] and other publications in the medical and dental literature. The recommendations in this document have been accepted by the Council on Dental Materials, Instruments and Equipment, the Council on Dental Therapeutics, the Council on Dental Research, and the Council on Dental Practice. The Councils strongly urge practitioners and dental laboratories to comply with these infection control practices. With the enactment of the OSHA Standard on Occupational Exposure to Bloodborne Pathogens in December 1991,[13] many of these infection control procedures are now required by law.

Dentists should recognize *an important distinction* between OSHA requirements and acceptable infection control practices. OSHA has a Congressional mandate to institute work place procedures which protect the *employee,* and, by law, is able to write regulations and enter the work place to conduct inspections and impose financial penalties. The 1991 OSHA Standard on Occupational Exposure to Bloodborne Pathogens is thus written to protect employees. OSHA does *not* have the mandate to institute practices which protect the *patient* or the *employer.* The OSHA Standard, although providing some patient and employer protection, does not encompass all the infection control practices recommended by the U.S. Public Health Service (Centers for Disease Control) and the American Dental Association to protect patients, employees, and employers from occupational transmission of infectious disease. Conversely, it is also important to note that OSHA has many requirements in the Bloodborne Pathogen Standard that neither the U.S. Public Health Service nor the Association include in their infection control recommendations (eg, where contaminated laundry should be done, the requirement to retain an employee's medical records for the duration of employment plus 30 years, the requirement that the employer pay for hepatitis B vaccination and for medical follow-up after an exposure incident).

Therefore, although dentists have a legal requirement to comply with the OSHA Standard, the Association believes that they should also be aware of and practice proper infection control procedures designed for the safety of everyone. These infection control procedures are detailed in this report, and, also, in various publications from the CDC and ADA referenced at the end of this report. Since this document is not intended to cover every aspect of infection control compliance, the dentist, his or her staff and that of dental laboratories should refer to the referenced publications.[2,4,10]

PREVENTION OF TRANSMISSION OF INFECTIOUS DISEASES

It is generally accepted that the dental health team is far more at risk to the hepatitis B virus (HBV) than to the human immunodeficiency virus (HIV) that causes AIDS. However, because of increasing acceptance of the HBV vaccine among practicing dentists in recent years (75%, Health Screening Data, 1991), the risk for HBV infection is generally limited to those who have not been vaccinated. Patients with hepatitis B or who are HBV carriers can be treated safely or with minimal risk of transmission of disease in the dental office when infection control procedures are used. As HIV appears to be much more difficult to transmit than HBV, there is confidence that the same procedures will prevent the transmission of HIV in the dental office.[14–15]

VACCINATION AGAINST HEPATITIS B

Dental health care workers are at a greater risk than the general population for acquiring hepatitis B through contact with patients. It is the policy of the ADA that all dentists and their staffs having patient contact should be vaccinated against hepatitis B.[16] The OSHA Standard now requires that employers make the hepatitis B vaccine available to occupationally exposed employees, at the employer's expense, within 10 working days of assignment of tasks that may result in exposure.[13]

INFECTION CONTROL PRACTICES FOR THE DENTAL OFFICE

Universal precautions

A thorough medical history should be obtained for all patients at the first visit and updated and reviewed at subsequent visits. However, since not all patients with infectious diseases can be identified by medical history, physical examination, or readily available laboratory tests, the CDC has introduced the concept of universal precautions.[17] This term refers to a method of infection control in which all human blood and certain human body fluids (saliva in dentistry) are treated as if known to be infectious for HIV, HBV, and other bloodborne pathogens. Universal precautions means that the same infection control procedures are used for all patients.

BARRIER TECHNIQUES

Gloves. Gloves must be worn when skin contact with body fluids or mucous membranes is anticipated, or when touching items or surfaces that may be contaminated with these fluids. After contact with each patient, gloves must be removed, hands must be washed, and then regloved before treating another patient. Repeated use of a single pair of gloves by disinfecting

xvi   The Williams & Wilkins' Dental Hygiene Handbook

them between patients is not acceptable. Exposure to disinfectants or other chemicals often causes defects in gloves, thereby diminishing their value as effective barriers.[18] Latex or vinyl gloves should be used for patient examinations and procedures. Heavy rubber gloves, also called utility gloves, should preferably be used for cleaning instruments and environmental surfaces. Dentists should be aware that allergic reactions to latex gloves or the cornstarch powder in gloves have been reported in health care workers and patients.[19–20] To reduce the possibility of such reactions, nylon glove liners for use under latex, rubber or plastic gloves are available. Polyethylene gloves, also known as food-handlers' gloves, may be worn over treatment gloves to prevent contamination of objects such as drawer or light handles or charts.

Protective clothing. Gowns, aprons, lab coats, clinic jackets, or similar outer garments, either reusable or disposable, must be worn when clothing or skin is likely to be exposed to body fluids. Professional judgment should be used to determine the degree of exposure anticipated in a given procedure. Protective clothing should be changed when visibly soiled or penetrated by fluids. OSHA requires that these garments not be worn outside the work area and that protective attire be removed and placed in laundry bags or containers that are properly marked after use. Contaminated articles should be laundered in a normal laundry cycle.[11]

Masks. Surgical masks or chin-length plastic face shields must be worn to protect the face, the oral mucosa, and the nasal mucosa when spatter of body fluids is anticipated. Masks should be changed when visibly soiled or wet. Face shields should be cleaned when necessary.

Protective eyewear. Protective eyewear in combination with a mask must be worn to protect the eyes when spatter and splash of body fluids is anticipated and a face shield is not chosen. The OSHA Standard specifies that protective eyewear be fitted with solid side shields.[13] Eyewear should be cleaned as necessary.

LIMITING CONTAMINATION

Three principal means of limiting contamination by droplets and spatter are the use of high-volume evacuation, proper patient positioning, and rubber dam. Dental personnel should also limit contamination by avoiding contact with objects such as charts, telephones, and cabinets during patient treatment procedures. A second pair of disposable gloves, such as foodhandlers' gloves, or a sheet of plastic wrap or foil may be used over gloves when it is necessary to prevent contamination of these objects.

HANDS

Handwashing. Hands must always be washed at the start of each day, before gloving, after removal of gloves, and after touching inanimate objects likely to be contaminated by body fluids from patients. For many routine dental procedures, such as examinations and nonsurgical procedures, handwashing with plain soap appears to be adequate, since soap and water will remove transient microorganisms acquired directly or indirectly from patient contact. For surgical procedures, an antimicrobial surgical handscrub should be used.[7] Hand washing facilities should be designed to avoid cross contamination at the scrub sink from water valve handles and soap dispensers.

Care of hands. Precautions should be taken to avoid hand injuries during procedures. If an injury, such as a needlestick, occurs or gloves are torn, cut, or punctured, gloves should be removed as soon as is compatible with the patient's safety. Hands should be washed thoroughly and regloved before completing the dental procedure.

HANDLING OF SHARP INSTRUMENTS AND NEEDLES

Needles, scalpel blades, and other sharp instruments should be handled carefully to prevent injuries. Syringe needles may be recapped after they are used. If a patient requires multiple injections over time from a single syringe, then the needle should be recapped between each use to avoid the possibility of a needlestick injury. Needles can be safely recapped by placing the cap in a special holder, by using a forceps or other appropriate instrument to grasp the cap, or by simply laying the cap on the instrument tray and then guiding the needle into the cap until the cap can be completely seated. Therefore, when recapping, the cap must not be held in the operator's hand as this poses a great risk of needlestick injury.

Disposable needles should not be bent or broken after use. Needles should not be removed manually from disposable syringes or otherwise handled manually. Forceps or other appropriate instruments may be used to handle sharp items. Disposable syringes, needles, scalpel blades, and other sharp items should be discarded into puncture-resistant biohazard (sharps) containers that are easily accessible.

STERILIZATION AND DISINFECTION

Sterilization is the process by which all forms of microorganisms are destroyed, including viruses, bacteria, fungi, and spores. Although methods of sterilization include the use of steam under pressure (autoclave), dry heat, chemical vapor, ethylene oxide gas, or immersion in chemical sterilant solutions, the use of the latter is discouraged. Immersion in a chemical sterilant solution instead of the use of physical means of sterilization is not recommended for several reasons: sterilization by chemical solutions cannot be monitored biologically; instruments sterilized by chemical solutions must be handled aseptically, rinsed in sterile water, and dried with sterile towels; and instruments sterilized by chemical solutions are not wrapped and, therefore, must be used immediately or stored in a sterile container.

Disinfection is generally less lethal to pathogenic organisms than sterilization. The disinfection process leads to a reduction in the level of microbial contamination and covers, depending on the disinfectant used and treatment time, a broad range of activity that may extend from sterility at one extreme to a minimal reduction in microbial contamination at the other.[21] Disinfection may be accomplished by using a chemical disinfectant according to the directions on the product label. When chemical solutions are used for disinfection, manufacturers' instructions must be followed carefully. Particular attention should be given to dilution requirements (if any), contact time, temperature requirements, antimicrobial activity spectrum and reuse life. A chemical agent for disinfection (other than sodium hypochlorite) in the dental setting must be registered by the Environmental Protection Agency (EPA) as a hospital disinfectant, and must be tuberculocidal. Virucidal efficacy must include, as a minimum, both lipophilic and hydrophilic viruses.

Table 1 summarizes appropriate sterilization and disinfection methods for dental instruments, materials, and other commonly used items. Consideration should be given to the effect of sterilization or disinfection on materials and instruments. The use of a rust inhibitor solution on instruments prior to autoclaving can be helpful in avoiding corrosion problems. Manufacturers should be consulted on appropriate sterilization or disinfection of specific products.

Instruments and equipment. Surgical and other instruments that normally penetrate soft tissue or bone (eg, forceps, scalpels, bone chisels, scalers, and surgical burs) must be sterilized after each use or discarded. Instruments that are not intended to penetrate oral soft tissues or bone (eg, amalgam condensers, and plastic instruments), but that may come into contact with oral tissues should also be sterilized after each use. Some plastic instruments will not withstand sterilization and should be discarded after each patient. Instruments that are metal or heat-stable should be sterilized between use by steam under pressure (autoclave), dry heat, or chemical vapor. If instruments are to be stored after sterilization, they should be wrapped or bagged before sterilizing, using a suitable wrap material such as muslin, clear pouches, or paper as recommended by the manufacturer of the sterilizer. The wrap or bag should be sealed with appropriate tape. Pins, staples, or paper clips should not be used as these make holes in the wrap that permit entry of microorganisms. After sterilization, the instruments should be stored in the sealed packages until they are used. Process indicators should be used with each load. Biological monitors should be used routinely to verify the adequacy of sterilization cycles. Weekly verification should be adequate for most dental practices.[10,22] Instruments that are not heat stable should be sterilized by immersion for 6 to 10 hours, in an EPA-registered chemical sterilant, according to manufacturers' instructions.

Instruments and equipment that come in contact with intact skin, that may be exposed to spatter or spray of body fluids, or that may have been touched by contaminated hands (eg, physical measurement devices, amalgamators) should be disinfected.

Instruments and equipment intended for sterilization or disinfection procedures must first be carefully prepared. Patient

TABLE 1.   Sterilization and Disinfection of Dental Instruments, Materials, and Some Commonly Used Items*

	Steam Autoclave	Dry Heat Oven	Chemical Vapor	Ethylene Oxide	Chemical Agents	Other Methods & Comments
Angle attachments*	+	+	+	++	+	
Burs						
Carbon steel	-	++	++	++	-	Discard
Steel	+	++	++	++	-	Discard
Tungston-carbide	+	++	++	++	-	Discard
Condensers	++	++	++	++	+	
Dapen dishes	++	+	+	++	+	
Endodontic instruments (broaches, files, reamers)	++	++	++	++	-	
Stainless steel handles	+	++	++	++	+	
Stainless w/plastic handles	++	++	-	++	-	
Fluoride gel trays						
Heat-resistant plastic	++	=	-	++	+	
Nonheat resistant plastic	=	=	-	++	-	Discard (++)
Glass slabs	++	++	++	++	+	
Hand instruments						
Carbon steel	-	++	++	++	-	

continued

		[Steam autoclave with chemical protection (2% sodium nitrite)]			
Stainless steel	++*	++	++	++		
Handpieces*	(++)*	–	(+)*	++		Discard (++)
Contra-angles	++	–	++	++		
Prophylaxis angles* (disposable preferred)	+	+	+	+		Discard
Impression trays						
Aluminum metal	++	+	++	++	–	
Chrome-plated	++	++	++	++	+	
Custom acrylic resin	=	=	=	++	+	Discard (++)
Plastic	=	=	++	++	=	Discard (++) preferred
Instruments in packs	++	Small packs	++	Small packs		
Instrument tray setups						
Restorative or surgical	Size limit	+	Size limit	++	=	
Mirrors	–	++	++	++	+	
Needles						Discard (++)
Disposable	=	=	=	=	=	Do not reuse

continued

TABLE 1.   Sterilization and Disinfection of Dental Instruments, Materials, and Some Commonly Used Items*

	Steam Autoclave	Dry Heat Oven	Chemical Vapor	Ethylene Oxide	Chemical Agents	Other Methods & Comments
Nitrous oxide						
Nose piece	(++)*	=	(++)*	++	(+)*	
Hoses	(++)*	=	(++)*	++	(+)*	
Orthodontic pliers						
High-quality stainless	++	++	++	++	-	
Low-quality stainless	-	++	++	++	-	
W/plastic parts	=	=	=	++	+	
Pluggers & Condensers	++	++	++	++	+	
Polishing wheels & disks						
Garnet and cuttle	=	-	-	++	=	
Rag	++	-	+	++	=	
Rubber	+	-	-	++	+	
Prostheses, removable	-	-	-	+	+	
Rubber dam equipment						
Carbon steel clamps	-	++	++	++	-	
Metal frames	++	++	++	++	+	
Plastic frames	-	-	-	++	+	

continued

	1	2	3	4	5	
Punches	–	++	++	++	+	
Stainless steel clamps	++	++	++	++	+	
Rubber items						
Prophylaxis cups	–	–	–	++	–	Discard (++)
Saliva evacuators, ejectors (plastic)	–	–	–	–		Discard (++) (single use/disposable)
Stones						
Diamond	+	+	++	++	–	
Polishing	++	+	++	++	–	
Sharpening	++	++	++	–	–	
Surgical instruments						
Stainless steel	++	++	++	++	–	
Ultrasonic scaling tips	+	=	=	++	+	
Water-air syringe tips	++	++	++	++	–	Discard (++)
X-ray equipment						
Plastic film holders	(++)*	=	(+)*	++	+	
Collimating devices	–	=	=	++	+	

++ Effective and preferred method.

+ Effective and acceptable method.

– Effective method, but risk of damage to materials.

= Ineffective method with risk of damage to materials.

* Since manufacturers use a variety of alloys and materials in these products, confirmation with the equipment manufacturers is recommended, especially for handpieces and their attachments.

debris and body fluids must be removed from the instruments and surfaces before sterilization or disinfection. This can be done by scrubbing the instruments with hot water and soap or detergent or by using a device such as an ultrasonic cleaner with an appropriate cleaning solution. After cleaning, the instruments should be dried before being wrapped or packaged, especially if dry heat or ethylene oxide sterilization is to be used. Dental personnel responsible for handling instruments should wear heavy-duty utility gloves to prevent hand injuries.

Handpieces. Although no documented cases of disease transmission have been associated with dental handpieces or prophy angles, sterilization between patients with acceptable methods which assure internal as well as external sterility is recommended. Disposable prophy angles are available and are to be discarded after one time use. The manufacturers' instructions must be followed for proper sterilization of handpieces and prophy angles and for the use and maintenance of waterlines and check valves. The first step, before sterilization, is to flush the handpiece with water by running it for 20 to 30 seconds, discharging the water into a sink or container. An ultrasonic cleaner should be used to remove any adherent material, but only if recommended by the handpiece manufacturer. Otherwise, the handpiece should be scrubbed thoroughly with a detergent and hot water. Many manufacturers recommend spraying a cleaner/lubricant into the assembled handpiece before and after sterilization. If in doubt as to whether a handpiece can be sterilized, contact the manufacturer. Some manufacturers will replace the handpiece components that cannot be sterilized, making the handpiece sterilizable. This is often automatically done when a handpiece is serviced.

Air/water syringes and ultrasonic scalers. Units should be flushed as described for handpieces. These attachments should be sterilized in the same manner as the handpieces, or in accordance with manufacturers' instructions. It is recommended that removable or disposable tips used only one time for one patient be used for these instruments.

X-ray equipment and films. Protective coverings or disinfectants should be used to prevent microbial contamination of position, indicating devices. Intraorally contaminated film packets should be handled in a manner to prevent cross contamination. Contaminated packets should be opened in the darkroom, using disposable gloves. The films should be dropped out of the packets without touching the films. The contaminated packets should be accumulated in a disposable towel. After all packets have been opened, they should be discarded and the gloves removed. The films can then be processed without contaminating darkroom equipment with microorganisms from the patient.[23] Alternatively, film packets can be placed in protective pouches before use. The uncontaminated packets can then be dropped out of the pouches before processing.

Operatory surfaces. Countertops and dental equipment surfaces such as light handles, X-ray unit heads, amalgamators, cabinet and drawer pulls, tray tables, and chair switches are likely to become contaminated with potentially infectious materials during treatment procedures. These surfaces can be either covered or disinfected. Surfaces can be covered with plastic wrap, aluminum foil, or impervious-backed absorbent paper. These protective coverings should be changed between patients, and when contaminated.

Alternatively, surfaces can be precleaned to remove extraneous organic matter and then disinfected with an EPA-registered disinfectant that is tuberculocidal following manufacturers' instructions. These include certain combination synthetic phenolics and iodophors, phenolic-alcohol combinations, and chlorine compounds. A solution of sodium hypochlorite (household bleach) prepared fresh daily is an effective germicide. Concentrations of sodium hypochlorite ranging from 5,000 ppm to 500 ppm, achieved by diluting household bleach in a ratio ranging from 1:10 to 1:100, is effective, depending on the amount of organic matter (blood and mucus) present on the surface to be cleaned and disinfected. Sodium hypochlorite should be used with caution because it is corrosive to some metals, especially aluminum. Corrosiveness is less of a problem with some commercial disinfectants. Glutaraldehydes of 2% and 3.2% strength are not suitable for this purpose. Surfaces should be disinfected between patients, and when they are visibly contaminated by splashes of body fluids.

Housekeeping surfaces, including floors, sinks, and related objects are not likely to be associated with the transmission of infection. Therefore, extraordinary attempts to disinfect these surfaces are not necessary. However, the removal of visible soil

TABLE 2. Disinfection of Prostheses, Casts, Wax Rims, Jaw Relation Records

Stone casts	Spray or immerse in hypochlorite or iodophor
Fixed (metal/porcelain)	Immerse in glutaraldehyde
Removable Dentures (acrylic/porcelain)	Immerse in iodophors or chlorine compounds
Removable Partials (metal/acrylic)	Immerse in iodophors or chlorine compounds
Wax rims/bites	Spray—wipe—spray with iodophors

and cleaning should be undertaken on a routine basis. Cleaners with germicidal activity may be used.

Impressions, prostheses, casts, wax rims, jaw relation records. Items such as impressions, jaw relation records, casts, prosthetic restorations and devices which have been in the patient's mouth should be properly disinfected prior to shipment to a dental laboratory (see Table 2). Disinfected impressions which are sent to the dental laboratory should be labeled as such in order to prevent duplication of the disinfection protocol.

Impressions must be rinsed to remove saliva, blood, and debris and then disinfected. Impressions can be disinfected by immersion in any compatible disinfecting product. Since the compatibility of an impression material with a disinfectant varies, the impression should be followed.[24] The use of disinfectants requiring times of no more than 30 minutes for disinfecting is recommended.

DISPOSAL OF WASTE MATERIALS

Disposable materials such as gloves, masks, wipes, paper drapes, and surface covers that are contaminated with body fluids should be carefully handled with gloves and discarded in sturdy, impervious plastic bags to minimize human contact. Blood, disinfectants, and sterilants may be carefully poured into a drain connected to a sanitary sewer system. Care should be taken to ensure compliance with applicable local regulations. It is recommended that drains be flushed or purged each night to reduce bacteria accumulation and growth. Sharp items, such as needles and scalpel blades, should be placed in puncture-resistant containers marked with the biohazard label. Human tissue may be handled in the same manner as sharp items, but should not be placed in the same container. Regulated medical waste (eg, sharps, tissues) should be disposed of according to the requirements established by local or state environmental regulatory agencies.

PRACTICES FOR THE DENTAL LABORATORY

Dental laboratories should institute appropriate infection control programs.[25] Such programs should be coordinated with the dental office.

Receiving area. A receiving area should be established separate from the production area. Countertops and work surfaces should be cleaned and then the area disinfected daily with an appropriate surface disinfectant used according to the manufacturer's directions.

Incoming cases. Unless the laboratory employee knows that the case has been disinfected by the dental office, all cases should be disinfected as they are received. Containers should be sterilized or disinfected after each use. Packing materials should be discarded to avoid cross contamination.

Disposal of waste materials. Solid waste that is soaked or saturated with body fluids should be placed in sealed, sturdy impervious bags. The bag should be disposed of following regulations established by local or state environmental agencies.

Production area. Persons working in the production area should wear a clean uniform or laboratory coat, a face mask, protective eyewear, and disposable gloves. Work surfaces and equipment should be kept free of debris and disinfected daily. Any instruments, attachments, and materials to be used with new prostheses/appliances should be maintained separately from those to be used with prostheses/appliances that have already been inserted in the mouth. Ragwheels can be washed and autoclaved after each case. Brushes and other equipment should be disinfected at least daily. A small amount of pumice should be dispensed in small disposable containers for individual use on each case. The excess should be discarded. A liquid disinfectant (1:20 sodium hypochlorite solution) can serve as a mixing medium for pumice.[26] Adding three parts green soap in the disinfectant solution will keep the pumice suspended.

Outgoing cases. Each case should be disinfected before it is returned to the dental office. Dentists should be informed about infection control procedures that are used in the dental laboratory.

REFERENCES

1. Council on Dental Materials and Devices and Council on Dental Therapeutics. Infection control in the dental office. JADA 97(4):673-677, 1978.

2. Council on Dental Therapeutics and Council on Prosthetic Services and Dental Laboratory Relations. Guidelines for infection control in the dental office and the commercial dental laboratory. JADA 110(6):969-972, 1985.

3. Council on Dental Materials, Instruments, and Equipment. Dentists' Desk Reference, 1983, and Council on Dental Therapeutics. Accepted Dental Therapeutics, 1984. Chicago, American Dental Association.

4. Council on Dental Materials, Instruments, and Equipment, Council on Dental Practice, and Council on Dental Therapeutics. Infection control recommendations for the dental office and the dental laboratory. JADA 116(2):241-248, 1988.

5. Division of Scientific Affairs. Facts about AIDS for the Dental Team, third ed. Chicago, American Dental Association, 1991.

6. Council on Dental Therapeutics and Council on Dental Materials, Instruments, and Equipment. Monograph on Safety and Infection Control, first ed. Chicago, American Dental Association, 1990.

7. Department of Veteran Affairs, American Dental Association, and Department of Health and Human Services. Infection Control in the Dental Environment, Video and training manual. American Dental Association, Chicago, 1989.

8. American Dental Association. The American Dental Association Regulatory Compliance Manual. American Dental Association, Chicago, 1990.

9. American Dental Association, OSHA: What You Must Know. American Dental Association, Chicago, 1992.

10. Centers for Disease Control. Recommended infection control practices for dentistry. MMWR 35:237-242, 1986.

11. Centers for Disease Control. Recommendations for prevention of HIV transmission in health care settings. MMWR 36:Suppl no. 2S, 1987.

12. Centers for Disease Control. Recommendations for preventing transmission of human immunodeficiency virus and hepatitis B virus to patients during exposure-prone invasive procedures. MMWR 40: 1-9, 1991.

13. Department of Labor, Occupational Safety and Health Administration. 29 CFR Part 1910.1030, Occupational exposure to bloodborne pathogens, final rule. Federal Register 56(235):64004-64182, 1991.

14. Centers for Disease Control. Protection against viral hepatitis. MMWR 39:1-26, 1990.

15. Henderson, D.K., Fahey, B.J., Willy, M., et al. Risk for occupational transmission of human immunodeficiency virus type 1 (HIV-1) associated with clinical exposures. Annals of Internal Medicine 113:740-746, 1990.

16. American Dental Association. Current Policies. Hepatitis B Vaccination and Post-Vaccination Testing for Dentists and Their Staffs (1987:509). American Dental Association, Chicago, 1988.

17. Centers for Disease Control. Recommendations for preventing transmission of infection with human T-lymphotropic virus type III/lymphadenopathy-associated virus in the workplace. MMWR 34:681-695, 1985.

18. Ready, M.A., Schuster, G.S., Wilson, J.T., Hanes, C.M. Effects of dental medicaments on examination glove permeability. J Prosthet Dent 61:499-503, 1989.

19. Food and Drug Administration. Allergic reactions to latex-containing medical devices. FDA Medical Alert MDA91-1, March 29, 1991.

20. Stewart, Jeff. Professional management of allergic hypersensitivity reactions to gloves. J Michigan Dental Assoc, March 1990.

21. Block, S.S. Disinfection, Sterilization and Preservation, ed 4. Philadelphia, Lea & Febiger, 1991.

22. Council on Dental Materials, Instruments, and Equipment, Council on Dental Practice, and Council on Dental Therapeutics. Biological indicators for verifying sterilization. JADA 117(5):653-654, 1988.

23. Council on Dental Materials, Instruments, and Equipment. Recommendations for radiographic darkrooms and darkroom practices. JADA 104(6):886-887, 1982.

24. Council on Dental Materials, Instruments and Equipment. Disinfection of impressions. JADA 122(3):110, 1991.

25. National Board for Certification of Dental Laboratories. Infection control requirements for certified dental laboratories. Alexandria, VA, National Association of Dental Laboratories, 1986.
26. Guidelines for Infection Control in the Dental Office and the Commercial Dental Laboratory. Quintessence of Dental Technology 9(9):603-607, 1985.

THE PROFESSIONAL DENTAL HYGIENIST

As a licensed primary healthcare professional, the dental hygienist provides a wide range of services in a variety of settings that will promote and contribute to the total well-being of the patient/client. The term "client" refers not only to an individual but extends to include the family and community. The role of the dental hygienist encompasses that of clinician/therapist, educator/health promoter, administrator/manager, consumer advocate, researcher, and change agent (1). As a professional, these roles are part of every day practice, whether in a private office, public health program, health maintenance organization, or institution.

TYPES OF SERVICES

Table 1.1 shows a few broad examples of the types of services dental hygienists may provide to patient/clients. Note that the areas overlap; indeed, each component is necessary for the entire treatment and maintenance plan to succeed. Preventive services are divided into primary (methods to prevent disease occurrence) and secondary (treatment of early disease or condition to prevent further progress) services. Educational services are strategies to guide behaviors toward health. Therapeutic services are clinical treatments designed to arrest or control disease and to maintain oral tissues in health.

TABLE 1.1. Sampling of Services Provided by Dental Hygienists

Types of Services	Individual	Family	Community
Preventive			
Primary	Sealants	Counsel parents on prevention of baby-bottle tooth decay	Promote water fluoridation
Secondary	Plaque/calculus removal	Counsel on harmful oral habits	Oral screenings and referrals
Educational	Home care instruction	Nutritional counseling	Oral health units in schools
Therapeutic	Scaling/root planing	Smoking cessation, counseling	Sealant programs
	Postoperative care		Fluoridation of water supply

DENTAL HYGIENE CARE

Dental hygiene care is the integration and coordination of preventive, educational, and therapeutic services to improve the oral health of the patient through the use of assessment, diagnosis, planning, implementation, and evaluation.

Factors Influencing Dental Hygiene Care

Legal: State, provincial, or national regulation and statutes delineate the scope of practice, settings, and licensure requirements for dental hygienists. The laws governing dental hygiene practice vary in different jurisdictions. It is imperative that each dental hygienist remain knowledgeable about the laws pertaining to the practice. Practice acts for states or provinces can be obtained from the governing agencies or bodies charged with regulating the profession.

Ethical: Professionals are held to a higher standard of ethics than is the general public. Dental hygienists are responsible, both morally and ethically, for providing care to all patients/clients. Numerous professional associations have defined ethical principles for their professions. The American Dental Hygienists' Association has ratified a Code of Ethics that serves the profession in this area (2).

Personal: The attitude, appearance, and demeanor of a dental hygienist reflect on the profession as a whole. These personal factors can and do influence the patient/client's attitude toward the healthcare professional and acceptance of treatment, and they affect the outcome of services provided.

OBJECTIVES FOR PRACTICE

Esther M. Wilkins, B.S., R.D.H., D.M.D., in her book *Clinical Practice of the Dental Hygienist*, seventh edition, cites the importance of self-assessment by the dental hygienist to continue self-improvement. With regard to patient care, she provides dental hygienists with a list of objectives to use in the goal of aiding *"individuals and groups in obtaining and maintaining optimum oral health."* These objectives are listed below (3).

1. Strive toward the highest degree of professional ethics and conduct.
2. Plan and carry out effective dental hygiene services essential to the total care program for each individual patient.
3. Apply knowledge and understanding of the basic and clinical sciences in the recognition of oral conditions and the prevention of oral diseases.
4. Apply scientific knowledge and skill to all clinical techniques and instructional procedures.
5. Recognize each patient as an individual and adapt techniques and procedures accordingly.
6. Identify and care for the needs of patients who have unusual general health problems that affect dental hygiene procedures.
7. Demonstrate interpersonal relationships that permit attending the patient/client with assurance and presenting dental health information effectively.
8. Provide a complete and personalized instructional service to each patient to become motivated toward changes in oral health behavioral practices.
9. Practice safe and efficient clinical routines for the application of universal precautions for infection control.
10. Apply a continuing process of self-development and self-evaluation in clinical practice throughout professional life.
    A. Be objective and critical of procedures used to perform the best possible service.
    B. Appreciate the need for acquiring new knowledge and skills by regularly enrolling in continuing education courses.

I would add one other objective: to belong to and take an active role in your professional association. Through interaction with colleagues and fellow professionals, your role as a healthcare provider is greatly enhanced.

INFORMATION TO SHARE WITH THE PATIENT/CLIENT

1. Function of the dental hygienist as a cotherapist
2. Your legal scope of practice
3. The role of the patient as an active participant in attaining and maintaining optimum oral health
4. The interaction of patient instructions and education in relation to clinical services

REFERENCES

1. American Dental Hygienist's Association, *Association Policy Manual*, 1995.
2. American Dental Hygienists' Association, House of Delegates: *Code of Ethics*, ratified, June, 1995.
3. **Wilkins**, E.M., ed: *Clinical Practice of the Dental Hygienist*, 7th ed. Baltimore, Williams & Wilkins, 1994, pp. 6–7.

INFECTION CONTROL: TRANSMISSIBLE DISEASES

2

Systematic procedures for maintaining strict infection control in oral health services facilities is vital for the protection of the patient, personnel, and others interacting in the facility. This chapter focuses on diseases that may be transmitted during treatment, factors that influence treatment, prophylactic measures and precautions, and characteristics of specific diseases.

The following table lists the influencing factors in the transmission of disease. At each phase, the cycle can be interrupted to control the spread of contamination. Exposure to infectious agents does not necessarily lead to an individual becoming infected or diseased. Other elements can influence the process. These elements include factors such as the amount of organisms and duration of exposure, virulence of the organism (its ability to survive interim exposure) and immune status of the host; antibody response; defense cell reaction; and general physical health and nutritional status of the host.

Autogenous Infection—occurs when normal defense mechanisms within a person are modified. The microflora within the oral cavity may become pathogenic when introduced into the tissues during treatment. Table 2.3 illustrates the sources, factors, and prevention of autogenous infection.

PATHOGENS TRANSMISSIBLE BY THE ORAL CAVITY

Many pathogens are transmitted through the oral cavity. Table 2.4 details the disease manifestation, mode of transfer, incubation, and communicability periods. Note

7

TABLE 2.1. Disease Transmission

Links in the Infectious Process	Control/Interruption of the Cycle
Infectious agent	Medical history
Bacteria	Universal precautions
Fungi	Clinical identification of
Viruses	lesions or symptoms
Protozoa	
Rickettsiae	
Reservoirs	Health of staff
People	Immunizations
Equipment	Universal precautions
Instruments	
Water (dental water lines)	
Port of exit	Universal precautions
Secretions: saliva, blood	Waste disposal
Skin and mucous membrane	
Droplets	
Transmission	Control of aerosols
Direct contact	Universal precautions
Indirect contact: fmite, vector	
Airborne	
Port of entry	Immunizations
Mucous membrane	Universal precautions
GI tract	
Respiratory tract	
Broken skin	
Eyes	
Susceptible host	Universal precautions
Immunosuppression	Treatment of secondary
Medically compromised	infection
Elderly	

TABLE 2.2.   Airborne Infection

Source	Prevention

Dust-borne organisms
  Brought in from outside
  Organisms from oral cavity of
    patient in contact with
    airborne dust via spatter
	Limitation of organisms
	  Postponement of elective
	    treatment for individuals
	    known to have
	    communicable organisms
	    in the oral cavity
	  Preoperative oral hygiene
	    measures

Aerosol production[a]
  Aerosols < 50 microns
  Spatter > 50 microns
	Toothbrushing
	  Antiseptic mouthrinse
	Interruption of transmission
	  Use of rubber dam
	  High-speed evacuation
	  More manual instrumentation
	  Air control methods for
	    adequate ventilation,
	    filtration, humidity
	  Vacuum cleaning (with
	    organism filter) rather than
	    dusting
	Clean water
	  Two minutes through all
	    tubings to handpieces,
	    ultrasonic scalers, air/
	    water syringes at least
	    2 minutes at the start
	    and end of the day and at
	    least 30 seconds after each
	    appointment during
	    the day
	Clinician protection
	  Masks and protective eyewear

[a] Greater concentration of aerosols and spatter are closest to instrumentation site. Aerosols can circulate with air currents and therefore travel from room to room (1–6).

TABLE 2.3. Autogenous Infection (7, 8)[a]

Source	Factors	Prevention
Bacteremia	Abnormal physical conditions	Complete medical and dental history
	Cardiac conditions	Antibiotic premedication
	Prosthetic joint replacement	
Injection site	Compromised immune system	Lowering of surface microbial count
	Systemic diseases	Bacterial plaque removal (floss, brushing)
	Alcoholism	Antibacterial rinsing
	Diabetes mellitus	Topical antiseptic application
	Glomerulonephritis	Preparation of injection site
	Leukemia	Drying of tissue site with sterile sponge
	Drug therapy	Adequate retraction of tissue
	Chemotherapeutic agents	Disposable needles
	Steroids	Needle contact with injection site only
	Prostheses/organ transplants	

[a]Patient with delayed healing may require additional doses of antibiotics.

that oral signs and symptoms may not be evident when pathogens are present. Stringent universal precautions, instrument sterilization, disposable materials, updated medical history, and consultation with the patient's physician, if necessary, should be used for every patient. In addition, every healthcare provider should be immunized for hepatitis B.

The following sections detail particular diseases that may be transmitted through the oral cavity.

TUBERCULOSIS (TB)

Clinical Management

1. Patient history (9): careful history taking, review of previous histories for comparison, and possible referral to physician
2. Extraoral and intraoral examination (10, 11): although TB is a primary lesion of the lungs, any organ or tissue may be involved
    A. Lymphadenopathy of regional lymph nodes
    B. Oral lesions: relatively rare but usually occur as ulcers; may be located on soft or hard palate, occasionally on tongue
3. Patient under treatment: chemotherapy can control contagious condition; isoniazid used for long periods, may be in combination with rifampin; infectivity decreased a few weeks after beginning therapy

VIRAL HEPATITIS

Viruses cause a variety of types of hepatitis (inflammation of the liver). Some of the specifically identified types of viral hepatitis are identified in this section. Tables 2.4 through 2.7 contain specific information on viral hepatitis, in addition to the following:

TABLE 2.4. Infectious Diseases

Infectious Agent	Disease or Condition	Route or Mode of Transmission	Incubation Period	Communicable Period	Vaccine
Human immunodeficiency virus (HIV)	Acquired immunodeficiency syndrome (AIDS) HIV infection	Blood and blood products (infected IV needles) Sexual contact Transplacental and perinatal	3 mo to 12 or more yr	From asymptomatic through life	*
Hepatitis A virus (HAV)	Type A hepatitis "infectious" hepatitis	Fecal-oral Food, water, shellfish	15–50 days (average 28–30 days)	2–3 weeks before onset (jaundice) through 8 days after	*
Hepatitis B virus (HBV)	Type B hepatitis "Serum" hepatitis	Blood Saliva and all body fluids	2–6 months (average 60–90 days)	Before, during, and after clinical signs	Yes

continued

		Sexual contact Perinatal		Carrier state: indefinite	
Hepatitis C virus (HCV) PT-NANB	Type C hepatitis Parenterally transmitted nonA, nonB	Percutaneous Blood Needles	2 weeks–6 months (6–9 weeks)	1 week before onset of symptoms Carrier state: indefinite	No
Delta hepatitis virus (HDV) Delta agent	Delta hepatitis	Coinfection with HBV Blood Sexual contacts Perinatal	2–10 weeks	All phases	HBV vaccine
Hepatitis E virus (HEV) ET-NANB	Type E hepatitis Enterically transmitted nonA, nonB	Fecal-oral Contaminated water	15–64 days	Similar to HAV	No

continued

TABLE 2.4. Infectious Diseases

Infectious Agent	Disease or Condition	Route or Mode of Transmission	Incubation Period	Communicable Period	Vaccine
Herpes simplex virus Type 1 (HSV-1) Type 2 (HSV-2)	Acute herpetic gingivostomatitis Herpes labialis Ocular herpetic infections Herpetic whitlow	Saliva Direct contact (lip, hand) Indirect contact (on objects, limited survival) Sexual contact	2–12 days	Labialis: 1 day before onset until lesions are crusted Acute stomatitis: 7 weeks after recovery Asymptomatic infection: with viral shedding Reactivation period: with viral shedding	No
Varicella-zoster virus (VZV)	Chickenpox Herpes zoster (shingles)	Direct contact Indirect contact Airborne droplet	2–3 weeks	5 days prior to onset of rash until crusting of vesicles	Yes

continued

Epstein-Barr virus (EBV)	Infectious mononucleosis	Direct contact Saliva	4–6 weeks	Prolonged Pharyngeal excretion 1 year after infection	No
Cytomegalovirus (CMV)	Neonatal cytomegalovirus infection Cytomegaloviral disease	Perinatal Direct contact (most body secretions) Blood transfusion Saliva	3–12 weeks after delivery 3–8 weeks after transfusion	Months to years	No
Mycobacterium tuberculosis	Tuberculosis	Droplet nuclei Sputum Saliva	4–12 weeks	As long as viable bacilli are discharged in sputum	BCG
Treponema pallidum	Syphilis Congenital syphilis	Direct contact Transplacental	10 days–3 months	Variable and indefinite May be 2–4 years	No
Neisseria gonorrhoeae	Gonorrhea Gonococcal pharyngitis	Direct contact Indirect (short survival of organisms)	2–7 days	During incubation Continued for months and years if untreated	No

continued

TABLE 2.4. Infectious Diseases

Infectious Agent	Disease or Condition	Route or Mode of Transmission	Incubation Period	Communicable Period	Vaccine
Bordetella pertussis	Whooping cough Pertussis	Direct contact with discharges	7–10 days	Not treated: from early catarrhal stage to 3 weeks after paroxysmal cough	Yes
Mumps virus (*Paramyxovirus*)	Infectious parotitis (mumps)	Direct contact (saliva) Airborne droplet	12–25 days (average 18 days)	12–25 days after exposure From 6–7 days before symptoms until 9 days after swelling	Yes
Poliovirus types 1, 2, 3	Poliomyelitis	Direct contact (saliva) Droplet Fecal-oral	7–14 days	Probably most infectious 7–10 days before and after onset of symptoms	Yes

continued

Influenza viruses (A, B, C)	Influenza	Nasal discharge Respiratory droplets	1–5 days	3 days from clinical onset	Yes
Measles virus (*Morbillivirus*)	Rubeola (measles)	Direct contact Saliva Airborne droplet	7–18 days to fever, 14 days to rash	Few days before fever to 4 days after rash appears	Yes
Rubella virus (Togavirus)	Rubella (German measles)	Nasopharyngeal secretions Direct contact Airborne droplets	16–23 days	From 1 week to at least 4 days after rash appears Highly communicable Infants shed virus for months after birth	Yes
	Congenital rubella syndrome	Maternal infection first trimester			
Group A streptococci (beta-hemolytic) *Streptococcus pyogenes*	Streptococcal sore throat Scarlet fever Impetigo Erysipelas	Respiratory droplets Direct contact	1–3 days	10–21 days, untreated Many nasal oropharyngeal carriers	No

continued

TABLE 2.4. Infectious Diseases

Infectious Agent	Disease or Condition	Route or Mode of Transmission	Incubation Period	Communicable Period	Vaccine
Staphylococcus aureus *Staphylococcus epidermidis*	Abscesses Boils (furuncle) Impetigo Bacterial pneumonia	Saliva Exudates Nasal discharge	4–10 days Variable and indefinite	While lesions drain and carrier state persists	No
Candida albicans	Candidiasis	Secretions Excretions (oral, skin, vagina)	Variable 2–5 days for "thrush" in children	While lesions are present	No
Streptococcus pneumoniae	Pneumonia Pneumococcal pneumonia	Droplet Direct contact Indirect	1–3 days Not well determined	While virulent organisms are discharged	Yes

*Vaccine progress.
BCG, Bacillus Calmette Guerin.

Hepatitis A

- Occurs more frequently in children and young adults (13)
- More severe in adults
- Early immunization is indicated (11, 12)

Hepatitis B

Individuals at risk or with risk behaviors for hepatitis B virus (HBV) (13, 16, 17) (a person may belong to more than one of the risk groups listed here):

- Infants born to HIV-infected mothers
- Users of parenteral drugs (needle sharing)
- Homosexually active men not using safe sex practices ("safe sex practices" is meant to include barrier protection with no exchange of body fluids [saliva, semen, vaginal secretions], in accord with recommended guidelines)
- Heterosexually active persons with multiple partners, including prostitutes, who are not using safe sex practices
- Persons who have repeatedly contracted sexually transmitted diseases
- Clients and staff in institutions for the mentally retarded and current or former residents, particularly individuals with Down's syndrome
- Patients and staff in hemodialysis units
- Recipients of blood products used for treating clotting disorders, particularly before 1985
- Clients with active or chronic liver diseases
- Healthcare workers with frequent blood contact, including emergency room staff, hospital surgical staff, dental hygienists, dentists, and blood bank and plasma fractionation workers
- Household contacts of HBV carriers
- Male prisoners
- Military populations stationed in countries with endemic HBV

- Travelers returned from areas of endemic HBV who stayed longer than 3 months or who were treated medically by transfusion while there
- Morticians and embalmers
- Immigrants/refugees from areas of endemic HBV

Prevention

Every healthcare individual should be immunized to reduce the possibilities of disease acquisition and transmission (12). (See Tables 2.6 and 2.7.)

Hepatitis C

- Associated with blood transfusion (13, 17)
- Plays a role in many cases of chronic liver disease
- Serologic test for antibody to HCV for blood donors
- Recommended measures for hepatitis B can be applied to hepatitis C

Hepatitis D

- Delta hepatitis virus (13), also called the delta agent
- Cannot cause infection except in the presence of HBV
- Most frequently the delta infection is superimposed on HBsAg carriers
- Occurs primarily in persons who have multiple exposures to HBV, particularly hemophiliacs and IV drug abusers
- Transmission similar to that of HBV
- Prevention of hepatitis B will prevent hepatitis D (immunization with hepatitis B vaccine protects recipient from delta hepatitis infection)

Hepatitis E

- Clinical course and distribution of HEV are similar to those of hepatitis A
- Transmitted by contaminated water or person-to-person by fecal-oral route

- High incidence after heavy rains where sewage disposal is inadequate
- High mortality rate in pregnant women; adults are affected more than children
- Prevention: sanitary disposal of wastes; handwashing, especially during food handling

Two hepatitis B vaccines are available for preexposure and postexposure prophylaxis. Both are administered intramuscularly in three doses: the first at the outset, then at 1 and 6 months. The vaccine should be given only in the deltoid muscle for adults and children and in the anterolateral thigh muscle for infants and neonates.

HERPESVIRUS DISEASES

Herpesvirus infections (21) cause a variety of diseases that are highly infectious. Table 2.9 lists the herpesviruses, their abbreviations, and some of the infections they cause. Table 2.10 lists the infections, characteristics, and facts pertinent to the infections. Below are factors pertaining to the clinical management of the patient in relation to herpesviruses.

Patient History

Ask specific questions regarding the patient's experiences with herpesviruses, using easily understood terms such as "fever blister" or "cold sores."

Active Lesion: Postponement of Appointment

    A. Transmission of infection:
        Contagiousness—possible transmission of infection to clinician or others
        Autoinoculation is possible that can be spread to eye or nose
    B. Irritation of lesions
        Can delay healing
        Increases the severity of the infection

TABLE 2.5. Viral Hepatitis Abbreviations

Abbreviation	Term	Significance
Hepatitis A		
HAV	Hepatitis A virus	Etiologic agent Hepatitis A
anti-HAV	Antibody to hepatitis A virus	Immunity to infection
IgM anti-HAV	IgM antibody to hepatitis A virus	Recent HAV infection
Hepatitis B		
HBV	Hepatitis B virus (Dane particle)	Etiologic agent hepatitis B
HBsAg	Hepatitis B surface antigen (Australian antigen)	Current HBV infection
		Surface marker in acute disease and carrier state
anti-HBs	Antibody to hepatitis B surface antigen	Indicates
		Active immunity to HBV (past infection)
		Passive immunity from HBIG
		Immune response from HB vaccine
HBeAg	Hepatitis B e antigen	High titer HBV in serum
		Indicates high infectivity
		Persists into carrier state
anti-HBe	Antibody to hepatitis B e antigen	Low-titer HBV
		Low degree infectivity
HBcAg	Hepatitis B core antigen	No test available

continued

anti-HBc	Antibody to hepatitis B core antigen	Indicates prior HBV infection
IgM anti-HBc	IgM class antibody to hepatitis B core antigen	Indicates recent HBC infection
Hepatitis C		
HCV	Hepatitis C virus (formerly parenterally transmitted non-A, non-B)	Etiologic agent for hepatitis C
anti-HCV	Antibody to hepatitis C virus	Indicates acute disease and chronic state Resembles hepatitis B
Hepatitis D		
HDV	Hepatitis D virus	Etiologic agent hepatitis D with HBsAg
anti-HDV	Antibody to hepatitis D virus	Indicates past or present infection
Hepatitis E		
HEV	Hepatitis E virus (formerly enterically transmitted non-A, non-B)	Etiologic agent hepatitis E
anti-HEV	Antibody to hepatitis E virus	Resembles hepatitis A
Immune globulins		
IG	Immune globulin	Contains antibodies to HAV and low-titer HBV antibodies
HBIG	Hepatitis B immune globulin	Contains high-titer antibodies to HBV

TABLE 2.6. Active Immunization: The Vaccines (13, 16, 18)

Types	Characteristics	Factors for Both
Plasma-derived HB vaccine[a]	Original vaccine was prepared using purified and formalin-treated HBsAg from plasma of HBsAg carriers Treatment steps in preparation of vaccine inactivate all classes of viruses so that transmission of any other disease becomes impossible	Both vaccines act in a comparable manner to stimulate antibody Both convey the same degree of immunity In healthy 20–39-year-old adults, immunity is conferred in more than 95% In children, protective antibodies are shown in 99%
Recombinant DNA HB vaccine[b]	Recombinant DNA technology has been used to synthesize HBsAG in a culture of *Saccharomyces cerevisiae*, a yeast. The HBsAg is purified and sterilized.	Postvaccination testing for anti-HBs within 1–6 months is recommended for a hemodialysis patient or other at-risk person having frequent exposure, including dental personnel No effect on carrier or person who has the antibody (20)

continued

Immunization is not contraindicated during pregnancy; in fact, HBV infection during pregnancy can be severe and the newborn can become a permanent carrier

Lower responses noted in older persons and hemodialysis patients and when injections are given in the buttock versus the deltoid (19)

Booster (16, 18)

Higher initial peak of response usually means longer persistence of antibody; antibody level drops can still provide protection

A 7-year booster is suggested; however, antibody levels can be tested to determine individual needs

For certain risk patients, particularly hemodialysis patients, annual antibody testing has been recommended (16)

[a]Heptavax, Merck Sharp & Dohme.
[b]Recombivax HB, Merck Sharp & Dohme; Enegerix B, Smith Kline Biologicals.

TABLE 2.7. Postexposure Prophylaxis (16)

Indications for prophylaxis
  Newborn of HBsAg-positive mother
  Significant hepatitis B exposure to HBsAg-positive blood
Treatment
  Hepatitis B immune globulin (HBIG)
    High-titer anti-HBs immune globulin (HBIG) is primarily used for
      postexposure prophylaxis
  Immune globulin (IG)
    Contains low-titer anti-HBs of varying amounts
    Lesser degree of effectiveness than HBIG; should be used if HBIG
      is not available
    Used for the prevention or modification of hepatitis A exposure
      and when protection for exposure to hepatitis C and E is
      needed

TABLE 2.8. HIV and HBV Postexposure Management

Patient (Source)	Exposed DHCW	Treatment
HBsAg positive or refuses testing or cannot be identified	Not HBV immunized	Start vaccine series Give HBIG (single-dose)
	HBV vaccine received	Test for anti-HB Adequate titer level: no treatment Inadequate titer level: give vaccine booster HBIG (single dose)
HBsAg negative	Not HBV immunized	Start vaccine series

continued

TABLE 2.8.   HIV and HBV Postexposure Management

Patient (Source)	Exposed DHCW	Treatment
Has AIDS or is HIV seropositive or refused testing or cannot be identified	HBV vaccine received	No treatment necessary
	Counsel concerning the risk	Negative for anti-HIV:
	Test for anti-HIV	Test again in 6 weeks, 12 weeks, 6 months, 1 year
		Counsel:
		Do not donate blood
		Use appropriate protection during sexual intercourse

DHCW, dental health-care worker; HBsAg, hepatitis B surface antigen; HBIG, hepatitis B immune globulin; Anti-HBs, antibody to hepatitis B surface antigen; Anti-HIV, antibody to human immunodeficiency virus.

C. Prodomal state
   May be the most contagious state
   Request patient to reschedule appointment when it is known a lesion is developing

Universal Precautions

• Universal precautions should be consistently applied for all patients, as it is not known whether the patient is infected

- Always use disposable and sterilizable materials, regardless if active lesions are present

HIV INFECTION

Acquired immunodeficiency syndrome (AIDS), caused by the human immunodeficiency virus (HIV), is a severe condition with varied manifestations ranging from asymptomatic mild abnormalities in immune response to extensive immunosuppression that can lead to a multitude of life-threatening infections and rare malignant conditions.

Many early indicators of HIV appear in the oral cavity, head, or neck. A thorough medical history along with the oral examination could lead to early recognition of HIV and referral for medical evaluation and testing for the patient. The goal of primary prevention (for those not infected) is to lower the rate at which new cases of HIV appear. The goals of secondary prevention (for seropos-

TABLE 2.9. Herpesvirus

Abbreviation	Name of Virus	Infections
VZV	Varicella-zoster	Varicella (chickenpox)
		Herpes zoster (shingles)
EBV	Epstein-Barr	EBV mononucleosis
HCMV	Human cytomegalovirus	Cytomegalovirus disease
		Fetal infection
HSV-1	Herpes simplex virus	Herpes labialis
HSV-2		Herpetic gingivostomatitis
		Herpetic keratoconjunctivitis
		Herpetic whitlow
		Encephalitis
		Neonatal herpes
HHV-6	Human herpesvirus 6	Mononucleosis-like rash

TABLE 2.10. Herpes Simplex Virus Infections (21, 22)

Infection	Characteristics	Factors
Primary herpetic gingivostomatitis	Gingivostomatitis and pharyngitis fever, malaise, inability to eat Lymphadenopathy for 2–7 days Painful oral vesicular lesions may occur on the gingiva, mucosa, tongue, and lips	May be asymptomatic—a subclinical carrier May excrete virus in saliva Both HSV-1 and HSV-2 can cause pharyngitis
Herpes labialis (cold sore, fever blister)	Prelesion stage may be a burning or stinging sensation in the area Most frequently in the vermillion border of the lips but can occur intraorally on the gingiva or hard palate Group of vesicles forms, rupture, and coalesce: crusting follows May take up to 10 days to heal Lesions are infectious	Both HSV-1 and HSV-2 can cause genital and oral-facial infection that cannot be distinguished clinically (23) Recurrent (HSV) lesions occur at or near the primary lesion at indefinite intervals Usually triggered by stress, sunlight, illness, or trauma Can be caused by dental appointment: emotional stress, oral trauma Autoinfection, transmission to others is possible *continued*

TABLE 2.10. Herpes Simplex Virus Infections (21, 22)

Infection	Characteristics	Factors
Herpetic whitlow	Herpes simplex infection of the fingers Most frequent location is around fingernail	Virus enters through minor skin abrasions Direct contact with vesicular lesion on lips or saliva that contains the viruses Lesions are infectious and transmissible before the whitlow is diagnosed Recurrences are not unusual (24)
Ocular herpes (21)	Fever, pain, blurring of vision, swelling, excess tearing, and secondary bacterial infection Herpes keratoconjunctivitis can cause deep inflammation and, if untreated, is a leading cause of loss of sight	Transmitted by the splashing of saliva or fluid from a vesicle lesion directly into an unprotected eye; extension of infection from a facial lesion; infection of an infant's eye in utero or during birth

itive individuals) are to reduce the rate of transmission and to introduce treatment early. HIV cuts across all levels of our community. Patient/clients in the oral health-care settings may be families, friends, significant others, or personal care givers; as a professional, our attitude and conduct should reflect support, acceptance, and empathy.

Tables 2.11 through 2.18 provide information pertinent to HIV infection and its management.

TABLE 2.11.   HIV and AIDS: Abbreviations/Definitions

AIDS: acquired immunodeficiency syndrome

AZT (ZDV): zidovudine, retrovir; drug used for the treatment of HIV infection and AIDS; first antiviral drug approved by the United States Food and Drug Administration (FDA)

CD4+: T-helper lymphocyte; primary target cell for HIV infection; CD4+ count decreases with the severity of HIV-related illness

DNA: deoxyribonucleic acid; a nucleic acid found in a cell nucleus; is a carrier of genetic information

HIV: human immunodeficiency virus; causes AIDS

HIV-1 antibody: antibody to human immunodeficiency virus type 1; antibody can be detected in the blood 6 to 8 weeks after infection

HL: hairy leukoplakia

IDU: injecting drug user

KS: Kaposi's sarcoma; a malignant vascular tumor; an opportunistic neoplasm that may occur in people with HIV infection

LAV: lymphadenopathy-associated virus; one of the former names for HIV

MMWR: *Morbidity and Mortality Weekly Report;* publication of the United States Centers for Disease Control and Prevention (**CDCP**), Atlanta, GA

PCP: pneumocystis pneumonia; caused by *Pneumocystis carinii;* an opportunistic infection that occurs in people with HIV infection

PGL: persistent generalized lymphadenopathy

PWA: person with AIDS

RNA: ribonucleic acid; a nucleic acid found in cytoplasm and in the nuclei of certain cells; RNA directs the synthesis of proteins, and replaces DNA as a carrier of genetic codes in some viruses

TABLE 2.12. 1992 Revised Classification System for HIV Infection and Expanded AIDS Surveillance Case Definition for Adolescents and Adults[a]

	Clinical Categories		
CD4+ Cell Categories	**[A] Asymptomatic, or PGL[b]**	**[B] Symptomatic, not [A] or [C] Conditions**	**[C] AIDS-indicator Conditions[c]**
≥ 500/mm³	A1	B1	C1
200–499/mm³	A2	B2	C2
< 200/mm³ AIDS-indicator cell count	A3	B3	C3

[a]All but A1, A2, B1, and B2 illustrate the expansion of the AIDS surveillance case definition. Persons with AIDS-indicator conditions (category C) are currently reportable to the health department in every state and U.S. territory. In addition to persons with clinical category C conditions (categories C1, C2, and C3), persons with CD4+ lymphocyte counts of less than 200/mm³ (categories A3 or B3) also have been reportable as AIDS cases in the United States and its territories since April 1, 1992.
[b]PGL, persistent generalized lymphadenopathy. Clinical category A includes acute (primary) HIV infection.
[c]See text.

TABLE 2.13. Stages, Characteristics/Factors, and Progression of HIV Infection

Stage	Characteristics/Factors
Individuals at risk	Those most likely to contract HIV infection (see Table 2.18)
HIV positive	Seropositive, no signs or symptoms This stage may extend for many years—12 or more years for some individuals
HIV-related conditions	Physical and neurologic effects of immune system deterioration
AIDS	Determined by the formal definition provided by the United States Centers for Disease Control and Prevention (see Table 2.14) (25)

TABLE 2.14. Clinical Categories of HIV Classification System (25)

Category	Conditions
A: Asymptomatic (acute primary) HIV or PGL	One or more of the following: Asymptomatic HIV infection Persistent generalized lymphadenopathy (PGL) Acute (primary) HIV infection or history of acute HIV infection Conditions in categories B and C must not have occurred[a]
B: Symptomatic (not A or C)	Attributed to HIV infection, indicative of a defect in cell-mediated immunity, and not listed under category C Bacillary agniomatosis Candidiasis, oropharyngeal (thrush) Candidiasis, vulvovaginal; persistent, frequent, or poorly responsive to therapy Cervical dysplasia (moderate or severe) cervical carcinoma in situ Constitutional symptoms, such as fever (38.5° C) or diarrhea lasting > 1 month Hairy leukoplakia, oral Herpes zoster (shingles), involving at least two distinct episodes or more than one dermatome Idiopathic thrombocytopenic purpura Listeriosis Pelvic inflammatory disease, particularly if complicated by tubo-ovarian abscess Peripheral neuropathy

continued

C: AIDS-Indicator — Strongly associated with severe immunodeficiency, occurs frequently in HIV-infected individuals, and can cause serious morbidity or mortality

Candidiasis of bronchi, trachea, or lungs

Candidiasis, esophageal

Cervical cancer, invasive

Coccidioidomycosis, disseminated or extrapulmonary

Cryptosporidiosis, chronic intestinal (> 1 month duration)

Cytomegalovirus disease (other than liver, spleen, or nodes)

Cytomegalovirus retinitis (with loss of vision)

Encephalopathy, HIV-related

Herpes simplex: chronic ulcer(s) (> 1 month duration) or bronchitis, pneumonitis, or esophagitis

Histoplasmosis, disseminated or extrapulmonary

Isosporiasis, chronic intestinal (> 1 month duration)

Kaposi's sarcoma

Lymphoma (or equivalent term)

Lymphoma, immunoblastic (or equivalent term)

Lymphoma, primary, of brain

continued

TABLE 2.14. Clinical Categories of HIV Classification System (25)

Category	Conditions
	Mycobacterium avium complex or *M. kansaii*, disseminated or extrapulmonary
	Mycobacterium tuberculosis, any site (pulmonary[a] or extrapulmonary)
	Mycobacterium, other species or unidentified species, disseminated or extrapulmonary
	Pneumocystis carinii pneumonia
	Pneumonia, recurrent[a]
	Progressive multifocal leukoencephalopathy
	Salmonella septicemia, recurrent
	Toxoplasmosis of brain
	Wasting syndrome caused by HIV

[a]Added in the 1993 expansion of the AIDS surveillance case definition.

TABLE 2.15. Clinical Course of HIV Infection

Transmission	AIDS virus (HIV) found in most body fluids
	Transmission primarily by way of blood, semen, vaginal secretions, breast milk
	Routes: principal routes are sexual, blood, and perinatal contacts
	1. Intimate unprotected sexual contact (both homosexual and heterosexual)
	2. Exposure to infected blood or blood products
	Intravenous drug use: sharing of needles, syringes, etc.
	Transfusion and use of blood products by individuals with blood disorders
	3. Maternal fetal or perinatal contact
	Viruses can be transmitted across the placenta
	Can occur in utero, during delivery, or after birth through breast milk or other close contact
	Individuals at risk (see Table 2.18)
	Serologic test for antibodies: detectable antibody levels within 3–12 weeks after exposure; there may not be clinical symptoms
Incubation period	Ranges from 3 months to 12 or more years (26)
Clinical progression	The HIV affects the immune system so that the infected person is vulnerable to a wide range of clinical disorders (see Table 2.13)
	1. Primary HIV infection—acute retroviral infection may be experienced within 12–18 weeks after exposure. Symptoms may not be identifed as specific for HIV infection. Transmission is possible because antibody development occurs during or following the infection.

continued

TABLE 2.15. Clinical Course of HIV Infection

2. Asymptomatic latent period—can be months to years after exposure, with no apparent symptoms. The virus can be transmitted to others.

3. Persistent generalized lymphadenopathy (PGL). May be noticed during routine extraoral clinical examination.

4. Symptomatic period—AIDS is the advanced stage of HIV infection. Four general categories are indicative of this stage:

    Opportunistic infections

    Constitutional disease: HIV wasting syndrome

    Encephalopathy: organic mental disorders

    Neoplasms

TABLE 2.16. HIV Oral Examination

Extraoral	Lymphadenopathy—palpation for enlarged lymph nodes (should be routine for all extraoral examinations) Skin lesions—see Table 2.17
Intraoral	Candidiasis (27), Kaposi's sarcoma (28, 29), and hairy leukoplakia (30) are highly correlated with the subsequent development of advanced HIV infection; all three lesions are highly observable during an oral examination
	Fungal infections (31)—oral candidiasis is the most frequently occurring infection; usually recognized clinically; exfoliative cytology may be used for differential distinction
	Viral infections (31)—Herpes simplex, hairy leukoplakia, oral lesions of chicken pox, verruca vulgaris, condyloma acuminatum, and cytomegalovirus ulcer are examples
	Bacterial infections—gingival and periodontal infections (32, 33); symptoms are more severe and progress more rapidly in immunosuppressed individuals
	Gingivitis: linear gingival erythema 2–3 mm red band along the gingival margin with petechia-like and/or diffuse red lesions of the attached gingiva
	Spontaneous bleeding and bleeding on probing
	(Increased bacterial plaque control and frequent maintenance programs are needed)
	Necrotizing ulcerative gingivitis (NUG); increased incidence in HIV-positive individuals; accelerated development of symptoms

continued

TABLE 2.16. HIV Oral Examination

	Periodontal infection (34)—a range of severity Characteristics of rapidly progressive periodontitis can occur in a few months; in extreme cases, loss of crestal alveolar bone has led to bone exposure and sequestration; severe pain and difficult mastication contribute to discomfort and malnutrition
Dental	Dental caries and dental erosion are problems for individuals medicated with zidovudin (AZT) or retrovir; nausea and vomiting are common side effects of AZT; vomiting can cause dissolution of the enamel in the form of dental erosion (daily personal and periodic professional fluoride must be included in the preventive oral hygiene program)
Xerostomia	Result of salivary gland diseases or side effects of medications; contributes to dental caries and discomfort from dry mucosa (diet review and instruction in selection of noncariogenic food and snack items should be given)

TABLE 2.17. Oral Lesions Associated with HIV Infection Classification

Group I. Lesions Strongly Associated with HIV Infection
Candidiasis
  Erythematous
  Pseudomembranous
Hairy leukoplakia
Kaposi's sarcoma
Non-Hodgkin's lymphoma
Periodontal disease
  Linear gingival erythema
  Necrotizing (ulcerative) gingivitis
  Necrotizing (ulcerative) periodontitis

Group II. Lesions Less Commonly Associated with HIV Infection
Bacterial infections
  Mycobacterium avium-intracellulare
  Mycobacterium tuberculosis
Melanotic hyperpigmentation
Necrotizing (ulcerative) stomatitis
Salivary gland disease
  Dry mouth due to decreased salivary flow rate
  Unilateral or bilateral swelling of major salivary glands
Thrombocytopenic purpura
Ulceration NOS (not otherwise specified)

Viral infections
  Herpes simplex virus
  Human papillomavirus (warty-like lesions)
  Condyloma acuminatum
  Focal epithelial hyperplasia
  Verruca vulgaris
Varicella-zoster virus
  Herpes zoster
  Varicella

Group III. Lesions Seen with HIV Infection
Bacterial infections
  Actinomyces israelii
  Escherichia coli
  Klebsiella pneumoniae
Cat scratch disease
Drug reactions (ulcerative, erythema multiforme, lichenoid, toxic epidermolysis)
Epithelioid (bacillary) angiomatosis
Fungal infection other than candidiasis
  Cryptococcus neoformans
  Geotrichum candidum
  Histoplasma capsulatum
  Mucoraceae (mucormycosis/zygomycosis)
  Aspergillus flavus

continued

TABLE 2.17.   Oral Lesions Associated with HIV Infection Classification

Neurologic disturbances	Viral infections
Facial palsy	Cytomegalovirus
Trigeminal neuralgia	Molluscum contagiosum
Recurrent aphthous stomatitis	

Reprinted with permission from European Commission Clearinghouse on Oral Problems Related to HIV Infection and World Health Organization Collaborating Centre on Oral Manifestations of the Human Immunodeficiency Virus, 1990, with revisions, 1992.

TABLE 2.18.   Individuals at High Risk for HIV Infection[a]

Sexually active homosexual and bisexual men having multiple sex partners without using safe sex practices[b]

Users or former users of intravenous drugs, when contaminated needles are shared

Recipients of blood transfusions or blood products prior to mandatory HIV antibody testing in 1985; this includes individuals with hemophilia or other coagulation disorders

Male and female prostitutes who do not use safe sex practices[b]

Healthcare workers who do not adhere to strict barrier procedures and do not follow essential blood and other body fluid precautions for infection control

Females artificially inseminated with HIV-infected semen

Recipients of HIV-infected organ transplants

Steady sexual partners of all those previously listed who do not use safe sex practices[b]

Steady sexual partners of those infected with AIDS or at risk for AIDS who do not use safe sex practices[b]

Infants born to HIV-infected mothers

Infants fed breast milk from HIV-infected mothers

[a] Compare this table with the list of individuals at risk for Hepatitis B.
[b] "Safe sex practices" is meant to include barrier protection and no exchange of body fluids (saliva, semen, vaginal secretions) in accord with recommended guidelines.

TABLE 2.19. HIV Infection in Children

Children at risk	Infants born to mothers infected with HIV (perinatal transmission)
	Intrauterine (vertical transmission)
	Intrapartum (passing through the birth canal)
	Postpartum—exposure to breast milk (36)
	Transfusions with infected blood or blood products
	Sexually abused by an infected perpetrator (37)
Clinical manifestations	Classified by three parameters (38):
	Infection status
	Clinical status
	Immunologic status
	Incubation or latent period—may be shorter than in adults, ranging from months after birth to several years
	Diagnosis—blood screening for the presence of virus or HIV antibody. When the mother is asymptomatic and has never been tested for HIV, the child's diagnosis may be the index case in the family. Testing of family members and parental counseling may reveal a parent in a risk category.

continued

TABLE 2.19. HIV Infection in Children

Clinical findings (39, 40)—Wide range of symptoms including disorders of nearly every body organ system. Oral lesions are common. Bacterial infections are more frequent and severe. Following is a partial list of frequently found conditions:

Failure to thrive, developmental delay

Hepatomegaly; splenomegaly

Generalized lymphadenopathy

Opportunistic infections

Persistent oral candidiasis; *Candida* esophageal

Localized infections (sinusitis, otitis media, impetigo)

Parotiditis

Herpetic gingivostomatitis; sore mouth and poor oral intake lead to malnutrition and dehydration

Pneumocystis carinii pneumonia and lymphocytic interstitial pneumonia

HIV Infection in Children

HIV infection in children younger than 13 years of age is increasing. Children aged 13 years and older are diagnosed and treated as adults (35). Table 2.19 presents factors pertinent to HIV infection in children. Many of the AIDS-indicator diseases of adult HIV infection are also found in the infected children.

REFERENCES

1. **Miller,** R.L. and Mick, R.E.: Air Pollution and Its Control in the Dental Office, *Dent. Clin. North Am., 22,* 453, July, 1978.
2. **Miller,** R.L.: Generation of Airborne Infection by High Speed Dental Equipment, *J. Am. Soc. Prev. Dent., 6,* 14, May-June, 1976.
3. **Larato,** D.C., Ruskin, P.F., and Martin, A.: Effect of an Ultrasonic Scaler on Bacterial Counts in Air, *J. Periodontol., 38,* 550, November-December, 1967.
4. **Holbrook,** W.P., Muir, K.F., MacPhee, I.T., and Ross, P.W.: Bacteriological Investigation of the Aerosol from Ultrasonic Scalers, *Br. Dent. J., 144,* 245, April, 18, 1978.
5. **Pokowitz,** W. and Hoffman, H.: Dental Aerobiology, *N.Y. State Dent. J., 37,* 337, June-July, 1971.
6. **Gross,** A., Devine, M.J., and Cutright, D.E.: Microbial Contamination of Dental Units and Ultrasonic Scalers, *J. Periodontol. 47,* 670, November 1976.
7. **Crawford,** J.J.: Sterilization, Disinfection and Asepsis in Dentistry, in Block, S.S., ed.: *Disinfection, Sterilization and Preservation,* 3rd ed. Philadelphia, Lea & Febiger, 1983, pp. 517–518.
8. **Malamed,** S.F.: *Handbook of Local Anesthesia,* 3rd ed. St Louis, The C.V. Mosby Co., 1990, p. 131.
9. **Benenson,** A.S., ed.: *Control of Communicable Diseases in Man,* 15th ed. Washington, D.C., American Public Health Association, 1990, pp. 457–465.
10. **Robinson,** H.B.G. and Miller, A.S.: *Colby, Kerr, and Robinson's Color Atlas of Oral Pathology,* 5th ed. Philadelphia, J.B. Lippincott Co., 1990, p. 91.

11. **Fehrenback**, M.J., Lemborn, U.E., and Phelan, J.A.: Immunity, in Ibsen, O.A.C. and Phelan, J.A., eds.: *Oral Pathology for the Dental Hygienist.* Philadelphia, W.B. Saunders Co., 1992, pp. 185–186.

12. **Szmuness**, W., Steven, C.E., Harley, E.J., Zang, E.A., Oleszko, W.R., William, D.C., Sadovsky, R., Morrison, J.M., and Kellner, A.: Hepatitis B Vaccine. Demonstration of Efficacy in a Controlled Clinical Trial in a High-risk Population in the United States, *N. Engl. J. Med., 303,* 833, October 9, 1980.

13. **Benenson**, A.S., ed.: *Control of Communicable Diseases in Man,* 15th ed. Washington, D.C., American Public Health Association, 1990, pp. 197–212.

14. **Werzberger**, A., Mensch, B., Kuter, B., Brown, L., Lewis, J., Sitrin, R., Miller, W., Shouval, D., Wiens, B., Calandra, G., Ryan, J., Provost, P., and Nalin, D.: A Controlled Trial of a Formalin-inactivated Hepatitis A Vaccine in Healthy Children, *N. Engl. J. Med., 327,* 453, August 13, 1992.

15. **Bancroft**, W.H.: Hepatitis A Vaccine (Editorial), *N. Engl. J. Med., 327,* 488, August 13, 1992.

16. **United States Centers for Disease Control:** Protection Against Viral Hepatitis. Recommendations of the Immunization Practices Advisory Committee (ACIP), *MMWR,* 39, 1-26, No. RR-2, February 9, 1990.

17. **United States Centers for Disease Control:** Public Service Interagency Guidelines for Screening Donors of Blood, Plasma, Organs, Tissues, and Semen for Evidence of Hepatitis B and Hepatitis C, *MMWR,* 40, 1–17, No. RR-4, April 19, 1991.

18. **United States Centers for Disease Control:** Hepatitis B Virus: A Comprehensive Strategy for Eliminating Transmission in the United States Through Universal Childhood Vaccination, *MMWR,* 40, 1–25, No. RR-13, November 22, 1991.

19. **United States Centers for Disease Control:** Suboptimal Response to Hepatitis B Vaccine Given by Injection into the Buttock, *MMWR,* 34, 105, March 1, 1985.

20. **Dienstag**, J.L., Stevens, C.E., Bhan, A.K., and Szumuness, W.: Hepatitis B Vaccine Administered to Chronic Carriers of Hepatitis B Surface Antigen, *Ann. Intern. Med., 96,* 575, May, 1982.

21. **Merchant,** V.A.: Herpesviruses and Other Microorganisms of Concern in Dentistry, *Dent. Clin. North Am., 35,* 283, April, 1991.

22. **Benenson,** A.S., ed.: *Control of Communicable Diseases in Man,* 15th ed. Washington, D.C., American Public Health Association, 1990, pp. 212–215.

23. **Lafferty,** W.E., Coombs, R.W., Benedetti, J., Critchlow, C., and Corey, L.: Recurrences After Oral and Genital Herpes Simplex Virus Infection. Influence of Site Injection and Viral Type, *N. Engl. J. Med., 316,* 1444, June 4, 1987.

24. **Manzella,** J.P., McConville, J.H., Valenti, W., Menegus, M.A., Swirkosz, E.M., and Arens, M.: An Outbreak of Herpes Simplex Virus Type 1 Gingivostomatis in a Dental Hygiene Practice, *JAMA, 252,* 2019, October 19, 1984.

25. **United States Centers for Disease Control:** Revised Classification System for HIV Infection and Expanded Surveillance Case Definition for AIDS Among Adolescents and Adults, *MMWR, 41,* 1–19, No. RR-17, December 18, 1992.

26. **Benenson:** A.S., ed.: *Control of Communicable Diseases in Man,* 15th ed. Washington, D.C., American Public Health Association, 1990, p.4.

27. **Klein,** R.S., Harris, C.A., Small, C.B., Moll, B., Lesser, M., and Friedland, G.H.: Oral Candidiasis in High-risk Patients as the Initial Manifestation of the Acquired Immunodeficiency Syndrome, *N. Engl. J. Med., 311,* 354, August 9, 1984.

28. **Silverman,** S., Migliorati, C.A., Lozada-Nur, F., Greenspan, D., and Conant, M.A.: Oral Findings in People With or at High Risk for AIDS: A Study of 375 Homosexual Males, *J. Am. Dent. Assoc., 112,* 187, February, 1986.

29. **Keeney,** K., Abaza, N.A., Tidwel, O., and Quinn, P.: Oral Kaposi's Sarcoma in Acquired Immune Deficiency Syndrome, *J. Oral Maxillofac. Surg., 45,* 815, September, 1987.

30. **Greenspan,** D., Greenspan, J.S., Hearst, N.G., Pan, L.Z., Conant, M.A., Abrams, D.I., Hollander, H., and Levy, J.A.: Relation of Oral Hairy Leukoplakia to Infection With the Human Immunodeficiency Virus and the Risk

of Developing AIDS, *J. Infect, Dis., 155,* 475, March, 1987.

31. **Greenspan,** D., Greenspan, J.S., Schiodt, M., and Pindborg, J.J.: *AIDS and the Mouth. Diagnosis and Management of Oral Lesions.* Copenhagen, Munksgaard, 1990, pp.91–102, 113–134.

32. **Drinkard,** C.R., Decher, L., Litle, J.S., Rhame, F.S., Balfour, H.H., Rhodus, N.L., Merry, J.W., Walker, P.O., Miller, C.E., Volberding, P.A., and Melnick, S.L.: Periodontal Status of Individuals in Early Stages of Human Immunodeficiency Virus Infection, *Community Dent. Oral Epidemiol., 19,* 281, October, 1991.

33. **Riley,** C., London, J.P., and Burmeister, J.A.: Periodontal Health in 200 HIV-positive Patients. *J. Oral Pathol. Med., 21,* 124, March, 1992.

34. **Winkler,** J.R. and Robertson, P.B.: Periodontal Disease Associated with HIV Infection, *Oral Surg. Oral Med. Oral Pathol., 73,* 145, February, 1992.

35. **MacDonald,** M.G., Ginzberg, H.M., and Bolan, J.C.: HIV Infection in Pregnancy: Epidemiology and Clinical Management, *J. Acquired Immune Deficiency Syndrome, 4,* 100, February, 1991.

36. **Ruff,** A.J., Halsey, N.S., Coberly, J., and Boulos, R.: Breastfeeding and Maternal-infant Transmission of Human Immunodeficiency Virus Type I, *J. Pediatr. 121,* 325, August, 1992.

37. **Gutman,** L.T., St. Claire, K.K., Weedy, C., Herman-Giddens, M.E., Lane, B.A., Niemeyer, J.C., and McKinney, R.E.: Human Immunodeficiency Virus Transmission by Sexual Abuse, *Am. J. Dis. Child., 145,* 137, February, 1991.

38. **United States Centers for Disease Control and Prevention:** 1194 Revised Classification System for Human Immunodeficiency Virus Infection in Children Less Than 13 Years of Age, *MMWR, 43,* 1–19, No. RR-12, September 30, 1994.

39. **Hoyt,** L.G. and Oleske, J.M.: The Clinical Spectrum of HIV Infection in Infants and Children: An Overview, in Yogev, R. and Connor, E., eds.: *Management of HIV Infection in Infants and Children.* St. Louis, The C.V. Mosby Co., 1992, pp. 227–245.

40. **Butler,** K.M. and Pizzo, P.A.: HIV Infection in Children, in Devita, V.T., Helman, S., and Rosenberg, S.A., eds.: *AIDS Etiology, Diagnosis, Treatment, and Prevention,* 3rd. ed. Philadelphia, J.B. Lippincott Co., 1992, pp. 285–312.

41. **Scott,** G.B.: HIV Infection in Children: Clinical Features and Management, *J. Acquired Immune Deficiency Syndrome, 4,* 109, February, 1991.

42. **Conner,** E., McSherry, G., and Yogev, R.: Antiviral Treatment of Pediatric HIV Infection, in Yogove, R. and Connor, E., eds.: *Management of HIV Infection in Infants and Children.* St. Louis, The C.V. Mosby Co., 1992, pp. 505–531.

43. **Gehrke,** F.S. and Johnsen, D.S.: Bottle Caries Associated with Anti-HIV Therapy (Letter), *Pediatr. Dent., 13,* 73, January-February, 1991.

44. **Howell,** R.B. and Houpt, M.: More Than One Factor Can Influence Caries Development in HIV-positive Children (Letter), *Pediatr. Dent. 13,* 247, July-August, 1991.

EXPOSURE CONTROL: BARRIERS

3

The use of *universal precautions* is essential to all exposure control protocols used in oral treatment situations. A written procedure/protocol manual is necessary to ensure standardization and consistency of activities pertinent to the health and safety of both the patient/client and the oral healthcare worker (1).

IMMUNIZATIONS

It is the responsibility of each healthcare worker to obtain and keep current all immunizations that will aid in preventing infectious disease transfer. Table 2.4 lists many of the transmissible diseases and their vaccines. Table 3.1 provides a summary of the vaccines and toxoids recommended for most adults by age groups (2). Hepatitis B vaccine is also recommended. Written records should be kept for all immunizations, boosters, and reimmunizations.

Exposure to certain infectious diseases should be followed by expedient testing and prophylactic immunization. Each exposure incident should be recorded. Annual testing for tuberculosis should also be done.

CLINICAL ATTIRE

The clinician's attire should present an adequate barrier to minimize cross-contamination. Table 3.2 gives a list of barrier attire for clinicians.

TABLE 3.1. Vaccines and Toxoids Recommended for Adults by Age Groups, United States

Age Group (Years)	Vaccine/Toxoid					
	Td[a]	Measles	Mumps	Rubella	Influenza	Pneumococcal Polysaccharide
18–24	X	X	X	X		
25–64	X	X[b]	X[b]	X		
≥65	X				X	X

From United States Centers for Disease Control: Update on Adult Immunization Recommendations of the Immunization Practices Advisory Committee (ACIP), *MMWR, 40,* 56, No. RR-12, November 15, 1991.

[a]Td, Tetanus and diphtheria toxoids, adsorbed (for adult use), which is a combined preparation containing < 2 flocculation units of diphtheria toxoid.

[b]Indicated for persons born after 1956.

TABLE 3.2.　Clinical Attire

Item	Characteristics
Outer garments: gowns, lab coats, scrub suits, uniforms	Adequate coverage of arms and clothing
	Disposable or commercially laundered (not to be taken home for cleaning or worn outside the clinic) (3)
Face mask	Filtration should block out particles at least as small as microns
	Fit should adequately cover nose, mouth, and fit under glasses comfortably
	Lining should be impenetrable to moisture
	Should be changed for each patient/client and worn no longer than 1 hour
	Glass fiber and synthetic fiber mat provide the most effective aerosol filter
Protective eyewear	Should be worn by both clinician and patient/client (6–9)
	Wide coverage, with side shields
	Shatterproof
	Lightweight
	Easily disinfected
Gloves	Effective barrier, minimal manufacturer's defects
	Impermeable to saliva, blood, and bacteria
	Strong and durable to resist tears and punctures
	Not adversely affected by materials used during clinical treatment
	Nonirritating or harmful to skin—allergies
	Proper fit for comfort, ease of motion, tactile sensitivity, and prevention of tearing
Jewelry	Ideally, no jewelry on hands and wrists to minimize microorganism areas

Hand Care/Gloving

Thorough handwashing is required to prevent the spread of microorganisms from the clinician and environment to the patient and control cross-contamination. The following is a list of basics for handwashing, hand care, and gloving.

1. Place mask and protective eyewear prior to handwashing.
2. Perform thorough handwashing with an antimicrobial soap before gloving and after glove removal.
3. Faucet handles should not be touched with bare hands; use disposable paper towels, foot pedal, or electronically controlled faucets for water-flow control.
4. There should be no contact with the inside of the sink during or after handwashing. (A separate sink and area away from the operatory should be used for instrument washing.)
5. Use paper towels from a dispenser that requires no contact except with the towel itself. Cloth towels must be used for only one patient.
6. Dry hands thoroughly.
7. Keep gloved hands from touching any surface that has not been disinfected and covered with a barrier material. This includes pencils, pens, charts/records, clothing, etc.
8. Remove gloves and wash hands if integrity of glove is disrupted (torn, cut, or punctured) and reglove with a new pair.
9. Remove gloves without contaminating hands from the exposed external surfaces of the used gloves.
10. Disposable, single-use gloves are not to be washed or reused.
11. Short fingernails and healthy cuticles are more suitable for hygienic purposes and clinical efficiency (10, 11).

REFERENCES

1. **United States Department of Labor,** Occupational Safety and Health Administration: Occupational Exposure to Bloodborne Pathogens; Final Rule, *Federal Register, 56,* No. 235, December 6, 1991.

2. **United States Centers for Disease Control:** Update on Adult Immunization. Recommendations of the Immunization Practices Advisory Committee (ACIP), *MMWR, 40,* 1–94, No. RR-12, November 15, 1991.

3. **Federation Dentaire Internationale,** Commission on Dental Practice: Technical Report: Recommendation for Hygiene in Dental Practice, *Int. Dent. J., 29,* 72, March, 1979.

4. **Micik,** R.E., Miller, R.L., and Leong, A.C.: Studies on Dental Aerobiology: III. Efficacy of Surgical Masks in Protecting Dental Personnel from Airborne Bacterial Particles. *J. Dent. Res., 50,* 626, May-June, 1971.

5. **Miller,** R.L. and Micik, R.E.: Air Pollution and Its Control in the Dental Office, *Dent. Clin. North Am., 22,* 453, July, 1978.

6. **Hartley,** J.L.: Eye and Facial Injuries Resulting from Dental Procedures, *Dent. Clin. North Am., 22,* 505, July, 1978.

7. **Colvin,** J.: Eye Injuries and the Dentist, *Aust. Dent. J., 23,* 453, December, 1978.

8. **Cooley,** R.L., Cottingham, A.J., Abrams, H., and Barkmeier, W.W.: Ocular Injuries Sustained in the Dental Office: Methods of Detection, Treatment, and Prevention, *J. Am. Dent. Assoc., 97,* 985, December, 1978.

9. **Wesson,** M.D. and Thornton, J.B.: Eye Protection and Ocular Complications in the Dental Office, *Gen. Dent. 37,* 19, January-February, 1989.

10. **Harfst,** S.A.: Personal Barrier Protection, *Dent. Clin. North Am., 35,* 357, April, 1991.

11. **Allen,** A.L. and Organ, R.J.: Occult Blood Accumulation Under the Fingernails: A Mechanism for the Spread of Bloodborne Infection, *J. Am. Dent. Assoc., 105,* 455, September, 1982.

INFECTION CONTROL: CLINICAL PROCEDURES

4

As stated in Chapter 3, a written procedure/protocol manual for effective exposure control should be present in every oral treatment facility. The manual should also include a written protocol for all clinical procedures. The protocol should have the objectives of reduction of pathogenic microorganisms to prevent infection, elimination of cross-contamination, and the use of universal precautions (1).

OPERATORY FACTORS

The treatment rooms should be free of clutter. Facilitate cleanliness and disinfection procedures. All surfaces that come in contact with the clinician or patient/client should be barrier-covered or operated by foot controls. Sinks should be large enough to accommodate thorough hand-washing procedures and not used for instrument cleaning. Supplies should be sterilizable or disposable and stored away from any possible contamination. Waste receptacles should have openings that allow for waste disposal without touching the sides of the container. The waste receptacles should be lined with heavy-duty plastic bags that can be sealed prior to disposal. Smaller individual patient/client bags near the treatment area that hold contaminated materials during clinical treatment should be used, tightly closed, and disposed in the larger waste receptacle.

INSTRUMENT MANAGEMENT

Handling of contaminated instruments should be minimized. The use of cassettes to hold instruments before, during, and after the sterilization process minimizes the risk of mishaps (2, 3). A separate area should be used for the cleaning and sterilization of all instruments. When handling instruments, heavy-duty, puncture-resistant gloves used only for this purpose should be worn along with a mask and protective eyewear. The use of transfer forceps to handle contaminated instruments is recommended if not using cassettes.

A presoak in disinfectant or detergent is indicated if the sterilization process is not initiated immediately after instrument use. Ultrasonic processing of instruments prior to sterilization is preferrable to manual cleaning. After drying, the cassette or group of instruments is placed in a see-through sterilization bag. The bag should have an indicator that changes color to signify that the sterilization process has been adequately completed. Note that regular testing of the sterilizer itself with a biologic indicator must be done to ensure that proper sterilization is achieved. Sterilized packets must be kept sealed until opened in front of the patient.

STERILIZATION

Tables 4.1 through 4.3 list information pertinent to the sterilization process.

CHEMICAL DISINFECTANTS

Disinfection is not a substitute for sterilization. Disinfection reduces the level of microbial contamination to a safe level, but it does not destroy all forms of microorganisms. Alcohols and quaternary ammonium compounds are not approved for instrument or environmental surface disinfection.

TABLE 4.1. Types of Sterilization

Type	Use	Advantages	Disadvantages
Moist heat steam under pressure	All material except oils, waxes, and powders impervious to steam or materials that cannot be subjected to high temperature	All microorganisms, spores, and viruses are destroyed quickly and efficiently Wide variety of materials may be treated Most economical method of sterilization	May corrode carbon steel instruments Unsuitable for oils or powders that are impervious to heat
Dry heat	Materials that cannot be subjected to steam under pressure Oils and powders when thermostabile at the required temperatures	For materials that cannot be subjected to steam under pressure Well suited for sharp instruments No corrosion as with steam under pressure	Long exposure required Slow and uneven penetration High temperature critical to some materials

continued

TABLE 4.1. Types of Sterilization

Type	Use	Advantages	Disadvantages
Chemical vapor sterilizer (4)	All materials except those that cannot withstand high temperatures or are chemically alterable	Corrosion and rust-free for carbon steel instruments Short sterilization cycle	Adequate ventilation needed Odor
Ethylene oxide (5)	All materials can be sterilized	All types of material can be sterilized with minimum or no damage Low temperature for operation	Not commonly found in dental practice settings High cost for equipment Verified ventilation is necessary Long operation time Airing needed for several hours for plastic, rubber, cloth materials

TABLE 4.2. Methods of Sterilization

Method	Sterilizing Requirement		
	Time	Temperature	Pressure
Moist heat steam under pressure (steam autoclave)	20 min	250° F 121° C	15 psi
Dry heat oven	60–120 min	320° F 160° C	
Unsaturated chemical vapor	20 min	270° F 132° C	20–40 psi
Ethylene oxide gas	10–16 hr	75° F 25° C	

TABLE 4.3. Spore Testing

When	Why
Once per week	To verify proper use and functioning
Whenever a new type of packaging material or tray is used	To ensure that the sterilizing agent is getting inside to the surface of the instruments
After training of new sterilization personnel	To verify proper use of the sterilizer
During initial uses of a new sterilizer	To make sure unfamiliar operating instructions are being followed
First run after repair of a sterilizer	To make sure that the sterilizer is functioning properly
With every implantable device; hold device until results of test are known	Extra precaution for sterilization of item to be implanted into tissues
After any other change in the sterilizing procedure	To make sure change does not prevent sterilization

Adapted from Miller, C.H. and Palenik, C.J.: Sterilization, Disinfection, and Asepsis in Dentistry, in Block, S.S., ed: *Disinfection, Sterilization, and Preservation,* 4th ed. Philadelphia, Lea & Febiger, 1991, p. 680.

Tables 4.4 through 4.6 provide information on chemical disinfectants.

TABLE 4.4. Chemical Disinfectants

Categories (classified by biocidal activity)
High level
    Inactivate spores, all forms of bacteria, fungi, and viruses
    Used as either a disinfectant or a sterilant according to time
       schedule
Intermediate level
    Inactivate all forms of microorganisms
    Does not destroy spores
Low level
    Inactivate vegetative bacteria and certain lipid-type viruses
    Does not destroy spores, tubercle bacilli, or nonlipid viruses
Uses
Environmental surfaces disinfection: operatory cleaning and
    disinfecting
Precleaning: holding solution for instruments before sterilization
Dental laboratory impressions and prostheses
Critical points
Disinfection is dependent on the correct concentration and length
    of exposure
Action of the agent is altered by foreign matter and dilution; areas
    and items should be clean and dry
Check manufacturer's labels and instructions to ensure optimum
    results

TABLE 4.5. Chemical Disinfecting Agents

Chemical Classification	Action	Factors

Glutaraldehydes
Glutaraldehyde 2% neutral
Glutaraldehyde 2% alkaline
Glutaraldehyde 2% alkaline with
  phenolic buffer
Glutaraldehyde 2% acidic
	High-level disinfectants	Caustic to skin
		Causes eye irritation
		Corrosive to some metal instruments
		Items must be rinsed in sterile water
		  after removal
		Not used as a surface disinfectant

Chlorine compounds
Chlorine dioxide
Sodium hypochlorite (5.25% household
  bleach)
	Water purification
	Denture cleaning
		Use life and stability necessitate fresh
		  preparation daily
		Instrument corrosion
		Can be harmful to eyes, skin, clothing
		Strong odor
		Economical

continued

TABLE 4.5. Chemical Disinfecting Agents

Chemical Classification	Action	Factors
Iodophors Iodophor (1% available iodine)	Broad-spectrum antimicrobial contained in surgical scrubs, liquid soaps, mouth rinses, and surface antiseptics before hypodermic injection	Hard water inactivates iodophors: 1 part iodophor concentrate to 213 parts soft or distilled water Amber color fades to clear as potency decreases
Phenolics o-phenylphenyl 9% with o-benzyl-p-chlorophenol 1%	High-concentration phenols destroy the cell wall and precipitate the protein Low concentrations are used as surface disinfectants and to inactivate enzyme systems	10-min disinfecting time, but immersion time for tuberculosis is 20 min

TABLE 4.6. Properties of an Ideal Disinfectant

1. Broad spectrum: should always have the widest possible antimicrobial spectrum
2. Fast acting: should always have a rapidly lethal action on all vegetative forms and spores of bacteria and fungi, protozoa, and viruses
3. Not affected by physical factors: active in the presence of organic matter, such as blood, sputum, and feces; should be compatible with soaps, detergents, and other chemicals encountered in use
4. Nontoxic
5. Surface compatibility: should not corrode instruments and other metallic surfaces; should not cause the disintegration of cloth, rubber, plastics, or other materials
6. Residual effect on treated surfaces
7. Easy to use
8. Odorless: an inoffensive odor would facilitate its routine use
9. Economical: cost should not be prohibitively high

Reprinted with permission from Molinari, J.A., Gleason, M.J., Cottone, J.A., and Barrett, E.D.: Comparison of Dental Surface Disinfectants, *Gen. Dent., 35,* 171, May-June, 1987.

UNIT WATER LINES

Tubings to handpieces, water syringes, and ultrasonic scalers harbor microorganisms that contribute to infection and bacteremia. The flushing of water lines is essential to reduce the microbial count (6).

The following procedures should be used:

1. 5–6-minute flushing of all water lines at the beginning and end of the day
2. 30-second flush of handpieces and waterspray before and after each patient's appointment
3. A check valve or antiretractor valve should be installed in handpiece lines (7)

OPERATORY PREPARATION

Every operatory should have an efficient plan to achieve cleanliness and order. Constant and continuous attention must be taken to ensure an immaculate environment for patient/client treatment. Table 4.7 serves as a guide for effective preparation of the operatory (8). The following list provides additional important points.

1. Contact should be limited to actual patient treatment. Materials pertinent to treatment should be ready to avoid touching of drawer handles or knobs to retrieve needed items.
2. Adequate supply of sterilized items such as handpieces and instruments should be available.
3. Disposable items should be used as much as possible.
4. Barriers/covers should be used on dental units, light handles, x-ray parts, and all areas where possible contamination can occur.
5. Be aware of items that may need chemical disinfection; if this is not feasible, the use of disposable or coverable items is indicated.
6. Clean and disinfect environmental surfaces, using a spray bottle to dispense the disinfectant.
7. Scrubbing of the area after spraying is necessary to remove microorganisms; spray again and leave surfaces wet.
8. Wear heavy-duty gloves, used only for these procedures.

PATIENT PREPARATION

Prevention of disease transmission for both the patient and the clinician can be further enhanced by preoperative procedures involving the patient. Table 4.8 outlines these procedures.

TABLE 4.7. Classification of Inanimate Objects (Spaulding)

Surface Category	Definition	Sterilization/Disinfection	Examples
Critical surfaces of instruments or devices	Penetrate/touch mucous membranes, oral fluids Contact normally sterile body areas	Sterilize or disposable	Needles Curets Explorers Probes
Semicritical surfaces of instruments or devices	Touch intact mucous membrane, oral fluids (No entrance to sterile body areas) Does not penetrate	Sterilize or high-level disinfection	Radiographic biteblock Ultrasonic handpiece Amalgam condenser
Noncritical surfaces of instruments or devices	Do not touch mucous membranes (only contact unbroken epithelium)	Cleaning and tuberculocidal intermediate-level disinfection	Light handles Certain x-ray machine parts Safety eyewear
Environmental surfaces	No contact with patient (or only intact skin)	Cleaning and intermediate to low disinfection	Counter tops Equipment surfaces Housekeeping surface

TABLE 4.8. Patient Preoperative Procedures

Procedure	Factor
Toothbrushing	Disturbs and removes microorganisms
	Contributes to surface degerming
Rinsing (antiseptic mouthrinse)	Reduction of the numbers of bacteria on the gingival and mucosal surfaces (9, 10)
	Reduction of aerosol contamination (11, 12)
	More favorable healing after treatment
Chlorhexidine rinse	Lowered bacterial count for more than 60 min
	Preprocedural rinsing before injections is advised (13)
Surface antiseptic application (14, 15)	Before injection of anesthetic
	Before scaling and other oral hygiene instrumentation

UNIVERSAL PROCEDURES/PREVENTION OF DISEASE TRANSMISSION

Chapters 2, 3, and this chapter provide information on the prevention of disease transmission. Table 4.9 gives more basic information on clinical management. Figure 4.1 illustrates needle recapping methods to prevent percutaneous injury.

TABLE 4.9. Universal Procedures/Prevention of Disease Transmission

Patient preparation	Comprehensive medical history
	Medical referral if needed
	Postponement of elective procedures if open lesions or communicable condition is present
	Germicidal rinsing
	Protective eyewear
Operatory preparation	See Table 4.7 and previous chapters
Dental team preparation	Current medical examinations, immunizations, and tests
	Clinical attire (mask, gloves, protective eyewear, appropriate overcovering)
	Thorough handwashing
	Avoidance of environmental contacts unrelated to planned procedures
Treatment considerations	
Hypodermic needles	Safe recapping method (see Fig. 4.1)
	Used needles in puncture-resistant container
	Disposal of partial and empty cartridges of anesthetic
Removable oral appliances	Handle with gloves
	Place in disposable cup with disinfectant, cover, and clean with ultrasonics
Posttreatment considerations	Follow protocol/procedures previously given

continued

TABLE 4.9.   Universal Procedures/Prevention of Disease Transmission

Occupational accidental exposure management	See Table 2.8 Procedure following exposure (16, 17): Immediately wash with soap and water, rinse, and dry Obtain permission for blood testing and arrange for counseling On the same day: Source person should be tested for HBsAg and anti-HIV Exposed person should be tested for anti-HBs and anti-HIV

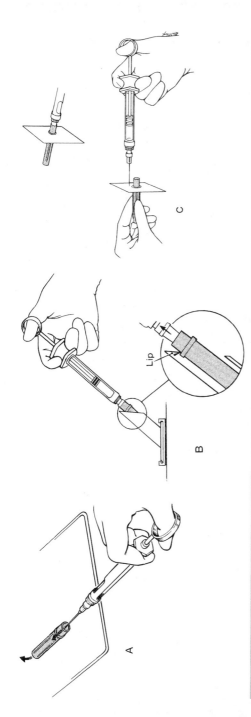

FIGURE 4.1. Prevention of percutaneous injury: needle recapping methods. One-handed recapping or recapping with a safety mechanical device is required. **A.** The "scoop" technique. A cap is placed on the tray and the needle is guided into it. **B.** An example of a commercially available holder for the cap. The device is fastened to the tray, and the cap is removed and recapped by directing the needle into the cap holder. **C.** Cardboard shield retained on the cap. During replacement of the cap, protection is provided as shown. Needles must be discarded in a puncture-resistant container.

REFERENCES

1. **Bassett,** K.: *Infection Control, Hazardous Waste Management, and Hazardous Materials: An Integrated Curriculum for the Dental Hygienist.* Tacoma, WA, Pierce College, Department of Dental Hygiene.

2. **Miller,** C.H.: Sterilization and Disinfection: What Every Dentist Needs to Know, *J. Am. Dent. Assoc., 123,* 46, March, 1992.

3. **D'Autremont,** P.: Instrument Sterilization, *Dentalhygienistnews, 5,* 17, Fall, 1992.

4. **Harvey Chemiclave,** MDT Biologics Corp., 19645 Rancho Way, Rancho Dominguez, CA 90220.

5. **Parisi,** A.N. and Young, W.E.: Sterilization with Ethylene Oxide and Other Gases, in Block, S.S., ed.: *Disinfection, Sterilization, and Preservation,* 4th ed. Philadelphia, Lea & Febiger, 1991, pp. 580–595.

6. **Gross,** A., Devine, M.J., and Cutright, D.E.: Microbial Contamination of Dental Units and Ultrasonic Scalers, *J. Periodontol. 47,* 670, November, 1976.

7. **Bagga,** B.S.R., Murphy, R.A., Anderson, A.W., and Punwani, I.: Contamination of Dental Unit Cooling Water with Oral Microorganisms and Its Prevention, *J. Am. Dent. Assoc., 109,* 712, November 1984.

8. **Favero,** M.S. and Bond, W.W.: Chemical Disinfection of Medical and Surgical Materials, in Block, S.S., ed.: *Disinfection, Sterilization, and Preservation,* 4th ed. Philadelphia, Lea & Febiger, 1991, pp. 617–641.

9. **Randall,** E. and Brenman, H.S.: Local Degerming with Povidone-Iodine. I. Prior to Dental Prophylaxis, *J. Periodontol. 45,* 866, December, 1974.

10. **Brenman,** H.S. and Randall, E.: Degerming with Povidone-Iodine. II. Prior to Gingivectomy, *J. Periodontol. 45,* 870, December, 1974.

11. **Litsky,** B.Y., Mascis, J.D., and Litsky, W.: Use of Antimicrobial Mouthwash to Minimize the Bacterial Aerosol Contamination Generated by the High-speed Drill, *Oral Surg. Oral Med. Oral Pathol., 29,* 25, January, 1970.

12. **Wyler,** D., Miller, R.L., and Micik, R.E.: Efficacy of Self-administered Preoperative Oral Hygiene Procedures in

Reducing the Concentration of Bacteria in Aerosols Generated During Dental Procedures, *J. Dent. Res., 50,* 509, March-April, 1971.

13. **Veksler,** A.E., Kayrouz, G.A., and Newman, M.G.: Reduction of Salivary Bacteria by Pre-procedural Rinses with Chlorhexidine 0.12%, *J. Periodontol., 62,* 649, November, 1991.

14. **Malamed,** S.F.: *Handbook of Local Anesthesia,* 3rd ed. St. Louis, The C.V. Mosby Co., 1990, pp. 103, 118.

15. **Connor,** J.P. and Edelson, J.G.: Needle Tract Infection, *Oral Surg. Oral Med. Oral Pathol., 65,* 401, April 1988.

16. **United States Centers for Disease Control:** Public Health Service Statement on Management of Occupational Exposure to Human Immunodeficiency Virus, Including Considerations Regarding Zidovudine Postexposure Use, *MMWR, 39,* 1–3, No. RR-1, January 26, 1990.

17. **United States Centers for Disease Control:** Protection Against Viral Hepatitis, Recommendations of the Immunization Practices Committee (ACIP), *MMWR, 39,* 20, No. RR-2, February 9, 1990.

PATIENT/CLIENT ASSESSMENT

5

The key elements in the successful treatment and rendering of services to all patients/clients are assessment, diagnosis, planning, implementation, and evaluation. This chapter provides the basic information necessary for each element. The collection and organization of data provides a coherent picture with which the clinician can base the best possible diagnosis and treatment plan specific to each patient.

PATIENT HISTORIES

The information gathered through patient histories is vital to providing any type of treatment. The total health and well-being of the patient may depend on the accuracy of histories. Treatment modalities will depend to a great extent on this data. Legal aspects are also an important consideration when recording histories (1). It should be noted that there are limitations to patient histories (2–4). Failure or reluctance to disclose all information, language barriers, the environment in which the history is taken, and the neutrality of the questioner may all influence the accuracy of histories.

Personal History

The data for the personal history is needed for the business and legal aspects of the office/clinic. Legal consents, consultation considerations, appointment planning, and financial arrangements are part of the personal history (1, 5). Table 5.2 gives an overview of the necessary items in a personal history.

TABLE 5.1.   Elements of Diagnostic Work-Up

Information	Components
Patient histories	Personal (see Table 5.2) Medical (see Tables 5.3–5.6) Dental (see Table 5.7)
Determination of vital signs	See Tables 5.8–5.10, Fig. 5.1
Extraoral and intraoral examination	See Tables 5.11–5.20, Figs. 5.2–5.10
Radiographic survey	Periapical survey Bitewing survey Occlusal survey—as needed Panoramic—as needed, not a substitute for a periapical survey See Tables 5.21–5.23
Study casts	As needed for diagnosis and treatment planning
Gingival and periodontal examination	Clinical signs of disease Probing depths, probes Soft tissue lesions, anomalies

continued

	Charting: missing teeth, restorations, recession, mobility, carious lesions, structural defects, tooth positions Dental or periodontal indices Bacterial plaque scores See Tables 5.24–5.27, Fig. 5.11
Tooth examination	Record findings of deposits, stains, carious lesions, pulp vitality, occlusion, attrition, abrasion, bruxing, habits affecting teeth, sealants See Tables 5.28–5.32, Figs. 5.12–5.21
Additional considerations	Photographs Biopsy or cytologic smear Referral for laboratory tests or medical referrals Consultations with specialists (medical or dental) See Table 5.17

TABLE 5.2. Items for the Personal History

Items to Record in Patient History	Considerations	Influences on Appointment Procedures
Name Addresses: residence and business Telephone numbers Sex Marital status For child: name of parent or guardian For parent: ages and sex of children	Accurate recording necessary for business aspects of dental practice	Aids in establishing rapport Instruction applicable to entire family Advice concerning fluorides for children
Birth date	Whether of age or a minor Oral conditions related to age changes; diseases, healing, and other possible characteristics	Approval of parent or guardian necessary for care of minor or person with a mental handicap; signature must be obtained Approach to patient instruction
Birthplace and residence in early years	Presence of fluoride in drinking water Food and eating patterns Conditions endemic to certain areas	Effects of fluoride on teeth Instruction in dietary needs adapted to cultural practices

continued

Occupation: present and former Spouse's occupation For children: parent's occupation	Instruction applied to specific needs May be a factor in etiology of certain diseases, dental stains, occlusal wear Dexterity in use of self-care devices related to dexterity gained from occupation May affect diet, oral habits, general health Influence on oral care of entire family For child: which parent will supervise and assist child in oral care

Physician	Name, address, and telephone number
	For consultation
	Consultation indicated:
	  for condition that may require premedication
	  when disease symptoms are suspected but patient does not state them
	  in an emergency

Referred by and address	To whom to send referral acknowledgment and appreciation Contribution to rapport with patient Patient referred by another patient may have a concept of the office procedures

Medical History

A medical history ascertains whether an individual has any disease or condition that requires special precautions or premedication or poses any complication or modification of treatment to be provided. In addition, the medical history alerts the clinician to any known drug allergies, medications that are being taken that affect the mouth, oral manisfestations of certain diseases, and communicable disease information and gives an insight to the physiologic state of the patient.

Thorough review of the history at the onset and an update at each appointment is necessary to ensure accurate information exists for continuing treatment. Consultation with the patient's physician concerning findings may be necessary (5). Any consultation, whether by phone or in person, must be followed up in writing to provide a legal record and clarify any misunderstanding that may arise. A formal request within a standardized form letter with fill-in-the-blank questions is an efficient method. Questions about prophylactic premedication, radiation therapy, or chemotherapy should be answered with consultation (6).

Prophylactic premedication is indicated for some cardiac conditions when any gingival bleeding will be induced by the performance of a dental procedure (7). In addition, other predisposing factors necessitate prophylactic premedication. Consultation with the patient's physician should be done to determine the need for preventive antibiotics. Table 5.3 lists some of the conditions that should be considered for premedication.

Dental History

The dental history adds another dimension to the diagnostic work-up. Through this history, the clinician is able

TABLE 5.3. Prophylactic Premedication Conditions

Category	Condition
Cardiac	Congenital heart disease; most congenital cardiac malformations
	Rheumatic heart disease
	Rheumatic fever and other febrile disease that predispose to valvular damage
	Heart murmur—physician should determine whether it is functional or organic and advise; functional murmur may not require premedication; organic murmur based on structural heart defect requires antibiotic premedication (8)
	Prosthetic cardiac valves (9)
	Vascular autographs generally do not need premedication (10)
	Previous history of infective endocarditis
	Indwelling transvenous cardiac pacemaker
	Mitral valve prolapse with insufficiency
	Surgically constructed systemic-pulmonary shunts
Orthopaedic	Prosthetic joint replacement (11–13)

continued

TABLE 5.3. Prophylactic Premedication Conditions

Category	Condition
Reduced capacity to resist infection	Corticosteroid or other immunosuppressive therapy Anticancer chemotherapy Blood diseases such as acute leukemia, agranulocytosis, and sickle cell anemia Uncontrolled, unstable diabetes mellitus (controlled diabetes can be treated as normal) Grossly contaminated traumatic facial injuries and compound fractures
Renal	Renal transplant Hemodialysis Glomerulonephritis or other active renal disorder (14)
Additional information	Individuals with delayed hearing may need additional antibiotics Bacteremia rarely persists for more than approximately 15 minutes after instrumentation is terminated Bacteremia incidence is reduced when periodontal tissues are maintained in optimum health

TABLE 5.4. Recommended Standard Prophylactic Regimen for Dental, Oral, or Upper Respiratory Tract Procedures in Patients Who Are At Risk[a]

Drug	Dosing Regimen
	Standard regimen
Amoxicillin	Adults: 2.0 g orally 1 hr before procedure
	Children: 50 mg/kg orally 1 hr before procedure
	Amoxicillin/penicillin-allergic patients
Clindamycin	Adults: 600 mg orally 1 hr before procedure
	Children: 20 mg/kg orally 1 hr before procedure
or	
Cephalexin or cefadroxil	Adults: 2.0 g orally 1 hr before procedure
	Children: 50 mg/kg orally 1 hr before procedure
or	
Azithromycin or claithromycin	Adults: 500 mg orally 1 hr before procedure
	Children: 15 mg/kg orally 1 hr before procedure
	Check with a physician for children under 16.

[a] Includes those with prosthetic heart valves and other high-risk patients. **Total pediatric dose should not exceed total adult dose.**

TABLE 5.5. Alternate Prophylactic Regimens for Dental, Oral, or Upper Respiratory Tract Procedures in Patients Who Are At Risk

Drug	Dosing regimen
	Patients unable to take oral medications
Ampicillin	Adults: 2 g IM or IV within 30 min before procedure
	Children: 50 mg/kg IM or IV within 30 min before procedure
	Amoxicillin/penicillin/ampicillin-allergic patients unable to take oral medications

continued

TABLE 5.5.   Alternate Prophylactic Regimens for Dental, Oral, or Upper Respiratory Tract Procedures in Patients Who Are At Risk

Clindamycin	Adults: 600 mg IV within 30 min before procedure
	Children: 20 mg/kg IV within 30 min before procedure
or	
Cefazolin	Adults: 1.0 g IM or IV within 30 min before procedure
	Children: 25 mg/kg IM or IV within 30 min before procedure

Total pediatric dose should not exceed total adult dose.

to learn about the patient's previous dental treatment, the present reason for seeking oral care, and attitudes and personal habits related to daily oral care. Table 5.6 lists the items in a dental history.

VITAL SIGNS

The recording of vital signs at the beginning of each appointment aids in the overall evaluation of the patient. Vital signs alert the practitioner to the health of the patient/client. Medical referral or consultation or postponement of procedures may be necessary if the vital signs deviate from normal. Tables 5.7 and 5.8 and Figure 5.1 list information pertinent to vital signs.

TABLE 5.6. Items for the Dental History

Items to Record in the History	Considerations	Influences on Appointment Procedures
Reason for present appointment	Chief complaint in patient's own words Pain or discomfort Onset, symptoms, duration of an acute condition	Need for immediate treatment Attitude toward dentistry and preventive care
Previous dental appointments	Date last treatment Services performed Regularity	Patient knowledge concerning regular dental care Cooperation anticipated
Anesthetics used	Local, general Adverse or allergic reactions	Choice of anesthetic
Radiation history	Type, number, dates of dental and medical radiographs Therapeutic radiation Availability of dental radiographs from previous dentist Amount of exposure considered with exposure for medical purposes	Amount of exposure; limitations Patient's appreciation for need and use of radiographs

continued

TABLE 5.6. Items for the Dental History

Items to Record in the History	Considerations	Influences on Appointment Procedures
Family dental history	Parental tooth loss or maintenance	Attitude toward saving teeth and preventive dentistry
Previous treatment	Type of treatment; frequency maintenance appointments	Attitude toward specialized care
	Whether referred to specialist	Previous familiarity with role of dental hygienist
Periodontal	History of acute infection (necrotizing ulcerative gingivitis)	Attitude toward self-care and disease control
	Surgery; postoperative healing	
Orthodontic	Age during treatment; completion	For current treatment, consultation with orthodontist needed to determine instructions
	Previous problem	
	Habit correction	
Endodontic	Dates, etiology	Periodic recheck
Prosthodontic	Types of prostheses	Care of prostheses and abutment teeth
Other	Extent of restorations	Understanding of prevention
	Tooth loss	
	Implants	

continued

Injuries to face or teeth	Causes and extent	Limitation of opening
	Fractured teeth or jaws	Special care during healing
Temporomandibular joint	History of injury, discomfort, disease, dislocation	Effect on opening; accessibility during instrumentation
	Previous treatment	
Habits	Clenching, bruxism, doodling	Tension of patient
	Mouth breathing	Instruction relative to effects of habits
	Biting objects: fingernails, pipe stem, thread, other	
	Cheek or lip biting	
	Patient awareness of habits	
Tobacco use	Form of tobacco, amount used	Instruction concerning oral effects
	Frequency	Need for frequent observation to detect tissue changes if patient continues at same rate (periodontal risk)
	Knowledge of effects on oral tissues	Dental stains; dentifrice selection
Fluorides	Systemic, topical, dates	Current preventive procedures and need for reevaluation
	Residences during tooth development years	
	Amount of fluoride in drinking water	

continued

TABLE 5.6. Items for the Dental History

Items to Record in the History	Considerations	Influences on Appointment Procedures
Plaque control procedures	Toothbrushing: current procedures Type of brush (manual or powered) Texture of filaments Frequency of use Age of brush; frequency of having a new brush Dentifrice Name How selected; reason Additional cleansing devices and frequency of use Dental floss Water irrigation Implants care Mouthrinse or other agents: frequency, purpose Source of instruction in care of oral cavity	Present practices and previous instruction New instruction needed; reception by patient Relation of techniques to prevention of dental caries and periodontal infections Supervision of child by parent: current practices Problems of habit change

TABLE 5.7. Adult Vital Signs

Vital Sign	Values of Significance in Dental and Dental Hygiene Appointments
Body temperature (oral)	Normal 37.0° C (98.6° F)
	Normal range 35.5°–37.5° C (96.0°–99.5° F)
Pulse rate	Normal range 60–100 per min
Respiration	Normal range 14–20 per min

Blood Pressure Category[a]	Systolic mm Hg	Diastolic mm Hg
Normal	< 130	< 85
High normal	130–139	85–89
Hypertension		
Stage 1 (mild)	140–159	90–99
Stage 2 (moderate)	160–179	100–109
Stage 3 (severe)	180–209	110–119
Stage 4 (very severe)	≥ 210	≥ 120

[a] Data from The Fifth Report of the Joint National Committee on Detection, Evaluation, and Treatment of High Blood Pressure. National Institutes of Health, National Heart, Lung, and Blood Institute, Publication 93–1088, January, 1993.

TABLE 5.8. Recommendations for Follow-up Based on Initial Set of Blood Pressure Measurements for Adults Age 18 and Older*

Initial Screening Blood Pressure (mm Hg)		
Systolic	Diastolic	Follow-up Recommended
< 130	< 85	Recheck in 2 yrs
130–139	85–89	Recheck in 1 yr
140–159	90–99	Confirm within 2 mos

continued

TABLE 5.8. Recommendations for Follow-up Based on Initial Set of Blood Pressure Measurements for Adults Age 18 and Older*

Initial Screening Blood Pressure (mm Hg)		Follow-up Recommended
Systolic	Diastolic	
160–179	100–109	Evaluate or refer to source of care within 1 mo
180–209	110–119	Evaluate or refer to source of care within 1 wk
≥ 210	≥ 120	Evaluate or refer to source of care immediately

[a] If the systolic and diastolic categories are different, follow recommendation for the shorter time follow-up (for example, 160/85 mm Hg should be evaluated or referred to source of care within 1 month).

TABLE 5.9. Blood Pressure Classification By Age in mm Hg (15)

Age	Mean Systolic	Mean Diastolic
3 yrs	108	70
6 yrs	114	74
12 yrs	122	78
16–18 yrs	136	84

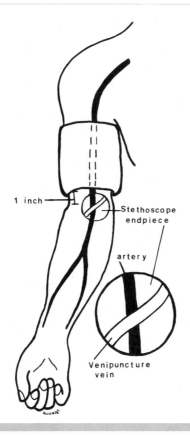

1 inch

Stethoscope endpiece

artery

Venipuncture vein

FIGURE 5.1. Blood pressure cuff in position. The lower edge of the cuff is placed approximately 1 inch above the antecubital fossa. The stethoscope endpiece is placed over the palpated brachial artery pulse point approximately 1 inch below the antecubital fossa and slightly toward the inner side of the arm.

EXTRAORAL AND INTRAORAL EXAMINATION

The extraoral and intraoral examination provides significant information about the patient that influences the general and oral health of the individual. Many disease processes may first be detected in the oral cavity. Malignant lesions of the oral cavity occur in 2–3%, female and male, respectively, of the United States' population. Each appointment should have a routine extraoral and intraoral examination. Early discovery of a lesion in the oral cavity may save a life. Tables 5.10 through 5.16 and Figures 5.2 through 5.10 pertain to the extraoral and intraoral examination.

The purpose of the examination is overall observation. Deviations from normal should be noted and addressed. Detection of lesions, conditions necessitating modification of treatment, prevention of oral disease, need for medical or specialist referrals, continuing evaluation of treatment progress, and recording of all changes and findings for legal purposes are all objectives of the examination.

The practitioner should develop a systematic sequence for the examination using direct observation and digital, bidigital, bimanual, and bilateral palpation (2).

CHILD ABUSE AND NEGLECT

It is the legal and ethical responsibility of every health-care practitioner to report suspected cases of child abuse and neglect. Elder abuse is also increasing (21–23). The intraoral and extraoral examination can provide key indicators that a patient is in jeopardy from a parent, guardian, or care giver. Table 5.17 gives the general and oral signs that may be suggestive of abuse or neglect.

TABLE 5.10. Descriptive Terms for Extraoral/Intraoral Examination (2)

Aphtha (af'thah): a little white or reddish ulcer

Crust: outer scab-like layer of solid matter formed by drying of a body exudate or secretion

Cyst (sist): a closed, epithelial-lined sac, normal or pathologic, that contains fluid or other material

Dorsal (dor'sal): back surface; opposite of ventral

Epidermis (ep˘ i der'mis): outermost and nonvascular layers of the skin composed of basal layer, spinous layer, granular layer, and horny layer

Corium (kō'rē-um): the dermis or true skin just beneath the epidermis; well supplied with nerves and blood vessels

Erosion (e-rō'zhun): soft tissue slightly depressed lesion in which the epithelium above the basal layer is denuded

Erythema (er˘i-the'mah): red area of variable size and shape; reaction to irritation, radiation, or injury

Exophytic (ek' so-fit'ik): growing outward

Exostosis (ek' sos-tō'sis): a benign bony growth projecting from the surface of bone

Fissure (fish'er): a narrow slit or cleft in the epidermis; when infected, ulceration, inflammation, and pain can result

Indurated (in'du-rāt'ed): hardened; abnormally hard

Lymphadenopathy (lim-fad'ĕ-nop'ah-the): disease of the lymph nodes; regional lymph node enlargement

Morphology (mor fol'ō-je): science that deals with form and structure

Palpation (pal-pa'shun): perceiving by sense of touch

Papilla (pah-pil'ah): small, nipple-shaped projection or elevation (**Papillary:** adjective)

Patch: circumscribed flat lesion larger than a macule; differentiated from surrounding epidermis by color and/or texture

Petechia (pe-te'ke-ah): minute hemorrhagic spot of pinpoint to pinhead size

continued

TABLE 5.10. Descriptive Terms for Extraoral/Intraoral Examination (2)

Polyp (pol'ip): any growth or mass protruding from a mucous membrane

Pedunculated (pē-dung'ku-lāt ed): polyp attached by a thin stalk

Sessile (ses'il): polyp with a broad base

Pseudomembrane (soo' do-mem'brān): a loose membranous layer or exudate containing microorganisms, precipitated fibrin, necrotic cells, and inflammatory cells produced during an inflammatory reaction on the surface of a tissue

Punctate (punk'tāt): marked with points or punctures differentiated from the surrounding surface by color, elevation, or texture

Purulent (pu'roo-lent): containing, forming, or discharging pus

Rubefacient (roo'bē-fa'shent): reddening of the skin

Scar (skar): cicatrix; mark remaining after healing of a wound or healing following a surgical intervention

Sclerosis (sklē-ro'sis): induration or hardening

Temporomandibular disorder (TMD): a collective term that includes a wide range of disorders of the masticatory system characterized by one or more of the following: pain in the preauricular area, temporomandibular joint (TMJ), and muscles of mastication, with limitation or deviation in mandibular motion and TMJ sounds during mandibular function

Torus (tō'rus): bony elevation or prominence, usually located on the midline of the hard palate (torus palatinus) and the lingual surface of the mandible in the premolar area (torus mandibularis)

Trismus (triz'mus): motor disturbance of the trigeminal nerve, especially spasm of the masticatory muscles with difficulty in opening the mouth

Ventral (ven'tral): anterior or inferior surface; opposite of dorsal

Verruca (vĕ-roo'kah): a wart-like growth

TABLE 5.11. Extraoral and Intraoral Examination

Order of Examination	To Observe	Influences on Appointments
1. Overall appraisal of patient	Posture, gait General health status; size	Response, cooperation, attitude toward treatment Length of appointment
2. Face	Hair; scalp Breathing; state of fatigue Voice, cough, hoarseness Expression: Evidence of fear or apprehension Shape; twitching; paralysis Jaw movements during speech Injuries; signs of abuse	Need for alleviation of fears Evidence of upper respiratory or other infections Enlarged masseter muscle (related to bruxism)
3. Skin	Color, texture, blemishes Traumatic lesions Eruptions, swellings Growths	Relation to possible systemic conditions Need for supplementary history Biopsy or other treatment Influences on instruction in diet

continued

TABLE 5.11. Extraoral and Intraoral Examination

Order of Examination	To Observe	Influences on Appointments
4. Eyes	Size of pupil Color of sclera Eyeglasses (corrective) Protruding eyeballs	Dilated pupils or pinpoint may result from drugs, emergency state Eyeglasses essential during instruction Hyperthyroidism
5. Nodes (palpate) Pre- and postauricular Occipital Submental; submaxillary Cervical chain Supraclavicular	Adenopathy; lymphadenopathy Induration	Need for referral Medical consultation Coordinate with intraoral examination
6. Temporomandibular joint (palpate)	Limitations or deviations of movement Tenderness; sensitivity Noises: clicking, popping, grating	Disorder of joint; limitation of opening Discomfort during appointment and during personal plaque control

continued

7. Lips		
Observe closed, then open	Color, texture, size	Need for further examination: referral
Palpate	Cracks, angular cheilosis	Immediate need for postponement of appointment when a lesion may be communicable or could interfere with procedures
	Blisters, ulcers	Care during retraction
	Traumatic lesions	Accessibility during intraoral procedures
	Irritation from lip-biting	Patient instruction: dietary, special plaque control for mouthbreather
	Limitation of opening; muscle elasticity; muscle tone	
	Evidences of mouthbreathing	
	Induration	

8. Breath odor		
	Severity	Possible relation to systemic condition
	Relation to oral hygiene, gingival health	Alcohol use history; special needs

9. Labial and buccal mucosa		
Left and right examined systematically	Color, size, texture, contour	Need for referral, biopsy, cytology
Vestibule	Abrasions, traumatic lesions, cheekbite	Frena and other anatomic parts that need special adaptation for radiography or impression tray
Mucobuccal folds	Effects of tobacco use	Avoid sensitive areas during retraction
Frena	Ulcers, growths	
Opening of Stenson's duct	Moistness of surfaces	
Palpate cheeks	Relation of frena to free gingiva	
	Induration	

continued

TABLE 5.11. Extraoral and Intraoral Examination

Order of Examination	To Observe	Influences on Appointments
10. Tongue		
Dorsal surface	Shape: normal, asymmetric	Need for referral, biopsy, cytology
Lateral borders	Color, size, texture, consistency	Need for instruction in tongue cleaning
Base of tongue (retract)	Fissures; papillae	
	Coating	
	Lesions: elevated, depressed flat	
	Induration	
11. Floor of mouth	Varicosities	Large muscular tongue influences
Ventral surface of tongue	Lesions: elevated, flat, depressed, traumatic	retraction, gag reflex, accessibility for
Palpate	Induration	instrumentation
Duct openings	Limitation of freedom of movement of	Film placement problems
Mucosa, frena	tongue	
Tongue action	Frena; tonguetie	
12. Saliva	Quantity; quality (thick, ropy)	Reduced in certain diseases, by certain
	Evidences of dry mouth: lip wetting	drugs
	Tongue coating	Special dental caries control program
		Influence on instrumentation
		Need for saliva substitute

continued

13. Hard palate	Height, contour, color	Need for referral, biopsy, cytology
	Appearance of rugae	Signs of tongue thrust, deviate swallow
	Tori, growths, ulcers	Influence on radiographic film placement
14. Soft palate, uvula	Color, size, shape	Referral, biopsy, cytology
	Petechiae	Large uvula influences gag reflex
	Ulcers, growths	
15. Tonsillar region, throat	Tonsils: size and shape	Referral, biopsy, cytology
	Color, size, surface characteristics	Enlarged tonsils encourage gag reflex
	Lesions, trauma	Throat infection, a sign for appointment
		postponement (refer to history)

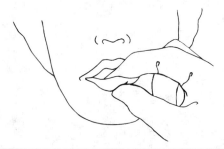

FIGURE 5.2. Bidigital palpation. Palpation of the lip to illustrate the use of a finger and thumb of the same hand.

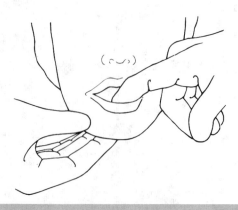

FIGURE 5.3. Bimanual palpation. Examination of the floor of the mouth by simultaneous palpation with fingers of each hand in apposition.

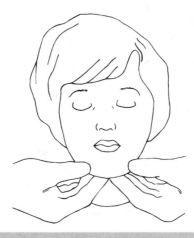

FIGURE 5.4. Bilateral palpation. Bilateral palpation is used to examine corresponding structures on opposite sides of the body.

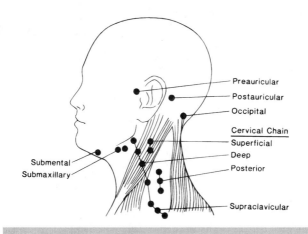

FIGURE 5.5. Lymph nodes. The location of the major lymph nodes into which the vessels of the facial and oral regions drain.

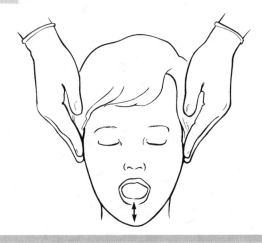

FIGURE 5.6. Assessment of the temporomandibular joint. The joint is palpated as the patient opens and closes the mouth.

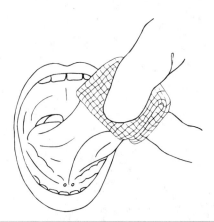

FIGURE 5.7. Examination of the tongue. To observe the posterior third of the tongue and the attachment to the floor of the mouth, hold the tongue with a gauze sponge, retract the cheek, and move the tongue out, first to one side and then the other, as each section of the mucosa is carefully examined.

Draw outlines of abnormalities in proper locations

MUCOSAL ABNORMALITIES

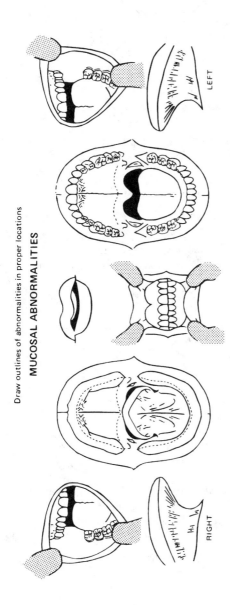

LEFT

RIGHT

FIGURE 5.8.   Record form for clinical findings. As part of a clinical examination record form, deviations from normal can be drawn to show the location and relative size. (Used with permission from the University of Southern California, School of Dentistry, Los Angeles, CA.)

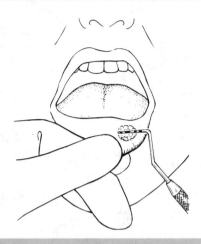

FIGURE 5.9. Use of a probe to measure a lesion. In addition to the exact location, the width and length of a lesion should be recorded. Using the probe is a convenient method of measuring the lesion.

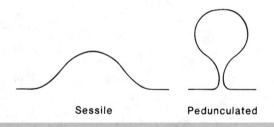

Sessile   Pedunculated

FIGURE 5.10. Attachment of nonblisterform lesions. The sessile lesion has a base as wide as the lesion itself; the pedunculated lesion is attached by a narrow stalk or pedicle.

TABLE 5.12. Description of Elevated Soft Tissue Lesions (18)

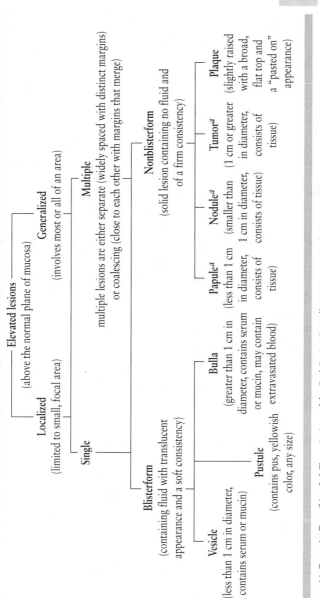

From McCann, A.: Describing Soft Tissue Lesions of the Oral Cavity, *Dental hygienistnews, 5, 9,* Spring, 1992.
[a]May be **pedunculated** (on a stem or stalk) or **sessile** (base or attachment is the greatest diameter of the lesion).

TABLE 5.13. Description of Depressed Soft Tissue Lesion (18)

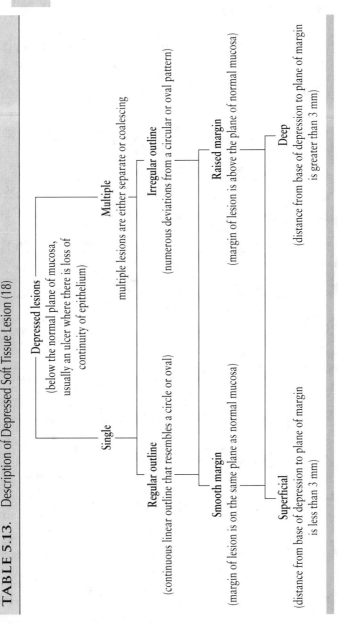

Depressed lesions
(below the normal plane of mucosa, usually an ulcer where there is loss of continuity of epithelium)

Single

Multiple
multiple lesions are either separate or coalescing

Regular outline
(continuous linear outline that resembles a circle or oval)

Irregular outline
(numerous deviations from a circular or oval pattern)

Smooth margin
(margin of lesion is on the same plane as normal mucosa)

Raised margin
(margin of lesion is above the plane of normal mucosa)

Superficial
(distance from base of depression to plane of margin is less than 3 mm)

Deep
(distance from base of depression to plane of margin is greater than 3 mm)

From McCann, A.: Describing Soft Tissue Lesions of the Oral Cavity, *Dentalhygienistnews*, 5, 10, Spring, 1992.

TABLE 5.14. Description of Flat Soft Tissue Lesions (18)

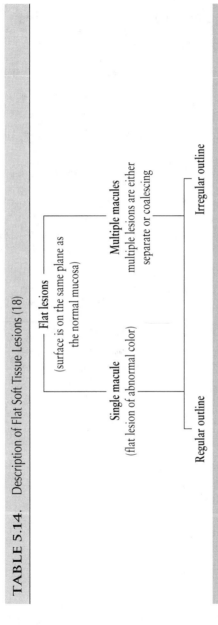

Flat lesions
(surface is on the same plane as the normal mucosa)

Single macule
(flat lesion of abnormal color)

Multiple macules
multiple lesions are either separate or coalescing

Regular outline

Irregular outline

From McCann, A.: Describing Soft Tissue Lesions of the Oral Cavity, *Dentalhygienistnews,* 5, 9, Spring, 1992.

TABLE 5.15. Description of Lesion Observations

Location and extent	Localized
	Generalized
	Single lesion
	Multiple lesions—separate or coalescing
Physical characteristics	Size (length and width measured in mm)
	Color:
	Most common: red, pink, white, red, and white
	Rarer: blue, purple, gray, yellow, black, brown
	Surface texture:
	smooth or irregular
	papillary, verrucus, fissure, corrugated, crusted
	Consistency: soft, spongy, resilient, hard, indurated
Morphologic categories (18)	Elevated, depressed, flat
History	Known or unknown to patient
	Duration
	Changes: size and appearance
	Symptoms

TABLE 5.16. Suspicious Lesion Follow-Up Procedures

Procedure	Indications
Biopsy (19, 20)	Any unusual oral lesion that cannot be identified with clinical certainty
	Any unhealed lesion evident for 2 wks
	Persistent, thick, white, hyperkeratotic lesion
	Any mass that does not break through the surface epithelium
	Surgically removed tissue
Cytologic smear[a] (19)	Lesion for which no biopsy is planned
	Keratotic lesions are not suitable for this procedure
	Refusal of patient to have a biopsy
	Follow-up examination for radiation-treated cancer
	Identifying *Candida albicans*, herpesvirus
	Cancer detection screenings (highly suspicious lesions should be referred for biopsy)
	Research studies in surface cell changes
Exfoliative Cytology	**Suspected Malignancy**
Laboratory results follow-up	All lesions should be followed up whether or not the reports are negative
	All lesions that are not healed must be continuously monitored and reevaluated

[a]Many limitations exist for the smear technique. Clearly pathologic lesions should be referred for immediate treatment and not delayed for cytologic smear analysis. Only surface lesions can be detected. Heavily keratinized lesions are not good candidates for this technique. Biopsy is needed for definitive diagnosis. Not diagnostically reliable; negative reports are not conclusive

TABLE 5.17. Recognition of Abuse/Neglect (24–26)

General signs	Behavioral:
	Extreme fear, excessive crying, no fear, unhappy and withdrawn
	Behavior changes when parent is present
	Language and motor skill development lag
	Overall appearance
	Failure to thrive; malnutrition
	Uncleanliness; signs of lack of care
	Inappropriate clothing for weather
	Wounds
	Abrasions and lacerations in various stages of healing, inconsistent with parental explanations
	Trauma
	Burns, bite marks, trauma signs on eyes, external ears, or neck
Oral signs	Lips: bruised or swollen; scars from previous trauma
	Mouth: abrasions at the corners of the mouth
	Lingual and labial frena: lacerations
	Teeth:
	Avulsed, fractured, darkened
	Radiographic signs of fractures present or previous

continued

Jaw: Fracture

Tongue: Injuries, evidence of scarring, recent healing

Dental neglect:

Untreated disease (rampant caries, pain, inflammation, bleeding gingiva)

Lack or irregularity of professional care

Appointments primarily for tooth extraction

Immaturity

Victim of abuse themselves

Drug or alcohol involvement

Disinterest or denial in relationship to the child

Critical, scolding, or belitting to child in front of others

Lack of interest in treatment plan for the child, only wants pain relief

Unavailable for consultation, does not accompany child to appointments

Provides inconsistent information about the sources and causes of damaged teeth, bruises, or other signs

of trauma

Parental attitude

SUBSTANCE ABUSE

The recognition of substance abuse by the oral healthcare practitioner is necessary because a medical or personal history may not reflect such information. Tables 5.18 and 5.19 will aid the practitioner in recognizing substance abuse.

DENTAL RADIOGRAPHS

Dental radiographs are a necessary diagnostic tool in the patient assessment. A thorough review of the patient's health and dental history and a clinical examination should be done before determining the number and types of radiographs to be taken (37). The clinician should obtain a history or the oral and body radiation from each patient (38). The objective in taking radiographs is to use the least amount of exposure to produce the best interpretive result (39). New technologies are in development and production that greatly reduce radiation exposure. Infection-control guidelines for all equipment and film need to be followed as well as radiation protection measures for patient and practitioner. Tables 5.20 through 5.22 provide information on radiation and radiographs.

STUDY CASTS

Study casts may be used as part of the patient's clinical assessment. The casts illustrate the various anomalies, teeth positions, occlusion, and anatomic characteristics of the oral cavity. They are also useful in presenting a visual aid for plaque control specific to the individual. Impressions should be disinfected before any laboratory procedures. The use of iodophore (1:213) and sodium hypochlorite (1:10) for 10–15 minutes on alginate impressions is effective (42–44).

TABLE 5.18.   Recognition of Signs of Substance Abuse (27–29)

General signs	Personal appearance
	Carelessness in appearance, personal hygiene (especially in one who was always groomed)
	Long sleeves to cover needle marks
	Blood stains on clothing or skin
	Dramatic weight loss
	Eyes
	Sunglasses for concealment of eyes
	Pupils dilated, constricted, red, inflamed, or bloodshot
	Arms
	Needle marks
	Unusual behavior
	Sneezing, itching
	Gazes into space, moody
	Drowsy; yawning; sleeping long hours
	Appearance of intoxication without alcohol odor; slurred speech
	Changes in habits, attitudes, and efficiency
	Irregular appointment attendance by previously conscientious and regular patient
	Possession of pills, capsules
	Hallucinations or convulsions

continued

TABLE 5.18. Recognition of Signs of Substance Abuse (27–29)

Oral signs	Poor oral hygiene; lack of personal care or interest in oral care
	High cariogenic-substance diet
	High dental caries incidence and tooth loss
	Few or any restorations on teeth needing treatment
	Xerostomia (drug-induced)
	High incidence of periodontal infections and gingival lesions
Appointment factors	Drug interactions
	Should not use products containing epinephrine with habitual marijuana and cocaine users (32)
	Methadone masks effects of narcotics, other drugs; must be used for pain relief
	Local anesthesia is less successful in addicts (33)
	Appointment postponement
	Patient under the influence of a drug
	Anesthesia or soft-tissue healing procedures

continued

Prophylactic antibiotic premedication (34)
 For addicts who inject their drugs
 Many IV drug abusers use prophylactic antibiotics regularly to prevent infections (35); specific questions
  should be directed to obtain this information
Increased disease incidence
 Hepatitis B, HIV infection (36)
Attempts to obtain prescriptions
 Caution is advised in writing prescriptions for pain medications without treatment of condition
 Prescription pads should be kept out of sight
 Drugs kept in the office or clinic should be locked up in an area inaccessible to patients

TABLE 5.19. Categories of Substances of Abuse with Street Names

Drug Category	Examples	Street Names
Opioids Analgesics	Heroin	H, Horse, junk, smack, Harry, chip, skag, hard or heavy goods
	Morphine	M, white stuff, Miss Emma, hocus, monkey
Central nervous system depressants Sedative-hypnotics	Barbiturates	Goofball, barbs, peanuts, downers, candy, yellows, yellow jackets, reds, red birds, red devils, blue devils, blue heavens, double trouble
Antianxiety	Alcohol	
	Diazepam (Valium)	
Central nervous system stimulants	Amphetamines	Bennies, peaches, splash, speed, crystal, uppers
	Cocaine	C, coke, Charlie, Cadillac, gold dust, stardust, joy powder, snow
	Freebase cocaine	Crack
Hallucinogens	LSD (d-lysergic acid diethylamide)	Acid, cubes, cupcake, blue dragon, sunshine
	Mescaline	Big chief, buttons, mesc
Phencyclidines	Phencyclidine	Hog, angel dust, peace pill, PCP
	Ketamine	PCE

continued

Cannabinoids	Marijuana	Grass, pot, hemp, Mary Jane, weed
	Hashish	Cigarettes: joint, reefer, roach
		Hash, soles
Inhalants	Acetone (paint thinner; model cement)	
	Benzene (adhesives; gasoline)	
	Ethyl acetate (paint thinner)	
	Nitrous oxide (anesthetic; propellant)	

TABLE 5.20. Types of Radiation Doses

Absorbed dose: the amount of energy imparted by ionizing radiation to a unit mass of irradiated material at a specific exposure point. The unit of absorbed dose is the rad or gray (Gy).

Cumulative dose: the total dose resulting from repeated exposures to radiation of the same region or of the whole body.

Dose: the amount of energy absorbed per unit mass of tissue at a site of interest.

Dose equivalent: the product of absorbed dose and modifying factors, such as the quality factor, distribution factor, and any other necessary factors; different types of radiation cause differing biologic effects; the traditional unit of dose equivalence is the rem (Sievert).

Erythema dose: the minimum quantity of x or gamma radiation that produces the appearance of redness (erythema).

Exit dose: the absorbed dose delivered by a beam of radiation to the surface through which the beam emerges from an object.

LLD50/30 dose: the dose of radiation that is lethal for 50% of a large population in a specified period of time, usually 30 days.

Lethal dose: the amount of radiation that is, or could be, sufficient to cause death of an organism.

Maximum permissible dose: the maximum dose equivalent that a person (or specified parts of that person) is allowed to receive in a stated period of time; the dose of radiation that would not be expected to produce any significant radiation effects in a lifetime.

Skin dose (surface absorbed dose): the absorbed dose delivered by a radiation beam and backscatter at the point where the central ray passes through the superficial layer of the object.

Threshold dose: the minimum dose that produces a detectable degree of any effect.

TABLE 5.21. Radiographic Surveys

Type	Purpose	Film
Periapical	View the entire tooth and its periodontal supporting structures Full mouth survey	Child—No. 0 (1.0) Anterior—No. 1 (1.1) Standard—No. 2 (1.2)
Bitewing (interproximal)	Horizontal—to show tooth crowns, alveolar crest, and interproximal area Vertical—to show more periodontal data, furcation involvement, bony defects	Standard—No. 2 Adult posterior—No. 3 Child survey—No. 2 Child survey—No. 1
Occlusal	Show large areas of the maxilla, mandible, or floor of the mouth	No. 4 Standard—No. 2
Panoramic	Supplement to periapical survey but not a substitute Oral pathology Edentulous patient/client Orthodontics Patient/clients with special circumstances that standard radiographs are not possible to obtain	Specialized equipment Film sizes: 5×12 or 6×12

continued

TABLE 5.21. Radiographic Surveys

Type	Purpose	Film
Child survey	Limited need in healthy children when oral cavity appears free from disease and teeth are spaced	
	Detection of congenital anomalies in mixed dentition (undergoing complete dental care or orthodontics)	
	Detection of proximal surface caries when contacts do not permit direct examination	
	Third molar assessment	
	Pulpal disease, infections	
	Trauma to teeth or jaws	
	Periodontal assessment reveals bone loss and periodontal pockets (40, 41)	
Edentulous	Detection of residual pathologic conditions, foreign bodies	
	Detection of retained teeth or root tips prior to denture construction	

TABLE 5.22.   Analysis of Radiographs: Causes of Inadequacies

	Inadequacy	Cause: Factors in Correction
Image	Elongation	Insufficient vertical angulation
	Foreshortening	Excessive vertical angulation
	Superimposition (overlapping)	Incorrect horizontal angulation (central ray not directed through interproximal space)
	Partial image	Cone-cut (incorrect direction of central ray or incorrect film placement)
		Incompletely immersed in processing tank
		Film touched other film or side of tank during processing
	Blurred or double image	Patient, tube, or packet movement during exposure
		Film exposed twice
		Bent film
	Stretched appearance of trabeculae or apices	Machine malfunction from time-switch to wall-plug
	No image	Failure to turn on the machine
		Film placed in fixer before developer

continued

TABLE 5.22. Analysis of Radiographs: Causes of Inadequacies

Inadequacy		Cause: Factors in Correction
Density	Too dark	Excessive exposure
		Excessive developing
		Developer too warm
		Unsafe safelight
		Accidental exposure to white light (may be completely black)
	Too light	Insufficient exposure
		Insufficient development or excessive fixation
		Solutions too cool
		Use of old, contaminated, or poorly mixed solutions
		Film placement: leaded side toward teeth
		Film used beyond expiration date
Fog	Chemical fog	Imbalance or deterioration of processing solutions

continued

Light fog	Unintentional exposure to light to which the emulsion is sensitive, either before or during processing
	Unsafe safelight
	Darkroom leak
	Holding unprocessed films too close to the safelight too long
Radiation fog	Improper storage of unused film
	Film exposed prior to processing
Reticulation (Puckered or pebbly surface)	Sudden temperature changes during processing, particularly from warm solutions to very cold water
Artifacts	Bent or creased film
	Static electricity
	Film removed from wrapper with excessive force
	Wrapper sticking to film, when opened with wet fingers; or if there was excessive moisture from patient's mouth
	Fingernail used to grasp film during placement on hanger
Herringbone pattern (light film)	Packet placed in mouth backward with foil next to teeth

continued

TABLE 5.22. Analysis of Radiographs: Causes of Inadequacies

	Inadequacy	Cause: Factors in Correction
Discoloration	Stains and spots	Unclean film hanger
		Splatterings of developer, fixer, dust
		Finger marks
		Insufficient rinsing after developing before fixing
		Splashing dry negatives with water or solutions
		Air bubbles adhering to surface during processing (insufficient agitation)
		Overlap of film on film in tanks or while drying
		Paper wrapper stuck to film (film not dried when removed from patient's mouth)
	At later date after storage of completed radiographs	Incomplete processing or rinsing
		Storage in too warm a place
		Storage near chemicals

GINGIVAL AND PERIODONTAL EXAMINATION

The gingival and periodonal examination is a vital part of assessment, diagnosis, and treatment planning. The examination uses visual assessment, periodontal probing, and exploring. Clinical attachment levels, recession, furcation involvement, mucogingival involvement, gingival probing depths, structural defects, lesions mobility and tooth mobility, radiographic findings (horizontal or vertical bone loss, periodontal ligament space, overhanging restorations, calculus), and any other characteristics influencing the oral condition should be recorded as part of the examination.

TOOTH EXAMINATION

The examination of the teeth includes noting deviations from normal plaque, calculus, caries, and occlusion, factors that are all part of the diagnostic work-up. This along with the other information gathered will aid in outlining the treatment plan for both hygiene and dental needs.

OCCLUSION

The occlusion of the patient contributes to the overall health of the oral cavity and determines the practitioner's treatment planning, oral hygiene instructions, instrumentation, and decisions for referral to specialists (orthodontist, TMJ). The static as well as functional occlusion should be observed and recorded. Occlusal trauma can exacerbate periodontal destruction when inflammatory disease is present (46). Figures 5.12 through 5.21 provide information on occlusion, malocclusion, and malrelations of groups of teeth.

TABLE 5.23. Examination of the Gingiva Clinical Markers

	Appearance in Health	Changes in Disease Clinical Appearance	Causes for Changes
Color	Uniformly pale pink or coral pink	Acute: bright red	Inflammation
	Variations in pigmentation related to complexion, race		Capillary dilation increased blood flow
		Chronic	
		Bluish pink,	Vessels engorged
		Bluish red	Blood flow sluggish
			Venous return impaired
			Anoxemia
			Increased fibrosis
		Pink	Deepening of pocket, mucogingival involvement
		Attached gingiva: color change may extend to the mucogingival line	
Size	Not enlarged	Enlarged	Edematous
	Fits snugly around the tooth		Inflammatory fluid
			Cellular exudate
			Vascular engorgement
			Hemorrhage

continued

Shape	Marginal gingiva Knife-edged, flat Follows a curved line about the tooth Papillae Normal contact: papilla is pointed and pyramidal; fills the interproximal area Space (diastema) between teeth: gingiva is flat or saddle-shaped	Fibrotic New collagen fibers Inflammatory changes Edema or fibrosis Marginal gingiva Rounded Rolled Papillae Bulbous Flattened Blunted Cratered Bulbous with gingival enlargement (see edematous and fibrotic, above) Cratered in necrotizing ulcerative gingivitis
Consistency	Firm	Soft, spongy: dents readily when pressed with probe Edematous: fluid between cells in connective tissue

continued

TABLE 5.23. Examination of the Gingiva Clinical Markers

	Appearance in Health	Changes in Disease Clinical Appearance	Causes for Changes
	Attached gingiva firmly bound down	Associated with red color, smooth shiny surface, loss of stippling, bleeding on probing	Fibrotic: collagen fibers
		Firm, hard: resists probe pressure Associated with pink color, stippling, bleeding only in depth of pocket	
Surface texture	Free gingiva: smooth	Acute condition: smooth, shiny gingiva	Inflammatory changes in the connective tissue; edema, cellular infiltration
	Attached gingiva: stippled	Chronic: hard, firm, with stippling, sometimes heavier than normal	Fibrosis
Position of gingival margin	Fully erupted tooth: margin is 1–2 mm above cementoenamel junction, at or slightly below the enamel contour	Enlarged gingiva: margin is higher on the tooth, above normal, pocket deepened	Edematous or fibrotic

continued

		Recession: margin is more apical; root surface is exposed	Junctional epithelium has migrated along the root; gingival margin follows
Position of junctional epithelium	During eruption: along the enamel surface Fully erupted tooth: the junctional epithelium is at the cementoenamel junction	Position, determined by use of probe, is on the root surface	Apical migration of the epithelium along the root
Mucogingival junctions	Make clear demarcation between the pink, stippled, attached gingiva and the darker alveolar mucosa with smooth shiny surface	No attached gingiva: Color changes may extend the full height of the gingiva; mucogingival line obliterated Probing reveals that the bottom of the pocket extends into the alveolar mucosa Frenal pull may displace the gingival margin from the tooth	Deepening of the pocket Apical migration of the junctional epithelium Attached gingiva decreases with pocket deepening Inflammation extends into alveolar mucosa

continued

TABLE 5.23. Examination of the Gingiva Clinical Markers

	Appearance in Health	Changes in Disease Clinical Appearance	Causes for Changes
Bleeding	No spontaneous bleeding or on probing	Spontaneous bleeding Bleeding on probing; bleeding near margin in acute condition; bleeding deep in pocket in chronic condition	Degeneration of the sulcular epithelium with the formation of pocket epithelium Blood vessels engorged Tissue edematous
Exudate	No exudate on pressure	White fluid, pus, visible on digital pressure Amount not related to pocket depth	Inflammation in the connective tissue Excessive accumulation of white blood cells with serum and tissue fluid makes up the exudate (pus)

TABLE 5.24. Types of Probes

Probe Markings (mm)	Examples	Description
Marks at 1-2-3-5-7-8-9-10	Williams	Round, tapered (available with color-code)
	University of Michigan with Williams marks	Round, narrow diameter, fine
	Glickman	Round with longer lower shank
	Merritt A and B	Round, single bend to shank
Marks at 3-3-2	University of Michigan O	Round, fine, tapered, narrow diameter
	Premier O	
	Marquis M-1	
Marks at 3-6-9-12, 3-6-8-11, and other variations	Hu-Friedy QULIX	Round, tapered, fine
	Marquis	Color-coded
	Nordent	
Marks at each mm to 15	Hu-Friedy PCPUNC 15	Round
		Color coded at 5-10-15
Marks at 3.5-5.5-8.5-11.5	WHO Probe (World Health Organization)	Round, tapered, fine, with ball end
		Color-coded
No marks	Gilmore	Tapered, sharper than other probes
	Nabors 1N, 2N	Curved, with curved shank for furcation examination

TABLE 5.25. Periodontal Case Types

Case Type 1—gingival disease

Inflammation of the gingiva characterized clinically by changes in color, gingival form, position, surface appearance, and presence of bleeding and/or exudate.

Case Type II—early periodontitis

Progression of the gingival inflammation into the deeper periodontal structures and alveolar bone crest, with slight bone loss. There is usually a slight loss of connective tissue attachment and alveolar bone.

Case Type III—moderate periodontitis

A more advanced stage of the preceding condition, with increased destruction of the periodontal structures and noticeable loss of bone support, possibly accompanied by an increase in tooth mobility. There may be furcation involvement in multirooted teeth.

Case Type IV—advanced periodontitis

Further progression of periodontitis with major loss of alveolar bone support usually accompanied by increased tooth mobility. Furcation involvement in multirooted teeth is likely.

Case Type V—refractory periodontitis

Includes those patients with multiple disease sites that continue to demonstrate attachment loss after appropriate therapy. These sites presumably continue to be infected by periodontal pathogens no matter how thorough or frequent the treatment provided. Also includes those patients with recurrent disease at single or multiple sites.

From American Academy of Periodontology: *Current Procedural Terminology for Periodontics and Insurance Reporting Manual,* 6th ed. Chicago, 1991.

TABLE 5.26.   Classification of Gingival and Periodontal Diseases[a]

Gingival Diseases

I. Plaque-associated gingivitis

  Chronic gingivitis

  Acute necrotizing ulcerative gingivitis

  Gingivitis associated with systemic conditions or
  medications. (These forms of gingivitis are plaque-
  associated, but the clinical presentation and therapeutic
  approaches may be modified by the systemic factors.)

  Hormone-influenced gingivitis

  Drug-induced gingivitis

  HIV gingivitis

II. Gingival manifestations of systemic diseases and
  mucocutaneous lesions

  Bacterial, viral, or fungal (e.g., acute herpetic
  gingivostomatitis)

  Blood dyscrasias (e.g., acute monocytic leukemia)

  Mucocutaneous diseases (e.g., lichen planus, cicatricial
  pemphigoid)

Rapidly progressive—most of the teeth are affected; the
  extent of clinical signs of inflammation may be less than
  expected; the age of onset is usually in the early 20s
  through the mid 30s.

Adult periodontitis

Periodontitis associated with systemic disease (e.g.,
  diabetes, HIV infection)—several systemic diseases
  appear to predispose the affected individuals to
  periodontitis, which may be of the early-onset type, but
  which may differ considerably from the early-onset
  form previously described.

Necrotizing ulcerative periodontitis—severe and rapidly
  progressive disease that has a distinctive erythema of
  the free gingiva, attached gingiva, and alveolar mucosa;
  extensive soft tissue necrosis; severe loss of periodontal
  attachment; deep pocket formation may not be evident.

continued

TABLE 5.26. Classification of Gingival and Periodontal Diseases[a]

Periodontal Diseases

I. Periodontitis

Early-onset periodontitis—age of onset is usually prior to 35 years; rapid rate of progression of tissue destruction; manifestation of defects in host defense; composition of the associated flora different from that of adult periodontitis.

Prepubertal—may be generalized or localized; onset between eruption of the primary dentition and puberty; may affect the primary and the mixed dentition; characterized by severe gingival inflammation, rapid bone loss, tooth mobility, and tooth loss.

Juvenile—may be generalized or localized; onset during the circumpubertal period; familial distribution; relative paucity of microbial plaque; less acute signs of inflammation than would be expected based on the severity of destruction; presence of abnormalities in leukocyte chemotaxis and bacteriocidal activity.

Refractory periodontitis—includes patients who are unresponsive to any treatment provided—whatever the thoroughness or frequency—as well as patients with recurrent disease at single or multiple sites.

II. Mucogingival conditions—the anatomy and position of the gingival tissues do not allow the control of inflammation or progressive recession.

III. Occlusal trauma—an injury to the attachment apparatus as a result of excessive occlusal forces.

Primary occlusal trauma—trauma resulting from excessive occlusal forces applied to a tooth or teeth with normal supporting structures.

Secondary occlusal trauma—trauma that occurs when normal occlusal forces are applied to the attachment apparatus of a tooth or teeth with inadequate support.

[a] Based on The American Academy of Periodontology: *Proceedings of the World Workshop in Clinical Periodontics*, Chicago, The American Academy of Periodontology, 1989, 1–23–24.

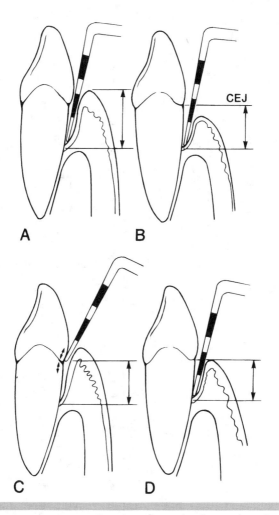

FIGURE 5.11. Clinical attachment level. **A.** Probing depth: the pocket is measured from the gingival margin to the attached periodontal tissue. **B.** Clinical attachment level in the presence of gingival recession is measured directly from the cementoenamel junction (CEJ) to the attached tissue. **C.** Clinical attachment level when the gingival margin covers the CEJ: first the CEJ is located as shown, then the distance to it is measured and subtracted from the probing depth. **D.** The clinical attachment level is equal to the probing depth when the gingival margin is at the level of the CEJ.

TABLE 5.27. Examination of the Teeth

Feature	To Observe	Dental Hygiene Implication
Morphology	Number of teeth (missing teeth verified by radiographic examination) Size, shape Arch form Position of individual teeth Injuries; fractures of the crown (root fractures observed in radiographs)	Selection and adaptation of instruments Areas prone to dental caries initiation, particularly the difficult-to-reach areas during plaque control Pulp test for vitality may be indicated
Development	Anomalies and developmental defects Pits and white spots	Distinguish hypoplasia and dental fluorosis from demineralization Identify pits for sealants
Eruption	Sequence of eruption: normal, irregular Unerupted teeth observed in radiographs	Care in using floss in the col area where the epithelium is usually less mature in young children Orthodontic needs Procedures for preservation of primary teeth

continued

Deposits
Food debris
Plaque
Calculus
  Supragingival
  Subgingival
	Overall evaluation of self-care and plaque-control measures
	Relation of appearance of teeth to gingival health
	Extent and location of plaque, debris, and calculus
	Calculus and the tooth surface pocket wall
		Need for instruction and guidance
		Frequency of follow-up and maintenance appointments

Stains Extrinsic Intrinsic	Extrinsic: colors relate to causes Intrinsic: dark, grayish Tobacco stain	Need for test for pulp vitality Stain removal procedures; selection of polishing agent Dentifrice recommendation Plaque-control emphasis for plaque-related stains Provide information concerning the oral effects of tobacco use
Regressive changes	Attrition: primary and permanent Abrasion: physical agents that may be a cause Erosion	Evaluate causes and treat or counsel for prevention Dietary analysis: for finding foods that may be related Selection of nonabrasive dentifrice Habit evaluation

continued

TABLE 5.27. Examination of the Teeth

Feature	To Observe	Dental Hygiene Implication
Exposed cementum	Relation to gingival recession, pocket formation	Special care areas where only slight attached gingiva remains
	Areas of narrow attached gingiva	Nonabrasive dentifrice advised
		Measures to prevent root-surface caries
		Care during instrumentation
	Hypersensitivity	Indication for application of desensitizing agent
Dental caries	Areas of demineralization	Charting
	Carious lesions (proximal lesions observed in radiographs)	Treatment plan
		Preventive program for caries control, fluoride, dietary factors
	Arrested caries	Follow-up and frequency of maintenance
	Root caries	
Restorations	Contour of restorations, overhangs	Chart and correct inadequate margins
	Proximal contact (see separate heading later in this table)	
	Surface smoothness	Selection of instruments and polishing agents
	Staining	Dentifrice selection to prevent discoloration

continued

Factors related to occlusion		
Tooth wear	Facets; worn-down cusp tips Health of supporting structures; observation of radiographs for signs of trauma from occlusion	Need for study of bruxism and other parafunctional habits
Proximal contacts	Use of floss to find open contact areas Areas of food retention	Chart inadequate contacts for corrective measures Use of floss by patient
Mobility	Degree; comparison of chartings	Need for reduction of inflammatory factors that may be related
	Possible causes	Dentist will identify and treat factors related to trauma from occlusion
Classification	Position of teeth Angle's classification	Relationship to orthodontic treatment needs
Habits	Nail or object biting; lip or cheek biting Observe effects on lip, cheek, teeth Tongue thrust; reverse swallow	Guidance for habit correction when indicated
Edentulous areas	Radiographic evaluation for impacted, unerupted teeth, retained root tips, other deviations from normal	Supplemental fulcrum selection during instrumentation Applied plaque-control procedures for abutment teeth

continued

TABLE 5.27. Examination of the Teeth

Feature	To Observe	Dental Hygiene Implication
Replacement for missing teeth	Teeth and tissue that support a prosthesis	Preventive measures for harm to supporting teeth and soft tissues
Dentures	Cleanliness of a prosthesis	Instruction in personal care of fixed and removable dentures; use of floss under fixed partial denture; other appropriate care
Partial dentures	Factors that contribute to food and debris retention	
Saliva	Amount and consistency	Relation to instruction for prevention of dental caries: more caries can be expected in a dry mouth
	Dryness of mouth	Use of saliva substitute; fluoride

TABLE 5.28. Tooth Development and Eruption: Primary Teeth

		Hard Tissue Formation Begins (Weeks In Utero)	Enamel Completed (Months After Birth)	Eruption (Months)	Root Completed (Year)
Maxillary	Central incisor	14	1½	10 (8–12)	1½
	Lateral incisor	16	2½	11 (9–13)	2
	Canine	17	9	19 (16–22)	3¼
	First molar	15½	6	16 (13–19 boys) (14–18 girls)	2½
	Second molar	19	11	29 (25–33)	3
Mandibular	Central incisor	14	2½	8 (6–10)	1½
	Lateral incisor	16	3	13 (10–16)	1½
	Canine	17	9	20 (17–23)	3¼
	First molar	15½	5½	16 (14–18)	2¼
	Second molar	18	10	27 (23–31 boys) (24–30) girls	3

Reprinted with permission from Lunt, R.C. and Law, D.B.: A Review of the Chronology of Eruption of Deciduous Teeth, *J. Am. Dent. Assoc.*, 89, 872, October, 1974.

TABLE 5.29. Tooth Development and Eruption: Permanent Teeth

		Hard Tissue Formation Begins	Enamel Completed (Years)	Eruption (Years)	Root Completed (Years)
Maxillary	Central incisor	3–4 mos.	4–5	7–8	10
	Lateral incisor	10 mos.	4–5	8–9	11
	Canine	4–5 mos.	6–7	11–12	13–15
	First premolar	1½–1¾ yrs.	5–6	10–11	12–13
	Second premolar	2–2¼ yrs.	6–7	10–12	12–14
	First molar	at birth	2½–3	6–7	9–10
	Second molar	2½–3 yrs.	7–8	12–13	14–16
	Third molar	7–9 yrs.	12–16	17–21	18–25
Mandibular	Central incisor	3–4 mos.	4–5	6–7	9
	Lateral incisor	3–4 mos.	4–5	7–8	10
	Canine	4–5 mos.	6–7	9–10	12–14
	First premolar	1¾–2 yrs.	5–6	10–12	12–13
	Second premolar	2¼–2½ yrs.	6–7	11–12	13–14
	First molar	at birth	2½–3	6–7	9–10
	Second molar	2½–3 yrs.	7–8	11–13	14–15
	Third molar	8–10 yrs.	12–16	17–21	18–25

Reprinted with permission from Ash, M.M.: *Wheeler's Dental Anatomy, Physiology, and Occlusion*, 6th ed. Philadelphia, W.B. Saunders Co., 1984, page 24.

TABLE 5.30. Dental Caries Charting: Classification of Cavities

Classification: Location	Appearance	Method of Examination
Class I Cavities in pits or fissures Occlusal surfaces of premolars and molars Facial and lingual surfaces of molars Lingual surfaces of maxillary incisors		Direct or indirect visual Exploration Radiographs not useful
Class II Cavities in proximal surfaces of premolars and molars		Early caries: by radiographs only Moderate caries not broken through from proximal to occlusal: Visual by color changes in tooth and loss of translucency Exploration from proximal Extensive caries involving occlusal: direct visual
Class III Cavities in proximal surfaces of incisors and canines that do not involve the incisal angle		Early caries: by radiographs or transillumination Moderate caries not broken through to lingual or facial: Visual by tooth color change Exploration Radiograph Extensive caries; direct visual

continued

TABLE 5.30. Dental Caries Charting; Classification of Cavities

Classification: Location	Appearance	Method of Examination
Class IV Cavities in proximal surfaces of incisors or canines that involve the incisal angle		Visual Transillumination
Class V Cavities in the cervical 1/3 of facial or lingual surfaces (not pit or fissure)		Direct visual: dry surface for vision Exploration to distinguish demineralization: whether rough or hard and unbroken Areas may be sensitive to touch
Class VI Cavities on incisal edges of anterior teeth and cusp tips of posterior teeth		Direct visual May be discolored

TABLE 5.31. Tooth Conditions

Condition	Definition	Etiology
Hypoplasia	Defect in the organic enamel matrix from disturbance during formation	Hereditary Systemic (environmental) example: fever fluorosis; prematurity; disease Local (single tooth)—trauma; periapical inflammation of primary tooth
Attrition	Tooth-to-tooth contact causing wearing away of tooth surface	Bruxism Usage (habits, aging, occupational factors)
Erosion	Loss of tooth substance by chemical process unrelated to bacterial action	Idiopathic (unknown) Chronic vomiting (pregnancy; eating disorders) Extrinsic Industrial (chemical exposure) Dietary (lemons; carbonated beverages)
Abrasion	Wearing away of tooth structure by means other than mastication	Abrasive agents (dentifrice; over-brushing) Oral habits (holding objects with teeth such as pipes, bobby pins, nails)

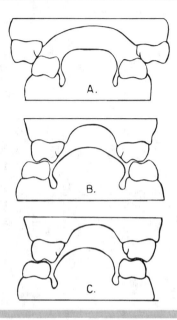

FIGURE 5.12. Posterior crossbite. **A.** The mandibular teeth lingual to the normal position. **B.** The mandibular teeth facial to the normal position. **C.** Unilateral crossbite: the right side is normal; on the left side, the mandibular teeth are facial to the normal position.

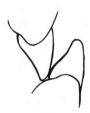

FIGURE 5.13. Anterior crossbite. The maxillary anterior teeth are lingual to the mandibular anterior teeth. Anterior crossbite occurs in Angle's class III malocclusion.

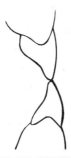

FIGURE 5.14. Edge-to-edge bite. The incisal surfaces occlude.

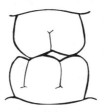

FIGURE 5.15. End-to-end bite. Molars in cusp-to-cusp occlusion as viewed from the facial.

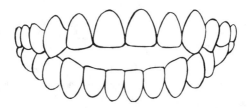

FIGURE 5.16. Open bite. A lack of incisal contact. The posterior teeth are in normal occlusion.

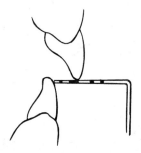

FIGURE 5.17. Overjet. The maxillary incisors are labial to the mandibular incisors. A measurable horizontal distance is evident between the incisal edge of the maxillary incisors and the incisal edge of the mandibular incisors. A periodontal probe can be used to measure the distance.

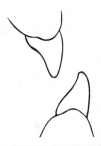

FIGURE 5.18. Underjet. Maxillary incisors are lingual to the mandibular incisors. A measurable horizontal distance is evident between the incisal edges of the maxillary incisors and the incisal edges of the mandibular incisors.

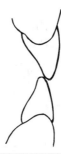

FIGURE 5.19.   Normal overbite. A profile view to show the position of the incisal edge of the maxillary tooth within the incisal third of the facial surface of the mandibular incisor.

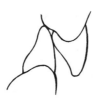

FIGURE 5.20.   Deep (severe) anterior overbite. The incisal edge of the maxillary tooth is at the level of the cervical third of the facial surface of the mandibular anterior tooth.

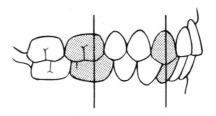

Normal (Ideal) Occlusion

Molar relationship: mesiobuccal cusp of maxillary first permanent molar occludes with the buccal groove of the mandibular first permanent molar.

Malocclusion

Class I: Neutroclusion. Molar relationship same as Normal, with malposition of individual teeth or groups of teeth.

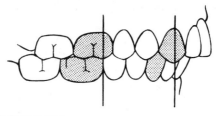

Class II: Distoclusion.

Molar relationship: buccal groove of the mandibular first permanent molar is distal to the mesiobuccal cusp of the maxillary first permanent molar by at least the width of a premolar.

Division 1: mandible is retruded and all maxillary incisors are protruded.

FIGURE 5.21. Normal occlusion and classification of malocclusion.

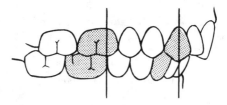

Class II: Distoclusion.

Division 2: mandible is retruded and one or more maxillary incisors are retruded.

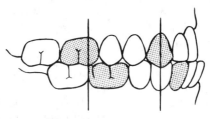

Class III: Mesioclusion.

Molar relationship: buccal groove of the mandibular first permanent molar is mesial to the mesiobuccal cusp of the maxillary first permanent molar by at least the width of a premolar.

FIGURE 5.21—*continued.*

REFERENCES

1. **Robbins,** K.S.: Medicolegal Considerations, in Malamed, S.F.: *Medical Emergencies in the Dental Office,* 4th ed. St. Louis, The C.V. Mosby Co., 1993, pp.91–101.
2. **Brady,** W.F. and Martinoff, J.T.: Validity of Health History Data Collected from Dental Patients and Patient Perception of Health Status, *J. Am. Dent. Assoc., 101,* 642, October, 1980.
3. **Geobel,** W.M.: Reliability of the Medical History in Identifying Patients Likely to Place Dentists at an Increased Hepatitis Risk, *J. Am. Dent. Assoc., 98,* 907, June, 1979.

4. **Comfort,** M.B. and Wu, P.C.: The Reliability of Personal and Family Medical Histories in the Identification of Hepatitis B Carriers, *Oral Surg. Oral Med. Oral Pathol., 67,* 531, May, 1989.

5. **Chiodo,** G.T. and Rosenstein, D.I.: Consultation Between Dentists and Physicians, *Gen. Dent., 32,* 19, January-February, 1984.

6. **United States Department of Health and Human Services,** Food and Drug Administration, Center for Devices and Radiological Health: *Selection of Patients for X-ray Examinations: Dental Radiographic Examinations.* Washington, D.C., Superintendent of Documents, HHS Publication FDA 88-8274, 1988, p. 10.

7. **Dajani,** A.S., Bisno, A.L., Chung, K.J., Durack, D.T., Freed, M., Gerber, M.A., Karchmer, A.W., Millard, H.D., Rahimtoola, S., Shulman, S.T., Watanakunakorn, C., and Taubert, K.A.: Prevention of Bacterial Endocarditis. Recommendations by the American Heart Association, *JAMA, 264,* 2919, December 12, 1990.

8. **Little,** J.W. and Falace, D.A.: *Dental Management of the Medically Compromised Patient,* 4th ed. St. Louis, The C.V. Mosby Co., 1993, p. 134.

9. **Baumgartner,** J.C. and Plack, W.F.: Dental Treatment and Management of a Patient with a Prosthetic Heart Valve, *J. Am. Dent. Assoc., 104,* 181, February, 1982.

10. **Lindemann,** R.A. and Henson, J.L.: The Dental Management of Patients with Vascular Grafts Placed in the Treatment of Arterial Occlusive Disease, *J. Am. Dent. Assoc., 104,* 625, May, 1982.

11. **Jacobsen,** P.L. and Murray, W.: Prophylactic Coverage of Dental Patients with Artificial Joints: A Retrospective Analysis of Thirty-three Infections in Hip Prostheses, *Oral Surg. Oral Med. Oral Pathol., 50,* 130, August, 1980.

12. **Howell,** R.M. and Green, J.G.: Prophylactic Antibiotic Coverage in Dentistry: A Survey of Need for Prosthetic Joints, *Gen. Dent., 33,* 320, July-August, 1985.

13. **Mulligan,** R.: Late Infections in Patients with Prostheses for Total Replacement of Joints: Implications for the

Dental Practitioner, *J. Am. Dent. Assoc., 101,* 44, July, 1980.

14. **Naylor,** G.D., Hall, E. H., and Terezhalmy, G.T.: The Patient with Chronic Renal Failure Who Is Undergoing Dialysis or Renal Transplantation: Another Consideration for Antimicrobial Prophylaxis, *Oral Surg. Oral Med. Oral Pathol., 65,* 116, January, 1988.

15. **United States National High Blood Pressure Education Program,** *The Fifth Report of the Joint National Committee on Detection, Evaluation, and Treatment of High Blood Pressure,* Washington, D.C., National Institutes of Health, National Heart, Lung, and Blood Institute, N.I.H. Publication No. 93-1088, January, 1993, pp. 1–49.

16. **Cancer Statistic, 1993,** *CA, 43,* 9, January/February, 1993.

17. **Engelman,** M.A. and Schackner, S.J.: *Oral Cancer Examination Procedure.* Published by Oral Cancer Prevention and Detection Center, St. Francis Hospital, Poughkeepsie, NY. Distributed by American Cancer Society, New York.

18. **McCann,** A.L. and Wesley, R.K.: A Method for Describing Soft Tissue Lesions of the Oral Cavity, *Dent. Hyg., 61,* 219, May, 1987.

19. **Sandler,** H.C. and Stahl, S.S.: Exfoliative Cytology as a Diagnostic Aid in the Oral Neoplasms, *J. Oral Surg., 16,* 414, September, 1958.

20. **Sabes,** W.R.: *The Dentist and Clinical Laboratory Procedures,* St. Louis, The C.V. Mosby Co., 1979, pp. 109–113.

21. **Holtzman,** J.M. and Bomberg, T.: A National Survey of Dentists' Awareness of Elder Abuse and Neglect, *Spec. Care Dentist., 11,* 7, January/February, 1992.

22. **Kelly,** M.A., Grace, E.G., and Wisnom, C.: Abuse of Older Persons: Detection and Prevention by Dental Professionals, *Gen. Dent., 40,* 30, January-February, 1992.

23. **Jorgensen,** J.E.: A Dentist's Social Responsibility to Diagnose Elder Abuse, *Spec. Care Dentist, 12,* 113, May/June, 1992.

24. **Giangrego,** E., ed.: Child Abuse: Recognition and Reporting, *Spec. Care Dent., 6,* 62, March-April, 1986.

25. **Schmitt,** B.D.: Physical Abuse: Specifics of Clinical Diagnosis, *Pediatr. Dent., 8,* 83, May, 1986.

26. **Maier,** C.: Save the Children, *Dent. Teamwork, 5,* 20, May-June, 1992.

27. **Aston,** R.: Drug Abuse, in Neidle, E.A. and Yagiela, J.A., eds.: *Pharmacology and Therapeutics for Dentistry,* 3rd ed. St. Louis, The C.V. Mosby Co., 1989, pp. 642–658.

28. **Roberts,** D.J.: Drug Abuse, in Rakel, R.E., ed.: *Conn's Current Therapy,* 45th ed. Philadelphia, W.B. Saunders Co., 1993, pp. 1097–1103.

29. **O'Brien,** C.P.: Drug Abuse and Dependence, in Wyngaarden, J.B., Smith, L.H., and Bennett, J.C., eds.: *Cecil Texbook of Medicine,* 19th ed. Philadelphia, W.B. Saunders Co., 1990, pp. 47–55.

30. **Dello russo,** N.M. and Temple, H.V.: Cocaine Effects on Gingiva (Letters to the Editor), *J. Am. Dent. Assoc. 104,* 13, January, 1982.

31. **Yukna,** R.A.: Cocaine Periodontitis, *Int. J. Periodontics Restorative Dent., 11,* 73, No. 1, 1991.

32. **Lee,** C.Y.S., Mohammad, H., and Dixon, R.A.: Medical and Dental Implications of Cocaine Abuse, *J. Oral Maxillofac. Surg., 49,* 290, March, 1991.

33. **Scheutz,** F.: Drug Addicts and Local Analgesia—Effectivity and General Side Effects, *Scand. J. Dent. Res., 90,* 299, August, 1982.

34. **Rosenbaum,** C.H.: Dental Precautions in Treating Drug Addicts: A Hidden Problem Among Teens and Preteens, *Pediatr. Dent., 2,* 94, June, 1980.

35. **Schaffer,** S.R. and Schaffr, S.K.: Use of Prophylactic Antibiotics by Drug Users, *JAMA, 252,* 1410, September 21, 1984.

36. **Friedland,** G.H., Harris, C., Butkus-Small, C., Shine, D., Moll, B., Darrow, W., and Klein, R.S.: Intravenous Drug Abusers and the Acquired Immunodeficiency Syndrome (AIDS). Demographics, Drug Use, and Needle-sharing Patterns, *Arch. Intern. Med., 145,* 1413, August, 1985.

37. **United States Food and Drug Administration,** Center for Devices and Radiological Health: *Selection of Patients*

*for X-ray Examinations: Dental Radiographic
Examinations.* Washington, D.C., Government Printing
Office, No. 017-015-00236-5.

38. **United States National Research Council:** *Health Effects
of Exposure to Low Levels of Ionizing Radiation. BEIR-V,*
Washington, D.C., National Academy Press, 1990.

39. **American Dental Association,** Council on Dental
Materials, Instruments, and Equipment:
Recommendations in Radiographic Practices:
An Update: 1988, *J. AM. Dent. Assoc., 118,* 115,
January, 1989.

40. **Myers,** D.R., O'Dell, N.L., Clark, J.W., and Cross, R.L.:
Localized Prepubertal Periodontitis: Literature Review
and Report of Case, *ASDC J. Dent. Child., 56,* 107,
March-April, 1989.

41. **Watanabe,** K.: Prepubertal Periodontitis: A Review
of Diagnostic Criteria, Pathogenesis, and Differential
Diagnosis, *J. Periodont. Res., 25,* 31, January, 1990.

42. **American Dental Association,** Council on Dental
Materials, Instruments, and Equipment, Council on
Dental Therapeutics, Council on Dental Research,
and Council on Dental Practice: *Infection Control
Recommendations for the Dental Office and Dental
Laboratory. J. Am. Dent. Assoc., 123,* Supplement,
August, 1992.

43. **Merchant,** V.A., Radcliffe, R.M., Herrera, S. P., and
Stroster, T.G.: Dimensional Stability of Reversible
Hydrocolloid Impressions Immersed in Selected
Disinfectant Solutions, *J. Am. Dent. Assoc., 119,*
533, October, 1989.

44. **Wood,** P.R.: *Cross Infection Control in Dentistry: A
Practical Illustrated Guide.* St. Louis, The C.V. Mosby
Co., 1992, pp. 159–163.

45. **Blackwell,** R.E.: *G.V. Black's Operative Dentistry,*
Volume II, 9th ed. Milwaukee, Medico-Dental
Publishing Co., 1955, pp. 1–4.

46. **Allen,** D.L., McFall, W.T., and Jenzano, J.W.:
Periodontics for the Dental Hygienist, 4th ed.
Philadelphia, Lea & Febiger, 1987, pp. 85–86.

47. **Angle,** E.H.: *Malocclusion of the Teeth,* 7th ed.
Philadelphia, S.S. White, 1907.

PLAQUE, CALCULUS, STAIN

6

This chapter discusses the deposits on tooth surfaces and their composition and distribution characteristics. The tables are for quick reference. Also included are tables for the removal of stain by polishing.

POLISHING

The decision to remove stain by means of polishing should be made on an individual basis. Selective polishing in which only stained areas of a tooth are polished when indicated should be utilized. Table 6.9 provides factors, considerations, and contraindications for the use of abrasives with a rubber cup for stain removal. Many stains can be removed during scaling, minimizing the need to use abrasives. Commercial toothpastes with low abrasiveness can be used instead of professional pastes when stain is minimal. Table 6.10 provides recommendations and precautions for airbrasive polishing.

Pit and fissure sealants can be placed successfully without prior polishing (26–28). If polishing is necessary, a fine pumice with water is preferable to commercial pastes, which may interfere with the integrity of the sealant.

Polishing prior to a professional application of fluoride is only necessary if there is stain remaining after scaling. Use of a prophylaxis paste with fluoride and low abrasiveness is indicated, which may help replace the fluoride removed by the abrasive (29).

Proximal surfaces can be polished to remove stain with dental floss or tape with a polishing agent. The use

TABLE 6.1. Tooth Deposits (1–3)

Category	Tooth Deposit	Description	Derivation
Nonmineralized	Acquired pellicle	Translucent, homogenous, thin, unstructured film covering and adherent to the surfaces of the teeth, restorations, calculus, and other surfaces in the oral cavity	Supragingival: saliva Subgingival: gingival sulcus fluid
	Microbial (Bacterial) plaques	Dense, organized bacterial systems embedded in an intermicrobial matrix that adhere closely to the teeth, calculus, and other surfaces in the oral cavity Water irrigation removes only the outer layer of loose organisms	Colonization of oral microorganisms
	Materia alba	Loosely adherent, unstructured, white or grayish-white mass of oral debris and bacteria that lies over bacterial plaque Vigorous rinsing and water irrigation can remove materia alba	Incidental accumulation

continued

Food Debris		Unstructured, loosely attached particulate matter	Food retention following eating
		Self-cleansing activity of tongue and saliva and rinsing vigorously remove debris	
Mineralized	Calculus	Calcified bacterial plaque; hard, tenacious mass that forms on the clinical crowns of the natural teeth and on dentures and other appliances	Plaque mineralization
	Supragingival	Occurs coronal to the margin of the gingiva; is covered with bacterial plaque	Supragingival: source of minerals is saliva
	Subgingival	Occurs apical to the margin of the gingiva; is covered with bacterial plaque	Subgingival: source of minerals is gingival sulcus fluid

Adapted from Schroeder, H.E.: Formation and Inhibition of Dental Calculus. Vienna, Hans Huber, 1969, pp. 14–15.

TABLE 6.2. Characteristics of Supragingival and Subgingival Plaque (4–7)

Characteristic	Supragingival Plaque	Subgingival Plaque
Location	Coronal to the margin of the free gingiva	Apical to the margin of the free gingiva
Origin	Salivary glycoprotein forms pellicle Microorganisms from saliva are selectively attracted to pellicle	Downgrowth of bacteria from supragingival plaque
Distribution	Starts on proximal surfaces and other protected areas Heaviest collection on Areas not cleaned daily by patient Cervical third, especially facial Lingual mandibular molars Proximal surfaces Pit and fissure plaque	Shallow pocket: similar to supragingival plaque Undisturbed; held by pocket wall Attached plaque covers calculus Unattached plaque extends to the periodontal attachment
Adhesion	Firmly attached to acquired pellicle, other bacteria, and tooth surfaces Surface bacteria (unattached): loose; washed away by saliva or swallowed	Adheres to tooth surface, subgingival pellicle, and calculus Subgingival flora: loose, floating, motile organisms in deep pocket do not adhere; they are between the adherent plaque on the tooth and the pocket epithelium

continued

Retention	Rough surfaces of teeth or restorations
	Malpositioned teeth
	Carious lesions
	Pocket holds plaque against tooth
	Overhanging margins of fillings that extend into pockets
Shape and size	Friction of tongue, cheeks, lips limits shape and size
	Molded by pocket wall to shape of the tooth surface
	Thickness: thicker at the cervical third and on proximal surfaces
	Follows form created by subgingival calculus
	Healthy gingiva: thin plaque, 15–20 cells thick
	May become thicker as the diseased pocket wall becomes less tight
	Chronic gingivitis: thick plaque, 100–300 cells thick
Structure	Adherent, densely packed microbial layer over pellicle on tooth surface
	Intermicrobial matrix
	Onset: small isolated colonies 2–5 days; colonies merge to form a covering of plaque
	Three layers
	Tooth-surface-attached plaque: many gram-positive rods and cocci
	Unattached plaque in middle: many gram-negative, motile forms; spirochetes; leukocytes
	Epithelium-attached plaque: gram-negative, motile forms predominate; many leukocytes migrate through epithelium

continued

TABLE 6.2. Characteristics of Supragingival and Subgingival Plaque (4–7)

Characteristic	Supragingival Plaque	Subgingival Plaque
Microorganisms	Early plaque: primarily gram-positive cocci Older plaque (3–4 days): increased numbers of filaments and fusiforms 4–9 days undisturbed: more complex flora with rods, filamentous forms 7–14 days: vibrios, spirochetes, more gram-negative organisms	Environment conducive to growth of anaerobic population Diseased pocket: primarily gram-negative, motile, spirochetes, rods See Table 6.3
Sources of nutrients for bacterial proliferation	Saliva Ingested food	Tissue fluid (gingival sulcus fluid) Exudate Leukocytes
Significance	Etiology of Gingivitis Supragingival calculus Dental caries	Etiology of Gingivitis Periodontal infections Subgingival calculus

TABLE 6.3. Major/Dominant Microorganisms in Periodontal Infections[a]

Periodontal Condition	Bacterial and Immunologic Features	Bacterial Species
Periodontal health	Gram-positive Coccal and rod forms Few gram-negative	Streptococcus species Actinomyces species Rothia dentocariosa
Gingivitis	Gram-positive and gram-negative bacteria Few motile rods and spirochetes Total numbers 10–20 times those in healthy tissue	Streptococcus species Actinomyces species Veillonella species Treponema species Fusobacterium nucleatum
Pregnancy gingivitis	Changes may relate to hormonal changes	Prevotella intermedia Capnocytophaga species
Necrotizing ulcerative gingivitis	Spirochetes invade tissue Gram-negative bacteria primarily	Treponema species Fusobacterium nucleatum Prevotella intermedia
Prepubertal periodontitis	Gram-negative bacteria predominate Capnophilic and anaerobic Impaired neutrophil function	Actinobacillus actinomycetemcomitans Capnocytophaga species Prevotella intermedia

continued

TABLE 6.3. Major/Dominant Microorganisms in Periodontal Infections[a]

Periodontal Condition	Bacterial and Immunologic Features	Bacterial Species
Juvenile periodontitis	Gram-negative Capnophilic and anaerobic Soft tissue invasion of bacteria Impaired neutrophil function	Actinobacillus actinomycetemcomitans Eikenella corrodens Prevotella intermedia Capnocytophaga species
Rapid progressive periodontitis	Gram-negative Anaerobic organisms Impaired neutrophil function	Porphyromonas gingivalis Actinobacillus actinomycetemcomitans Prevotella intermedia Fusobacterium nucleatum Eikenella corrodens Campylobacter rectus
Adult periodontitis	Gram-negative Anaerobic organisms Complex flora: coccoid, spiral, and rod forms Motile	Porphyromonas gingivalis Actinobacillus actinomycetemcomitans Prevotella intermedia

continued

Refractory periodontitis	*Bacteroides forsythus*
	Treponema denticola
	Treponema socranskii
	Campylobacter rectus
	Fusobacterium nucleatum
	Streptococcus intermedius
	Eikenella corrodens
	Actinomyces species
	Eubacterium species
Gram-negative	*Bacteroides forsythus*
Anaerobic organisms	*Fusobacterium nucleatum*
Defective host defenses	*Porphyromonas gingivalis*
Resistance to usual therapy	*Campylobacter rectus*
	Prevotella intermedia
	Peptostreptococcus
	Actinobacillus actinomycetemcomitans
	Capnocytophaga species
	Spirochetes
	Motile rods
	Candida

[a]See special listing of references for this table at end of chapter.

TABLE 6.4. Clinical Characteristics of Dental Calculus (10, 11)

Characteristic	Supragingival Calculus	Subgingival Calculus
Color	White, creamy-yellow, or gray May be stained by tobacco, food, or other pigments Slight deposits may be invisible until dried with compressed air	Light to dark brown, dark green, or black Stains derived from blood pigments from diseased pocket
Shape	Amorphous, bulky Gross deposits may Form interproximal bridge between adjacent teeth Extend over the margin of the gingiva Shape of calculus mass is determined by the anatomy of the teeth, contour of gingival margin, and pressure of the tongue, lips, cheeks	Flattened to conform with pressure from the pocket wall Combinations of the following calculus formations occur:[10] Crusty, spiny, or nodular Ledge or ring-like formations Thin, smooth veneers Finger- and fern-like formations Individual calculus islands
Consistency and texture	Moderately hard	Brittle, flint-like

continued

	Newer deposits less dense and hard Porous Surface covered with nonmineralized plaque	Harder and more dense than supragingival calculus Newest deposits near bottom of pocket are less dense and hard Surface covered with plaque Related to pocket depth Increased amount with age because of accumulation Quantity is related to personal care, diet, and individual tendency as it is with supragingival. Subgingival is primarily related to the development and progression of periodontal disease
Size and quantity	Quantity has direct relationship to Personal oral care procedures and plaque control measures Physical character of diet Individual tendencies Function and use Increased amount in tobacco smokers	
Distribution on individual tooth	Coronal to margin of gingiva May cover a large portion of the visible clinical crown, or may form fine thin line near gingival margin	Apical to margin of gingiva Extends to bottom of the pocket and follows contour of soft tissue attachment With gingival recession, subgingival calculus may become supragingival and become covered with typical supragingival calculus

continued

TABLE 6.4. Clinical Characteristics of Dental Calculus (10, 11)

Characteristic	Supragingival Calculus	Subgingival Calculus
Distribution on teeth	Symmetrical arrangement on teeth except when influenced by Malpositioned teeth Unilateral hypofunction Inconsistent personal care Abrasion from food Occurs with or without associated subgingival deposits Location related to openings of the salivary gland ducts: Facial surface of maxillary molars Lingual surface mandibular anterior teeth	May be generalized or localized on a few teeth Heaviest on proximal surfaces, lightest on facial surfaces Occurs with or without associated supragingival deposits

TABLE 6.5. Classification of Stains

By location	Extrinsic
	    External tooth surface
	    Removable by toothbrushing, scaling, and/or polishing
		Intrinsic
		    Within tooth substance
		    Not removable by scaling or polishing

By source	Exogenous
	    From sources outside the tooth
	    May be extrinsic or become intrinsic
		Endogenous
		    Originate within the tooth
		    Always intrinsic

TABLE 6.6. Extrinsic Stains (12–23)

Type	Clinical Appearance	Occurrence	Etiology
Yellow	Dull, yellowish discoloration of bacterial plaque	All ages Individuals with poor oral hygiene	Usually food pigments
Green	Light or yellowish green to dark green	Any ages; primarily in children Permanent and primary teeth	Poor oral hygiene Chromogenic bacteria Gingival hemorrhage Chlorophyll preparations Industrial metallic dusts (12) Certain drugs
Black Line	Follows contour of gingival crest	All ages; more common in children More common in females	Microorganisms embedded in an intermicrobial substance Does not cause oral disease (13–15)
	Bases of pits and fissures	Frequently found in clean mouths	
Tobacco	Light to dark brown, black	Any surface pits and fissures	Tobacco and smokeless tobacco

continued

	May be incorporated into calculus deposits May become exogenous intrinsic stain	Most frequently on lingual Cervical third, primarily Amount of stain may not be related to amount of tobacco used	
Other brown stains			
Brown pellicle	Smooth and structureless Takes on various colors	Recurs readily after removal (16)	Chemical alteration of pellicle (17)
Stannous fluoride (18–20)	Light brown, yellowish	After repeated use of stannous fluoride gel or other product After topical fluoride application	Formation of stannous oxide or brown tin oxide from the reaction of the tin ion in the fluoride compound
Foodstuffs	Brownish stained pellicle Brownish stained teeth		Coffee, tea, cola, certain foods
Anti-plaque agents (chlorhexidine, alexidine) (21, 22)		Dependent on oral hygiene More pronounced on proximal surfaces Exposed roots more easily stained	
Betel leaf (23)	Dark brown, almost black Thick, hard, both smooth and rough surfaces	Eastern countries; all ages	Microorganisms and mineralized material

continued

TABLE 6.6. Extrinsic Stains (12–23)

Type	Clinical Appearance	Occurrence	Etiology
Orange and red	Cervical third More frequent on anterior teeth (both facial and lingual surfaces)	Rare	Chromogenic bacteria
Metallic stains Industrial sources			
Copper or brass: green or bluish green		Bacterial plaque	Mouth inhalation of dust particles
Iron: brown to greenish-brown		Primarily anterior teeth	May become exogenous intrinsic
Nickel: green		Commonly, the cervical third	
Cadium: yellow or golden brown			
Drug sources			
Iron: black (iron sulfide), brown		All tooth surfaces	Drug enters plaque and imparts color
Manganese (from potassium permanganate): black			Pigment may attach directly to tooth surfaces

TABLE 6.7. Endogenous Intrinsic Stains (24, 25)

Cause	Factors
Pulpless teeth	Root canals
	Necrosis and decomposition of the pulp tissue
	Hemorrhages in the pulp chamber
Tetracyclines (24, 25)	Can be transferred through the placenta and enter fetal circulation
	Can cause discoloration of child's teeth if given in the third trimester of pregnancy to the mother
	Can cause discoloration if given during infancy or early childhood
Imperfect tooth development (24, 25)	Hereditary: genetic
	Amelogenesis Imperfecta
	Dentinogenesis Imperfecta
	Enamel hypoplasia
	Systemic hypoplasia
	Local hypoplasia (single tooth)
Dental fluorosis	Ingestion of excessive fluoride during the period of mineralization
	Severe effects may produce cracks or pitting
Other systemic causes	Prolonged jaundice early in life
	Erythoblastosis fetalis (Rh incompatibility)

TABLE 6.8. Exogenous Intrinsic Stains (18)

Causes	Factors
Restorative materials	Discoloration of tooth around a silver amalgam (gray to black)
	Copper amalgam (used in restorations of primary teeth) can produce bluish-green discoloration
Endodontic therapy and restorative materials	Silver nitrate: bluish-black
	Volatile oils: yellowish-brown
	Strong iodine: brown
	Aureomycin: yellow
	Silver-containing root canal sealer: black
Drugs	Stannous fluoride topical application: light to dark brown
	Ammoniacal silver nitrate: dark brown to black (18)
Stain in dentin	e.g., carious lesion discoloration

of finishing strips should be used only with discrimination and great caution, when other polishing methods have not succeeded, and only on enamel surfaces.

The use of a porte polisher may also be considered for selected areas to be polished or when, because of contraindications or other reasons, a prophylaxis angle and rubber cup are not feasible.

TABLE 6.9. Effects of Polishing (30–43)

Factor	Considerations/Contraindications
Bacteremia (30)	Antibiotic prophylaxis for individuals at risk (Chapter 5)
	Postpone until plaque is controlled and gingiva does not bleed when brushing
Environmental	
Aerosol production (31):	Potential disease transmission
	Limited use of rotary instruments on individuals with known communicable disease (Chapters 3, 4)
	Individuals with respiratory problems such as emphysema or asthma contraindicate the use of power-driven instruments
Spatter (32):	Protective eyewear for both clinician and patient
	Commercial prophylaxis paste chemicals may cause inflammatory responses
Teeth	
Removal of tooth structure	Repeated over a period of years, substantial tooth substance can be lost (33)
	Exposed cementum should not be polished (34, 35)
	Demineralization areas should be avoided (36)
	Greater amounts of dentin, cementum, and demineralized enamel are lost than from intact enamel (36)
	Newly erupted teeth have incomplete mineralization of the tooth surface, which abrasives can damage

continued

TABLE 6.9. Effects of Polishing (30–43)

Factor	Considerations/Contraindications
Increased roughness	Coarse abrasives can create a rougher tooth surface than before polishing (37, 38)
Areas of thin enamel	Create sensitivity
	Can expose dentinal tubules
	Outermost layer of tooth structure contains the greatest amount of fluoride (39)
Removal of fluoride-rich surface	Individuals with xerostomia from any cause should not be polished—if stain removal must be done, replenishment of the fluoride by means of topical fluoride application (gel or solution) should follow (40).
	Prophylaxis paste with fluoride is not a substitute. Individuals at risk for dental caries: rampant, nursing, or root caries; radiation to head (especially involving the salivary glands); xerostomia; thin enamel; ameliogenesis imperfecta. Demineralized areas should be evaluated for postponement or not polished.
Heat production	Can cause pain and discomfort
Effect on gingiva	Trauma to gingival tissue
	Possible removal of epithelium, causing soreness and sensitivity and lengthening healing time, which may cause inadequate plaque removal, severe inflammation, and calculus reformation (41)

continued

	Particles of polishing agent can be forced into the subepithelial tissues causing irritation
	Polishing after scaling, root planing, and curettage is not recommended on the same day
	Delayed healing from foreign-body reactions (42)
Effect on restorations	Can leave rough surfaces on gold, amalgam, and composites (43)
	Titanium implants may be scratched
Postponement or contraindicated	No stain is present
	Plaque control instructions have not been given
	Inadequate plaque control is demonstrated
	Bleeding tissue upon brushing
	Immediately following deep subgingival scaling, root planing or curettage
	Communicable disease potentially disseminated by aerosol
	Any of the aforementioned contraindications

TABLE 6.10. Airbrasive Polishing: Recommendations/Precautions/Contraindications (44–53)

Recommendations/ precautions (44, 45)	Preoperative antibacterial mouthrinse
	Use high-volume evacuation rather than saliva ejector (45)
	Patient should remove contact lenses and wear protective eyewear
	Lubricate patient's lips
	Patient should be covered, including hair
	Follow universal precautions
	Review medical history
	Antibiotic premedication for individuals at risk for any dental hygiene procedure
Contraindications	Individuals on a restricted sodium diet (46)
	Individuals with respiratory disease
	Individuals with conditions that limit swallowing or breathing
	Individuals with communicable infection that can contaminate the aerosols produced
	Not for use on root surfaces (47–49)
	Soft, spongy gingiva (postpone until gingiva is healthy) (50)
	Not for use on restorations (damage) (51–53)

REFERENCES

1. **Schroeder,** H.E.: *Formation and Inhibition of Dental Calculus,* Vienna, Hans Huber Publishers, 1969, pp. 14–15.
2. **Meckel,** A.H.: Formation and Properties of Organic Films on Teeth, *Arch. Oral Biol., 10,* 585, July-August, 1965.

3. **Meckel,** A.H.: The Nature and Importance of Organic Deposits on Dental Enamel, *Caries Res., 2,* 104, No. 2, 1968.

4. **Loe,** H., Theilade, E., and Jensen, S.B.: Experimental Gingivitis in Man, *J. Peridontol., 36,* 177, May-June, 1965.

5. **Carranza,** F.A., Saglie, R., Newman, M.G., and Valentin, P.L.: Scanning and Transmission Electron Microscopic Study of Tissue-invading Microorganisms in Localized Juvenile Periodontitis, *J. Periodontol., 54,* 598, October, 1983.

6. **Mandel,** I.D.: Relation of Saliva and Plaque to Caries, *J. Dent. Res., 53,* 246, March-April, Supplement, 1974.

7. **Gron,** P., Yao, K., and Spinelli, M.: A Study of Inorganic Constituents in Dental Plaque, *J. Dent. Res., 48,* 799, September-October, 1969.

8. **Artun,** J. and Osterberg, S.K.: Periodontal Status of Secondary Crowded Mandibular Incisors. Long-term Results After Orthodontic Treatment, *J. Clin. Periodontol., 14,* 261, May, 1987.

9. **Van Houte,** J., Sansone, C., Joshipura, K., and Kent, R.: Mutans Streptococci and Nonmutans Streptococci Acidogenic at Low pH, and In Vitro Acidogenic Potential of Dental Plaque in Two Different Areas of the Human Dentition, *J. Dent. Res., 70,* 1503, December, 1991.

10. **Everett,** F.G. and Potter, G.R.: Morphology of Submarginal Calculus, *J. Periodontol., 30,* 27, January, 1959.

11. **Mandel,** I.D.: Dental Calculus (Calcified Dental Plaque), in Genco, R.J., Goldman, H., and Cohen, D.W., eds.: *Contemporary Periodontics.* St. Louis, The C.V. Mosby Co., 1990, pp. 135–146.

12. **Shay,** D.E., Haddox, J.H., and Richmond, J.L.: An Inorganic Qualitative and Quantitative Analysis of Green Stain, *J. Am. Dent. Assoc., 50,* 156, February, 1955.

13. **Theilade,** J., Slots, J., and Fejerskov, O.: The Ultrastructure of Black Stain on Human Primary Teeth, *Scand. J. Dent. Res., 81,* 528, No. 7, 1973.

14. **Slots,** J.: The Microflora of Black Stain on Human

Primary Teeth, *Scand. J. Dent. Res., 82,* 484, No. 7, 1974.

15. **Theilade,** J.: Development of Bacterial Plaque in the Oral Cavity, *J. Clin. Periodontol., 4,* 1, December, 1977.

16. **Mecket,** A.H.: The Formation and Properties of Organic Films on Teeth, *Arch. Oral Biol., 10,* 585, July-August, 1965.

17. **Eriksen,** H.M. and Nordbo, H.: Extrinsic Discoloration of Teeth, *J. Clin. Periodontol., 5,* 229, November, 1978.

18. **Horowitz,** H.S. and Chamberlin, S.R.: Pigmentation of Teeth Following Topical Applications of Stannus Fluoride in a Nonfluoridated Area, *J. Public Health Dent., 31,* 32, Winter, 1971.

19. **Shannon,** I.L.: Stannous Fluoride: Does It Stain Teeth? How Does It React with Tooth Surfaces? A Review, *Gen. Dent., 26,* 64, September-October, 1978.

20. **Leverett,** D.H., McHugh, W.D., and Jensen, O.E.: Dental Caries and Staining After Twenty-eight Months of Rinsing with Stannous Fluoride or Sodium Fluoride, *J. Dent. Res. 65,* 424, March, 1986.

21. **Flotra,** L., Gjermo, P., Rolla, G., and Waerhaug, J.: Side Effects of Chlorhexidine Mouthwashes, *Scand. J. Dent. Res., 79,* 119, April, 1971.

22. **Formicola,** A.J., Deasy, M.J., Johnson, D.H., and Howe, E.E.: Tooth Staining Effects of an Alexidine Mouthwash, *J. Periodontol. 50,* 207, April, 1979.

23. **Reichart,** P.A., Lenz, H., Konig, H., Becker, J., and Mohr, U.: The Black Layer on the Teeth of Betel Chewers: A Light Microscopic, Microradiographic, and Electromicroscopic Study, *J. Oral Pathol., 14,* 466, July, 1985.

24. **Robinson,** H.B.G. and Miller, A.S.: *Color Atlas of Oral Pathology,* 5th ed. Philadelphia, J.B. Lippincott Co., 1990, pp. 41–47, 55.

25. **Haring,** J.I. and Ibsen, O.A.C.: Developmental Disorders, in Ibsen, O.A.C. and Phelan, J.A., eds.: *Oral Pathology for the Dental Hygienist.* Philadelphia, W.B. Saunders Co., 1992, pp. 267–271, 395–399.

26. **Mertz-Fairhurst,** E.J., Fairhurst, C.W., Williams, J.E., Della-Giustina, V.E., and Brooks, J.D.: A Comparative Clinical Study of Two Pit and Fissure Sealants: 7-year

Results in Augusta, GA, *J. Am. Dent. Assoc., 109,* 252, August, 1984.

27. **Simonsen,** R.J.: The Clinical Effectiveness of a Colored Pit and Fissure Sealant at 36 Months, *J. Am. Dent. Assoc., 102,* 323, March, 1981.

28. **Simonsen,** R.J.: Retention and Effectiveness of Dental Sealant after 15 Years, *J. Am. Dent. Assoc., 122,* 34, October, 1991.

29. **Knutson,** J.W.: Sodium Fluoride Solutions: Technique for Application to the Teeth, *J. Am. Dent. Assoc., 36,* 37, January, 1948.

30. **DeLeo,** A.A.: The Incidence of Bacteremia Following Oral Prophylaxis on Pediatric Patients, *Oral Surg., 37,* 36, January, 1974.

31. **Micik,** R.E., Miller, R.L., Mazzarella, M.A., and Ryge, G.: Studies on Dental Aerobiology: I. Bacterial Aerosols Generated During Dental Procedures, *J. Dent. Res., 48,* 49, January-February, 1969.

32. **Hartley,** J.L.: Eye and Facial Injuries Resulting from Dental Procedures, *Dent. Clin. North Am., 22,* 505, July, 1978.

33. **Vrbic,** V., Brudevold, F., and McCann, H.G.: Acquisition of Fluoride by Enamel from Fluoride Pumice Pastes, *Helv. Odontol. Acta, 11,* 21, April, 1967.

34. **Kontturi-Narhi,** V. Markkanen, S., and Markkanen, H.: Effects of Airpolishing on Dental Plaque Removal and Hard Tissues as Evaluated by Scanning Electron Microscopy, *J. Periodontol., 61,* 334, June, 1990.

35. **Stookey,** G.K.: In Vitro Estimates of Enamel and Dentin Abrasion Associated with a Prophylaxis, *J. Dent. Res., 57,* 36, January, 1978.

36. **Zuniga,** M.A. and Caldwell, R.C.: The Effect of Fluoride-containing Prophylaxis Pastes on Normal and "White-Spot" Enamel, *ASDC J. Dent. Child., 36,* 345, September-October, 1969.

37. **Brasch,** S.V., Lazarou, J., Van Abbe, N.J., and Forrest, J.O.: The Assessment of Dentifrice Abrasivity In Vivo, *Br. Dent. J., 127,* 119, August 5, 1969.

38. **Jefferies,** R.W.: Polishing Dental Enamel, *N.Z. Dent. J., 69,* 167, July, 1973.

39. **Brudevold,** F., Gardner, D.E., and Smith, F.A.: The

Distribution of Fluoride in Human Enamel, *J. Dent. Res., 35,* 420, June, 1956.

40. **Vrbic, V.** and Brudevold, F.: Fluoride Uptake from Treatment with Different Fluoride Prophylaxis Pastes and from the Use of Pastes Containing a Soluble Aluminum Salt Followed by Topical Application, *Caries Res., 4,* 158, No. 2, 1970.

41. **Loe,** H. Reactions of Marginal Periodontal Tissues to Restorative Procedures, *Int. Dent. J., 18,* 759, December, 1968.

42. **Miller,** W.A.: Experimental Foreign Body Reactions to Toothpaste Abrasives, *J. Periodontol., 47,* 101, February, 1976.

43. **Roulet,** J.F. and Rolet-Mehrens, T.K.: The Surface Roughness of Restorative Materials and Dental Tissues after Polishing with Prophylaxis and Polishing Pastes, *J. Periodontol., 53,* 257, April, 1982.

44. **Glenwright,** H.D., Knibbs, P.J., and Burdon, D. W.: Atmospheric Contamination During Use of an Air Polisher, *Br. Dent. J., 159,* 294, November 9, 1985.

45. **Worrall,** S.F., Knibbs, P.J., and Glenwright, H.D.: Methods of Reducing Bacterial Contamination of the Atmosphere Arising from Use of an Airpolisher, *Br. Dent. J., 163,* 118, August 22, 1987.

46. **Rawson,** R.D., Nelson, B.N., Jewell, B.D., and Jewell, C.C.: Alkalosis as a Potential Complication of Air Polishing Systems. A Pilot Study, *Dent. Hyg., 59,* 500, November, 1985.

47. **Willmann,** D.E., Norling, B.K., and Johnson, W.N.: A New Prophylaxis Instrument: Effect on Enamel Alterations, *J. Am. Dent. Assoc., 101,* 923, December, 1980.

48. **Atkinson,** D.R., Cobb, C.M., and Klloy, W.J.: The Effect of an Air-powder Abrasive System on In Vitro Root Surfaces, *J. Periodontol., 55,* 13, January, 1984.

49. **Galloway,** S.E. and Pashley, D.H.: Rate of Removal of Root Structure by the Use of the Prophy-jet Device, *J. Periodontol, 58,* 464, July, 1987.

50. **Miskin,** D.J., Engler, W.O., Javed, T., Darby, T.D., Cobb, R.L., and Coffman, M.A.: A Clinical Comparison

of the Effect on the Gingiva of the Prophy-jet and the Rubber Cup and Paste Techniques, *J. Periodontol., 57,* 151, March, 1986.

51. **Cooley,** R.L., Lubow, R.M., and Patrissi, G.A.: The Effect of an Air-powder Abrasive Instrument on Composite Resin, *J. Am. Dent. Assoc., 112,* 362, March, 1986.

52. **Lubow,** R.M. and Cooley, R.L.: Effect of Air-powder Abrasive Instrument on Restorative Materials, *J. Prosthet. Dent., 55,* 462, April, 1986.

53. **Felton,** D.A., Bayne, S.C., Kanoy, B.E., and White, J.T.: Effect of Air Abrasives on Marginal Configurations of Porcelain-Fused-To-Metal Alloys: An SEM Analysis, *J. Prosthet. Dent., 65,* 38, January, 1991.

References for Table 6.3

Choi, J.I., Nakagawa, T., Yamada, S., Takazoe, I., and Okuda, K.: Clinical, Microbiological and Immunological Studies on Recurrent Periodontal Disease, Part I, *J. Clin. Periodontol., 17,* 426, August, 1990.

Christersson, L.A., Fransson, C.L., Dunford, R.G., and Zambon, J.J.: Subgingival Distribution of Periodontal Pathogenic Microorganisms in Adult Periodontitis, *J. Periodontol., 63,* 418, May, 1992.

Dzink, J.L., Socransky, S.S., and Haffajee, A.D.: The Predominant Cultivable Microbiota of Active and Inactive Lesions of Destructive Periodontal Diseases, *J. Clin. Periodontol., 15,* 316, May, 1988.

Falkler, W.A., Martin, S.A., Vincent, J.W., Tall, B.D., Nauman, R.K., and Suzuki, J.B.: A Clinical, Demographic and Microbiologic Study of ANUG Patients in an Urban Dental School, *J. Clin. Periodontol., 14,* 307, July, 1987.

Haffajee, A.D., Socransky, S.S., Dzink, J.L., Taubman, M.A., and Ebersole, J.L.: Clinical, Microbiological Features of Subjects with Refractory Periodontal Diseases, *J. Clin. Periodontol., 15,* 390, July, 1988.

Kornman, K.S. and Loesche, W.J.: The Subgingival Microbial Flora During Pregnancy, *J. Periodont. Res., 15,* 111, March, 1980.

Kornman, K.S. and Robertson, P.B.: Clinical and Microbiological Evaluation of Therapy for Juvenile Periodontitis, *J. Periodontol.,* 56, 443, August, 1985.

Listgarten, M.A.: Electron Microscopic Observations on the Bacterial Flora of Acute Necrotizing Ulcerative Gingivitis, *J. Periodontol.,* 36, 328, July-August, 1965.

Listgarten, M.A., Lai, C.H., and Young, V.: Microbial Composition and Pattern of Antibiotic Resistance in Subgingival Microbial Samples From Patients with Refractory Periodontitis, *J. Periodontol.,* 64, 155, March, 1993.

Loesche, W.J., Syed, S.A., Schmidt, E., and Morrison, E.C.: Bacterial Profiles of Subgingival Plaques in Periodontitis, *J. Periodontol.,* 56, 447, August, 1985.

Loesche, W.J., Syed, S.A., Laughon, B.E., and Stoll, J.: The Bacteriology of Acute Necrotizing Ulcerative Gingivitis, *J. Periodontol.,* 53, 223, April, 1982.

Mandell, R.L., Ebersole, J.L., and Socransky, S.S.: Clinical Immunologic and Microbiologic Features of Active Disease Sites in Juvenile Periodontitis, *J. Clin. Periodontol.,* 14, 534, October, 1987.

Moore, W.E.C., Moore, L.H., Ranney, R.R., Smibert, R.M., Burmeister, J.A., and Schenkein, H.A.: The Microflora of Periodontal Sites Showing Active Destructive Progression, *J. Clin. Periodontol.,* 18, 729, November, 1991.

Page, R.C., Altman, L.C., Ebersole, J.L., Vandesteen, G.E., Dahlberg, W.H., Williams, B.L., and Osterberg, S.K.: Rapidly Progressive Periodontitis. A Distinct Clinical Condition, *J. Periodontol.,* 54, 197, April, 1983.

Preber, H., Bergstrom, J., and Linder, L.E.: Occurrence of Periopathogens in Smoker and Nonsmoker Patients, *J. Clin. Periodontol.,* 19, 667, October, 1992.

Slots, J.: The Predominant Cultivable Organisms in Juvenile Periodontitis, *Scand. J. Dent. Res.,* 84, 1, January, 1976.

Tanner, A.: Microbial Succession in the Development of Periodontal Disease, in Hamada, S., Holt, S.C., and McGhee, J.R., eds.: *Periodontal Disease: Pathogens and Host Immune Responses.* Tokyo, Quintessence, 1991, pp. 13–25.

Tanner, A. and Bouldin, H.: The Microbiota of Early Periodontitis Lesions in Adults, *J. Periodontol.,* 16, 467, August, 1989.

INDICES AND SCORING METHODS

7

This chapter gives a brief overview of indices and scoring methods that are used in clinical practice and community programs for oral health assessments. The indices presented here are the most commonly used. Please note that Table 7.2 provides general information only; for scoring method details, refer to the references listed at the end of this chapter.

TABLE 7.1. Types of Indices

Type	Purpose	Uses
Individual assessment score	Evaluation/monitoring progress and maintenance of oral health Measures effects of personalized disease control programs Monitors progress of disease healing Patient education, motivation	Aids patient in recognizing oral problems Evaluates effectiveness of current oral hygiene habits Patient motivation toward preventive oral health practices Provides comparison basis for evaluation over a period of time
Clinical trial	Determines the effect of an agent or procedure on the prevention, progression, or control of a disease Comparison of an experimental group with a control group	Baseline data prior to introduction of experimental factors Measures effectiveness of specific agents for the prevention, control, or treatment of oral conditions Measures effectiveness of mechanical devices for personal care
Epidemiologic survey	Survey for the study of disease characteristics of populations Not designed for evaluation of an individual patient	Shows prevalence and incidence of particular conditions occurring within a given population Provides baseline data of existing oral health practices Assesses the needs of a community Compares effects of community programs and evaluates the results

TABLE 7.2. Examples of Indices/Systems

Index/System	Purpose	Selection Area
Periodontal screening & recording (PSR) (American Academy of Periodontology and American Dental Association) (1)	Rapidly assess state of periodontal health	Dentition divided into sextants; each tooth is examined, but when a Code 4 is found in a sextant, the remaining teeth in the sextant are not probed
	Motivation of the patient to seek complete periodontal assessment and treatment	
	This is not a substitute for a complete periodontal probing	
Plaque index (PI I) (Silness and Loe) (2, 3)	Assess thickness of plaque at the gingival area	Entire dentition or selected teeth
		Four gingival areas examined per tooth (distal, facial, mesial, lingual)
		Modified procedure examines facial, mesial, and lingual areas
Plaque control record (O'Leary, Drake and Naylor) (4)	Record bacterial plaque on individual tooth surfaces to permit patient to visualize progress while learning plaque control	All teeth
		Four surfaces (facial, lingual, mesial, distal)
		Six areas may be recorded (5)
Plaque-free score (Grant, Stern, Everett) (6)	Determines location, number, and percent of plaque-free surfaces for motivation and instruction	All erupted teeth
		Four surfaces (facial, lingual or palatal, mesial, distal)

continued

TABLE 7.2. Examples of Indices/Systems

Index/System	Purpose	Selection Area
	Can also be used to record interdental bleeding	
Patient hygiene performance (PHP) (Podshadley and Haley) (7)	Assess extent of plaque and debris over a tooth surface	Teeth #3, 8, 14, 19, 24, 30
	Debris for the PHP: soft foreign material of bacterial plaque, materia alba, and food debris loosely attached to tooth surfaces	Facial surfaces of incisors and maxillary molars
		Lingual surface of mandibular molars
Oral hygiene index (OHI) (Greene and Vermillion, Waggener) (8, 9)	Measure existing debris and calculus as an indication of oral cleanliness	Dentition divided into sextants
	Two components: Debris Index and Calculus Index, used singly or combined	Fully erupted teeth (reached occlusal plane)
		12 surfaces (one facial, one lingual) in each sextant, that have the greatest amount of debris, plaque, and calculus
Simplified oral hygiene index (OHI-S) (Greene and Vermillion) (10, 11)	Assess oral cleanliness by estimating the tooth surface covered with debris	Same surfaces as PHP Index

continued

Index	Purpose	Units
	Two components: Simplified Debris Index (DI-S), Simplified Calculus Index (CI-S), used singly or combined	Four gingival units for each tooth: labial and lingual marginal gingiva (M units); mesial and distal papillary gingiva (P units)
Sulcus bleeding index (SBI) (Muhlemann and Son) (12)	Locate areas of gingival sulcus bleeding upon probing to recognize and record presence of early (initial) inflammatory gingival disease	
Gingival bleeding index (GBI) (Carter and Barnes) (13)	Record presence or absence of gingival inflammation determined by bleeding from interproximal gingival sulci	Two sulci in each interproximal area scored individually or as one interdental unit; Certain areas may be excluded because of accessibility, tooth position, diastema, or other factors
Papillary-marginal-attached gingival index (P-M-A) (Schour and Massler) (14, 15)	Assess the extent of gingival changes in large groups for epidemiologic studies	Three gingival units examined for each tooth: papillary, marginal, attached
Gingival index (GI) (Loe and Silness) (3, 16)	Assess the severity of gingivitis based on color, consistency, and bleeding on probing	Selected teeth or entire dentition; Four gingival areas: distal, facial, mesial, lingual

continued

TABLE 7.2. Examples of Indices/Systems

Index/System	Purpose	Selection Area
Periodontal index (PI) (Russell) (17, 18)	Assess and score the periodontal disease status of populations in epidemiologic studies	Each tooth scored according to the condition of the surrounding tissues
Periodontal disease index (PDI) (Ramfjord) (19, 20)	Show the periodontal status of an individual or group by assessing the prevalence and severity of gingivitis and periodontitis Combines evaluation of gingival status with probed attachment level A Calculus Index and plaque index are usually included but are not a part of the PDI	Six teeth are used to represent the six segments of the dentition: Nos. 3, 9, 12, 19, 25, 28
Calculus score (used with PDI) (Ramfjord) (20)	Evaluate the presence and extent of calculus Used in conjunction with the PDI Should be scored prior to PDI	Six teeth of the PDI; four surfaces: facial, lingual (or palatal), mesial, distal

continued

Index	Purpose	Details
Dental plaque score (used with PDI) (Ramfjord) (20)	Evaluate the extent of plaque on the basis of tooth surface coverage	Six teeth of the PDI; four surfaces: facial, lingual, mesial, distal
Community Periodontal Index of Treatment Needs (CPITN) (Federation Dentaire Internationale, Ainamo et al.) (21, 22)	Screen and monitor individual or group periodontal needs	Adults (20 years and older): Dentition divided into sextants; evaluate all teeth. Children and adolescents: Dentition divided into sextants; evaluate one tooth per sextant
Decayed, missing, and filled permanent teeth (DMFT) (23)	Determine total dental caries experience, past and present	Based on 28 teeth. Excluded teeth: Third molars; Unerupted teeth; Congenitally missing; Supernumerary; Extracted teeth for reasons other than caries; Teeth restored for other than caries; Primary tooth retained with the permanent successor erupted

continued

TABLE 7.2. Examples of Indices/Systems

Index/System	Purpose	Selection Area
Decayed, missing, and filled permanent tooth surfaces (DMFS)	Determine total dental caries experience, past and present, by recording tooth surfaces instead of teeth	Teeth excluded same as DMFT Total surface count = 128 Posterior—five surfaces: facial, lingual, mesial, distal, occlusal Anterior—four surfaces: facial, lingual, mesial, distal Missing posterior teeth = five surfaces
Decayed, indicated for extraction, and filled teeth or surfaces (dft and dfs) (deft and defs) (24)	Determine dental caries experience as shown for the primary teeth present in the oral cavity by evaluating teeth or surfaces	Teeth evaluated = 20 Surfaces evaluated = 88 Teeth excluded: missing teeth, supernumerary teeth restored for reasons other than dental caries Mixed dentition requires separate indices
Decayed, missing, and filled (dmft or dmfs)	Determine dental caries experience, past and present, for children older than 7; 7 years and up to 11 or 12 years old	dmft: 12 teeth (eight primary molars, four primary canines) dmfs: 56 surfaces Mixed dentition requires separate indices

REFERENCES

1. **American Academy of Periodontology and American Dental Association:** *Periodontal Screening & Recording.* Sponsored by Procter & Gamble, Chicago, IL, June, 1992.
2. **Silness,** J. and Loe, H.: Periodontal Disease in Pregnancy. II. Correlation Between Oral Hygiene and Periodontal Condition, *Acta Odontol. Scand., 22,* 121, No. 1, 1964.
3. **Loe,** H.: The Gingival Index, the Plaque Index and the Retention Index Systems, *J. Periodontol., 38,* 610, November-December, 1967 (Part II).
4. **O'Leary,** T.J., Drake, R.B., and Naylor, J.E.: The Plaque Control Record, *J. Periodontol., 43,* 38, January, 1972.
5. **Ramfjord,** S.P. and Ash, M.M.: *Periodontology and Periodontics.* Philadelphia, W.B. Saunders Co., 1979, pp. 529–531.
6. **Grant,** D.A., Stern, I.B., and Everett, F.G.: *Periodontics,* 5th ed. St. Louis, C.V. Mosby Co., 1979, pp. 529–531.
7. **Podshadley,** A.G. and Haley, J.V.: A Method for Evaluating Oral Hygiene Performance, *Public Health Rep., 83,* 259, March, 1968.
8. **Greene,** J.C. and Vermillion, J.R.: Oral Hygiene Index: A Method for Classifying Oral Hygiene Status, *J. Am. Dent. Assoc., 61,* 172, August, 1960.
9. **Waggener,** E.W.: Community Dentistry, in Steele, P.F., ed.: *Dimensions of Dental Hygiene,* 2nd ed. Philadelphia, Lea & Febiger, 1975, pp.13–16.
10. **Greene,** J.C. and Vermillion, J.R.: The Simplified Oral Hygiene Index, *J. Am. Dent. Assoc., 68,* 7, January, 1964.
11. **Greene,** J.C.: The Oral Hygiene Index—Development and Uses, *J. Periodontol., 38,* 625, November-December, 1967 (Part II).
12. **Muhlemann,** H.R. and Son, S.: Gingival Sulcus Bleeding—A Leading Symptom in Initial Gingivitis, *Helv. Odontol. Acta, 15,* 107, October, 1971.
13. **Carter,** H.G. and Barnes, G.P.: The Gingival Bleeding Index, *J. Periodontol., 45,* 801, November, 1974.

14. **Schour,** I. and Massler, M.: Prevalence of Gingivitis in Young Adults, *J. Dent. Res., 27,* 733, Abstract No. 33, December 1948.

15. **Massler,** M.: The P-M-A Index for the Assessment of Gingivitis, *J. Periodontol., 38,* 592, November-December, 1967 (Part II).

16. **Loe,** H. and Silness, J.: Periodontal Disease in Pregnancy. I. Prevalence and Severity, *Acta Odontol. Scand., 21,* 533, No. 6, 1963.

17. **Russell,** A.L.: A System of Classification and Scoring for Prevalence Surveys of Periodontal Disease, *J. Dent. Res., 35,* 350, June, 1956.

18. **Russell,** A.L.: The Periodontal Index, *J. Periodontol., 38, 585,* November-December, 1967 (Part II).

19. **Ramfjord,** S.P.: Indices for Prevalence and Incidence of Periodontal Disease, *J. Periodontol., 30,* 51, January, 1959.

20. **Ramfjord,** S.P.: The Periodontal Disease Index (PDI), *J. Periodontol. 38,* 602, November-December, 1967 (Part II).

21. **Federation Dentaire Internationale:** A Simplified Periodontal Examination for Dental Practices, FDI WG6 and Joint FDI/WHO WGI, Federation Dentaire Internationale, 64, Wimpole Street, London, WIM 8AL.

22. **Ainamo,** J., Barmes, D. Beagrie, G., Cutress, T., Martin, J., and Sardo-Infirri, J.: Development of the World Health Organization (WHO) Community Periodontal Index of Treatment Needs (CPITN), *Int. Dent. J., 32,* 281, September, 1982.

23. **Klein,** H., Palmer, C.E., and Knutson, J.W.: Studies on Dental Caries. I. Dental Status and Dental Needs of Elementary School Children, *Public Health Rep., 53,* 751, May 13, 1938.

24. **Gruebbel,** A.O.: A Measurement of Dental Caries Prevalence and Treatment Service for Deciduous Teeth, *J. Dent. Res., 23,* 163, June, 1944.

DENTAL HYGIENE
TREATMENT PLAN

8

Much discussion and controversy surrounds the concept of the dental hygienist's qualifications to "diagnose." Dental hygiene diagnosis does exist; it is done every day in all settings. The education of dental hygienists provides more than adequately the ability to recognize oral diseases and plan treatment modalities within the legal scope of dental hygiene practice.

Chapter 5 gives the basic information needed for the first part of a dental hygiene treatment plan: the assessment of the patient. With the data collected and analyzed, the next step is to develop a dental hygiene diagnosis based on the findings and clinical judgment of the practitioner. Components of the diagnosis must take into consideration the problem, the cause of the problem, and the signs and symptoms that are present. Collaboration with the dentist during diagnosis aids in the treatment-planning phase, helping to ensure a comprehensive and coordinated treatment plan for the patient.

The objectives of the treatment plan are to eliminate and control the etiologic and predisposing disease factors, eliminate the signs and symptoms of disease, restore the normal functions of the oral environment, maintain health, and prevent the recurrence of disease. Ideally, the treatment plan will be implemented as initially presented; however, other factors must be taken into consideration that may alter the "ideal" plan. This is to be expected. A treatment plan needs to be flexible to fit the individual and his or her needs or willingness to participate as a partner in restoring oral health. Clear explanations of proposed treatment, outlining treatment procedures, number of appointments, responsibilities of both the practitioner and the patient in the treatment, expense of treatment, insurance payments, expected outcomes and possible negative aspects, and alternative or optional treatment modalities need to be presented to the patient/client. This is part of informed consent, the agreement between the patient/client and the practitioners to begin the treatment as presented. Formal forms with carbon copies for all parties are available to keep in the record (1, 2).

Implementation of the treatment plan follows. Phases of implementation include preventive, preparatory, and definitive treatment, maintenance, and continuing evaluation.

Evaluation is ongoing throughout the treatment phase, upon the treatment's completion, and throughout follow-up appointments. Responsiveness of tissue, resolution of problem areas, effectiveness of the patient's home care, and effectiveness of the treatment rendered can all be monitored, with modifications made to the treatment plan if necessary.

TABLE 8.1.	Dental Hygiene Treatment Plan
Objectives	Eliminate and control etiologic and predisposing disease factors
	Eliminate the signs and symptoms of disease
	Restore normal function
	Maintain health
	Prevent recurrence of disease
Components	Assessment procedures (histories, probings, charting, etc.)
	Dental hygiene diagnosis
	Planning of treatment:
	Priority (pain, acute conditions, biopsies, tests)
	Preventive (self-care instructions, interventions to arrest and reverse early stages of disease)
	Preparatory (periodontal therapy, dental caries, endontice treatment, extractions, etc.)
	Treatment phase (gingival and periodontal treatment, restorative, prosthetics, orthodontics, tissue maintenance during therapy)
	Evaluation (ongoing throughout)
	Maintenance (daily plaque control, regularly scheduled maintenance and reevaluation appointments, updating of records, radiographs as needed)
	Implementation
	Evaluation

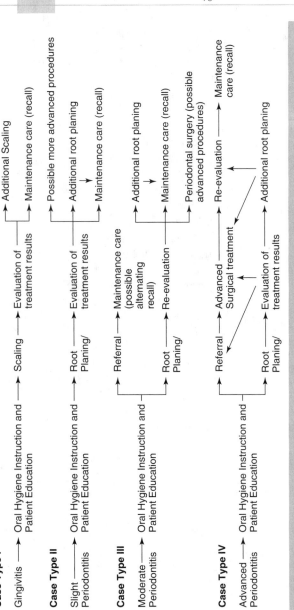

FIGURE 8.1. General treatment patterns by case type. Flowcharts show suggested treatment programs for the four basic case types from gingivitis to advanced periodontitis. Note that the first step in all programs is patient instruction. (Adapted from Karch, J.D.: Diagnosing and Managing the Periodontal Patient, *Risk Management Series*, p. 19. Copyright 1986, American Dental Association.)

Case Type I

Gingivitis → Oral Hygiene Instruction and Patient Education → Scaling → Evaluation of treatment results → Additional Scaling / Maintenance care (recall)

Case Type II

Slight Periodontitis → Oral Hygiene Instruction and Patient Education → Root Planing → Evaluation of treatment results → Possible more advanced procedures / Additional root planing / Maintenance care (recall)

Case Type III

Moderate Periodontitis → Oral Hygiene Instruction and Patient Education → Referral → Maintenance care (possible alternating recall) / Root Planing/ → Re-evaluation → Additional root planing / Maintenance care (recall) / Periodontal surgery (possible advanced procedures)

Case Type IV

Advanced Periodontitis → Oral Hygiene Instruction and Patient Education → Referral → Advanced Surgical treatment / Root Planing/ → Evaluation of treatment results → Re-evaluation → Additional root planing / Maintenance care (recall)

REFERENCES

1. **Robbins,** K.S.: Medical-legal Considerations, in Malamed, S.F., ed.: *Handbook of Medical Emergencies in the Dental Office,* 4th ed. St. Louis, The C.V. Mosby Co., 1993, pp. 91–101.
2. **Bailey,** B.L.: Informed Consent in Dentistry, *J. Am. Dent. Assoc., 110,* 709, May, 1985.

ORAL INFECTION CONTROL

9

The complete dental hygiene treatment plan must include a preventive treatment plan. This chapter provides a brief review of preventive measures and aids used in a preventive program.

TABLE 9.1. Preventive Treatment Plan

Phase	Factors
Patient needs assessment	Review of patient information (histories, radiographs, examination findings, chartings)
	Identify infection (presence and severity), predisposing factors
	Gather baseline data for future comparisons (indices, probings)
Intervention planning	Use personal information gathered to aid in plan formulation and customizing plan
	Consider any physical or mental disabilities
	Current personal oral care practices
	Outline recommended that lists oral hygiene goals and instructions
Implementation	Motivation, demonstration, and counseling for daily care
	Self-evaluation techniques for home care
Clinical preventive services	Scaling and debridement
	Caries-preventive agent application

continued

TABLE 9.1. Preventive Treatment Plan

Phase	Factors
Evaluation of changes	Gingival tissue, bleeding, plaque, self-care techniques
	Use indices to compare with baseline data
	Counseling for areas needing improvement
Long-term maintenance	Evaluation, monitoring of oral hygiene home-care practices
	When indicated, provide additional preventive techniques

TABLE 9.2. Factors for Toothbrush Selection (1)

Characteristic	Factors
Meets individual patient needs	Size, shape, and texture adapt to teeth positions; accessibility to problem areas
	Easy and efficient manipulation; handle design is comfortable
Functional properties	Flexibility, softness, diameter of the bristles or filaments
	Strength, rigidity, and lightness of handle
	Easily cleaned and aerated; impervious to moisture
	End-rounded filaments or bristles
	Designed for utility, efficiency, and cleanliness
	Durable and inexpensive

Natural bristle toothbrushes are not recommended because the bristles cannot be standardized; wear more rapidly and irregularly; are hollow, which allows microorganisms and debris to collect inside; and are water absorbent, which causes softening of the bristles (2).

TABLE 9.3. Oral Hygiene Aids

Types of Aids	Factors/Characteristics
Manual toothbrushes	See Table 9.2
Power-assisted toothbrushes	Selection of action modes: rotational, counter-rotational, oscillating-counter-rotational, sonic
	If used properly after instruction, power-assisted brushes are effective alternatives to the manual brush
	Good choice for individuals with limited manual dexterity or disabilities, those undergoing orthodontic treatment, or caregivers
	Caution or avoidance of pressure on synthetic restorations or exposed cementum or dentin
Tongue brushes/scrapers	A regular soft-bristle toothbrush can be used
	Commercially available tongue brushes and paste
	Tongue scrapers made of plastic or flexible metal
	Reduces oral debris, retards bacterial plaque formation and total plaque accumulation, reduces the number of microorganisms, contributes to overall cleanliness, lessens mouth odors
	Good for individuals with coated tongues or fissures; smokers

continued

TABLE 9.3. Oral Hygiene Aids

Types of Aids	Factors/Characteristics
Interdental brushes	Comes in a variety of styles
	Reusable handles with various sized and shaped brush inserts
	Brushes on a thin wire handle
	Single-tuft brush with either flat or tapered filament
	Angled or flat shanks
	Adequate space for insertion is needed
	To remove bacterial plaque from proximal surfaces adjacent to open embrasures, orthodontic appliances, fixed prostheses, dental implants, periodontal splints, space maintainers, areas not adequately accessible with a regular toothbrush, and concave areas that are not accessible with dental floss or other interdental aids (3, 4)
	For application of chemotherapeutic agents
	Exposed class III furcations
Interdental tip	Cone- or pyramid-shaped flexible rubber or plastic tip attached to a handle or at the end of a toothbrush
	Power-driven device now available
	Rubber tip is preferable to rigid plastic because of easier adaptation to the interdental area

continued

	For cleaning debris from the interdental area and bacterial plaque removal from tooth surfaces
	Plaque removal at and just below the gingival margin
	Round toothpick inserted into a plastic handle
Toothpick in holder	For periodontal patient to remove plaque at and just under the gingival margin; interdental cleaning, especially for concave proximal tooth surfaces, exposed furcation areas
	For orthodontic patient to remove plaque at the gingival margin above appliances and around fixed appliances
	Triangular-shaped 2-inch long device made of balsawood or birchwood
	For cleaning exposed proximal tooth surfaces when interdental gingiva is missing
Wood interdental cleaner	Adequate space is needed or the gingival tissue can be traumatized
	Must carefully follow instructions for use
	Wood can splay with use, so more than one may be needed each session
	Multitude of types: waxed, unwaxed, flavored, teflon, gortex, regular, thin, flat (there is no difference in the effectiveness of plaque removal between waxed and unwaxed floss, patient
Dental floss and tape	preference aids in compliance with plaque control) (5–9)
	Should be used prior to toothbrushing
	Removes bacterial plaque and reduces interproximal bleeding, thus contributing to gingival health

continued

TABLE 9.3. Oral Hygiene Aids

Types of Aids	Factors/Characteristics
Tufted dental floss	Floss/yarn combination
	Plaque removal from tooth surfaces adjacent to wide embrasures where interdental papilla have been lost
	Plaque removal from abutments and under pontics of fixed partial dentures
	Plaque removal around dental implants
Knitting yarn	Tooth surfaces adjacent to wide proximal spaces where dental floss does not adequately remove plaque
	Plaque removal under fixed partial dentures
	Plaque removal around dental implants
Gauze strip	Isolated teeth; teeth separated by diastema; distal surfaces of most posterior teeth
	6- to 8-in strip of 1-in gauze, folded in thirds or half
	For proximal surfaces of widely spaced teeth
	For surfaces of teeth next to edentulous areas
	For areas under posterior cantilevered section of a fixed appliance
Oral irrigation	Devices may be power driven or attached to a faucet
	Specific tips for supragingival and subgingival irrigation

continued

Effective for supragingival removal of loosely attached bacterial plaque and for reducing gingivitis (effect is enhanced if an antimicrobial agent is used) (15–17)

Reduces or alters microbial flora (17–19)

Penetrates into pocket, subgingival access (20–23)

Enhances effectiveness of antimicrobial agents vs. mouthrinsing

Researched agents for oral irrigation

Chlorhexidine gluconate (16, 17, 24, 25)

Stannous fluoride (24, 26–28)

Phenolic compounds (essential oils) (15, 29)

Sanguinaria (30, 31)

Effective for bacterial plaque removal from problem areas

Special need area care: prosthetic replacements, orthodontic appliances, intermaxillary fixation appliances for orthognathic surgery (32) and fractured jaw, complex restorations, and other extensive rehabilitation

May aid in the postponement of periodontal surgery if maintenance appointments are frequently scheduled and an antimicrobial agent is used

If the patient requires antibiotic premedication for dental treatment, consultation with patient's physician should be done before recommending use of adjunctive oral hygiene aids that can create bacteremias (33, 34)

continued

TABLE 9.3. Oral Hygiene Aids

Types of Aids	Factors/Characteristics
Mouthrinses (see Table 9.4)	Supragingival procedure (20, 35)
	Either therapeutic or cosmetic
	Clinical setting
	Pretreatment to reduce microorganisms (36, 37)
	Reduce aerosol contamination (38)
	Facilitate impression procedures
	Rinse and refresh the mouth during and following dental/hygiene procedures
	Home care:
	Mouth cleaning (dislodge debris, limited cleaning only)
	Postsurgical care
	Postnonsurgical periodontal therapy
	Treatment (pathologic conditions)
	Dental caries prevention (fluoride)
	Cosmetic: removes loose debris, temporary mechanical reduction of microorganisms, pleasant taste/sensation, temporary suppression of locally caused halitosis
Dentifrices (see Table 9.5)	For bacterial plaque, materia alba, and debris removal from the teeth and gingiva
	For cosmetic and sanitary purposes and/or preventive/therapeutic purposes

TABLE 9.4. Mouthrinses

Characteristic of effective mouthrinses (39)	Nontoxic
	No or limited absorption; action should be confined to bacterial plaque
	Substantivity (released over a period of time with potency retained)
	Bacterial specificity for organisms most pathogenic for a given infection
	Low induced drug resistance
Self-prepared mouthrinses	Used for postoperative care following dental/hygiene procedures
	May reduce edema
	Saline rinses should not be used by individuals on low-salt or sodium-free diets
	Types
	Plain water
	Isotonic sodium chloride: ½ tsp salt to 1 cup warm water
	Hypertonic sodium choride: ½ tsp salt to ½ cup warm water
	Sodium bicarbonate: ½ tsp "soda" to 1 cup warm water
	Sodium chloride-sodium bicarbonate
	½ tsp sodium chloride
	½ tsp sodium bicarbonate
	1 cup warm water

continued

TABLE 9.4. Mouthrinses

Commercial mouth-rinses (40)	Basic ingredients for both cosmetic and therapeutic; oral rinses include water, alcohol, flavoring oils, and coloring materials
	There are a variety of nonalcohol rinses available
	Active ingredients
	Oxygenating agents (41) (use of hydrogen peroxide as well as other oxygen-liberating drugs after treatment of disease can cause sponginess of gingiva, black hair tongue, hypersensitivity of exposed root surfaces, and demineralization of tooth surfaces) (42–44)
	Astringents: zinc chloride, zinc acetate, alum, tannic, acetic, and citric acids (repeated use can cause tooth demineralization and tissue irritation)
	Anodynes: phenol derivatives, essential oils
	Buffering agents; sodium borate solution NF (National Formulary), sodium perborate NF, sodium bicarbonate USP
	Deodorizing agents: chlorophyll and others
	Antimicrobial agents:
	bisbiguanides: chlorhexidine, alexidine
	bipyridines: octenidine
	pyrimidines: hexetidine

continued

halogens: iodine, iodophores, fluorides

phenolic compounds

    phenol; thymol, Hexylresorcinol, Listerine (thymol, eucalyptol, menthol; methylsalicylate)

    Triclosan (with zinc citrate)

Quaternary ammonium compounds: Cetylpyridinium chloride, Benzethonium chloride

Herbal extract: Sanguinarine

Chlorhexidine

Most effective antiplaque, antigingivitis chemotherapeutic agent available

0.2% chlorhexidine gluconate twice-daily use prevents bacterial plaque accumulation and gingivitis (46); extensive world-wide use except in the United States

0.12% chlorhexidine gluconate

    Approved for use in the United States

    Clinical effects compare favorably with those of the 0.2% mouthrinse (47)

Uses

    Decreases bacterial plaque formation, inhibits gingivitis development

    Short-term adjunctive therapy following surgical treatment

    Control inflammation in necrotizing ulcerative gingivitis (NUG)

    Suppresses *mutans Streptococcus*; prevents smooth surface dental caries (48)

continued

TABLE 9.4. Mouthrinses

Side effects

Brown stain on teeth

Temporary loss of taste

Bitter taste of the product

Burning sensation of the mucosa

Dryness, soreness of the mucosa

Epithelial desquamation

Discoloration of teeth, tongue, and restorations

Slight increase in supragingival calculus formation

TABLE 9.5. Dentifrices

Components (40)	Purpose	Criteria	Ingredients
Detergents	Lower surface tension; penetrate and loosen deposits and stains Emulsify debris Contribute to foaming action	Nontoxic, neutral in reaction Active in acid or alkaline media Compatible with other ingredients No distinctive flavor Foaming characteristics	Synthetic detergents Sodium lauryl sulfate USP (United States Pharmacopoeia) Sodium n-lauryl sarcosinate Sodium cocomonoglyceride sulfonate
Cleaning and polishing agents	Abrasive for cleaning Polishing agent to produce smooth tooth surface	Cleans well, no damage to tooth surface Provides high polish that prevents or delays reaccumulation of stains and deposits	Calcium carbonate Calcium pyrophosphate Dicalcium phosphate, dihydrate Dicalcium phosphate, anhydrous Insoluble sodium metaphosphate (IMP) Hydrated aluminum oxide Silica, silicates, and dehydrated silica gels Gel dentifrices (40) Synthetic amorphous silica zero-gel Synthetic amorphous complex aluminosilicate salt

continued

TABLE 9.5. Dentifrices

Components (40)	Purpose	Criteria	Ingredients
Binders	Prevent separation of solid and liquid detergents during storage	Stable, nontoxic; compatibility with other ingredients	Organic hydrophilic colloids Alginates Synthetic derivatives of cellulose Organic colloids require a preservative to prevent microbial growth
Humectants	Retain moisture; prevent hardening upon air exposure Stabilize the preparation	Stable, nontoxic	Glycerine Sorbitol Propylene glycol Require a preservative to prevent microbial growth
Preservatives	Prevent bacterial growth Prolong shelf life	Compatibility with other ingredients	Alcohols Benzoates Formaldehyde Dichlorinated phenols

continued

Sweetening agents	Pleasant flavor	Noncariogenic	Artificial noncariogenic sweetener
			Sorbitol and glycerin contribute to sweet flavor
Flavoring agents	Desirable taste	Remain unchanged during manufacturing and storage	Essential oils (peppermint, cinnamon, wintergreen, clove)
	Mask flavor of other ingredients	Compatibility with other ingredients	Menthol
			Artificial noncariogenic sweetener
Coloring agents	Attractiveness	Does not stain teeth or discolor other oral tissues	Vegetable dyes

TABLE 9.6. Prophylactic or Therapeutic Dentifrices

Type	Factors
Dental caries control/remineralization	Fluoride-containing dentifrices for fluoride deposition Recommended for all age groups Necessary for children and caries-prone adults Necessary for prevention of root caries in cases of gingival recession and root exposure after periodontal therapy
Gingival health: control of bacterial plaque	Chemotherapeutic agents added to the dentifrice may destroy or inhibit the growth of microorganisms in plaque
Calculus-prevention agents	Dentifrices contain either a pyrophosphate system or a zinc system Does not have an effect on existing calculus deposits Preventive measure in the formation of new calculus Use to supplement mechanical plaque removal efforts, motivational incentive (49)
Desensitization	Fluorides, potassium nitrate, strontium chloride, sodium citrate are effective agents Abrasiveness of the dentifrice must be considered to prevent further sensitivity from dentinal tubules that may be uncovered from the abrasive

TABLE 9.7. Utilization of Oral Hygiene Aids

Problem	Device/Method	Special Adaptations
Debris removal	Water irrigation Toothbrush	Wide embrasures Under fixed partial dentures
Sulcular brushing	Toothbrush with soft end-rounded filaments	Facial and lingual surfaces Distal surfaces of most-posterior teeth, particularly terminal abutment
Proximal surfaces plaque removal	Floss Floss with threader Yarn with floss and/or threader Toothpick holder Pipe cleaner Interdental brush Single-tuft brush	Abutment teeth Proximal root surfaces Pontic surfaces Narrowed embrasures
Proximal surfaces open contacts	Gauze strip Yarn	Terminal abutment of removable partial denture Distal surfaces of most-posterior teeth in the dental arch

continued

TABLE 9.7. Utilization of Oral Hygiene Aids

Problem	Device/Method	Special Adaptations
Exposed furcation molars	Pipe cleaner Floss/yarn in threader Interdental brush Interdental rubber tip	Rotated tooth
Exposed furcation maxillary first premolar	Interdental brush Interdental rubber tip	Fused root with groove
Exposed root surfaces	Fluoride dentifrice Dentifrice containing desensitizing agent	Desensitization Prevent abrasion of cementum or dentin
Fixed partial denture	Toothbrush (soft nylon) Floss threader with floss/yarn Any other proximal surface procedures as applicable	Gingival surfaces of pontics Proximal surfaces of pontics and retainers
Edentulous gingiva under removable denture	Toothbrush (soft nylon) (manual or power assisted)	Stimulation and plaque removal
Tongue cleaning	Toothbrush (soft nylon)	Deep fissures
Removable denture	Denture brush Clasp brush Chemical cleanser for immersion	Clasps

REFERENCES

1. **American Dental Association,** Council on Dental Therapeutics: *Accepted Dental Therapeutics,* 40th ed. Chicago, American Dental Association, 1984, pp. 386–387.
2. **Massassati,** A. and Frank, R.M.: Scanning Electron Microscopy of Unused and Used Manual Toothbrushes, *J. Clin. Periodontol,* 9, 148, March, 1982.
3. **Smukler,** H., Nager, M.C., and Tolmie, P.C.: Interproximal Tooth Morphology and Its Effect on Plaque Removal, *Quintessence Int.,* 20, 249, April, 1989.
4. **Kiger,** R.D., Nylund, K., and Feller, R.P.: A Comparison of Proximal Plaque Removal Using Floss and Interdental Brushes, *J. Clin. Periodontol.,* 18, 681, October, 1991.
5. **Lobene,** R.R., Soparkar, P.M., and Newman, M.B.: Use of Dental Floss. Effect on Plaque and Gingivitis, *Clin. Prev. Dent.,* 4, 5, January-February, 1982.
6. **Hill,** H.C., Levi, P.A., and Glickman, I.: The Effects of Waxed and Unwaxed Dental Floss on Interdental Plaque Accumulation and Interdental Gingival Health, *J. Periodontol.,* 44, 411, July, 1973.
7. **Lamberts,** D.M., Wunderlich, R.C., and Caffesse, R.G.: The Effect of Waxed and Unwaxed Dental Floss on Gingival Health. Part I. Plaque Removal and Gingival Response, *J. Periodontol.,* 53, 393, June, 1982.
8. **Wunderlich,** R.C., Lamberts, D.M., and Caffesse, R.G.: The Effect of Waxed and Unwaxed Dental Floss on Gingival Health. Part II. Crevicular Fluid Flow and Gingival Bleeding., *J. Periodontol.,* 53, 397, June, 1982.
9. **Beaumont,** R.H.: Patient Preference for Waxed or Unwaxed Dental Floss, *J. Periodontol.,* 61, 123, February, 1990.
10. **Finkelstein,** P. and Grossman, E.: The Effectiveness of Dental Floss in Reducing Gingival Inflammation, *J. Dent Res.,* 58, 1034, March, 1979.
11. **Abelson,** D.C., Parton, J.E., Maietti, G.M., and Cowherd, M.G.: Evaluation of Interproximal Cleaning by Two Types of Dental Floss, *Clin. Prev. Dent.,* 3, 19, July-August, 1981.

12. **Hanes,** P.J., O'Dell, N.L., Baker, M.R., Keagle, J.G., and Davis, H.C.: The Effect of Tensile Strength on Clinical Effectiveness and Patient Acceptance of Dental Floss, *J. Clin. Periodontol, 19,* 30, January, 1992.

13. **Graves,** R.C., Disney, J.A., and Stamm, J.W.: Comparative Effectiveness of Flossing and Brushing in Reducing Interproximal Bleeding, *J. Periodontol., 60,* 643, May, 1989.

14. **Killoy,** W.J., Chairman, Discussion Section II, Consensus Report: *Proceedings of the World Workshop in Clinical Periodontics.* American Academy of Periodontology, Princeton, N.J., 1989, pp. 11–15.

15. **Cianco,** S.G., Mather, M.L., Zambon, J.J., and Reynolds, H.S.: Effect of a Chemotherapeutic Agent Delivered by an Oral Irrigation Device on Plaque, Gingivitis, and Subgingival Microflora, *J. Periodontol., 60,* 310, June, 1989.

16. **Flemmig,** T.F., Newman, M.G., Doherty, F.M., Grossman, E., Meckel, A.H., and Bakdash, M.B.: Supragingival Irrigation with 0.06% Chlorhexidine in Naturally Occurring Gingivitis. I. 6-Month Clinical Observations, *J. Periodontol., 61,* 112, February, 1990.

17. **Brownstein,** C.N., Briggs, S.D., Schweitzer, K.L., Briner, W.W., and Kornman, K.S.: Irrigation with Chlorhexidine to Resolve Naturally Occurring Gingivitis., *J. Clin Periodontol., 17,* 588, September, 1990.

18. **Cobb,** C.M., Rodger., R.L., and Killoy, W.J.: Ultrastructural Examination of Human Periodontal Pockets Following the Use of an Oral Irrigation Device *In Vivo, J. Periodontol., 59,* 155, March, 1988.

19. **Newman,** M.G., Flemmig, R.F., Nachnani, S., Rodrigues, A., Calsina, G., Lee, Y.S., deCarmargo, P., Doherty, F.M., and Bakdash, B.: Irrigation with 0.06% Chlorhexidine in Naturally Occurring Gingivitis. II. 6-Month Microbiological Observations, *J. Periodontol., 61,* 427, July, 1990.

20. **Wunderlich,** R.C.: Subgingival Penetration of an Applied Solution, *Int. J. Periodontics Restorative Dent., 4,* 64, No. 5, 1984.

21. **Eakle,** W.S., Ford, C., and Boyd, R.L.: Depth of

Penetration in Periodontal Pickets with Oral Irrigation, *J. Clin. Periodontol., 13,* 39, January, 1986.

22. **Boyd,** R.L., Hollander, B.N., and Eakle, W.S.: Comparison of a Subgingivally Placed Cannula Oral Irrigator Tip with a Supragingivally Placed Standard Irrigator Tip, *J. Clin. Periodontol., 19,* 340, May, 1992.

23. **Braun,** R.E. and Ciancio, S.G.: Subgingival Delivery by an Oral Irrigation Device, *J. Periodontol., 63,* 469, May, 1992.

24. **Krust,** K.S., Drisko, C.L., Gross, K., Overman, P., and Tira, D.E.: The Effects of Subgingival Irrigation with Chlorhexidine and Stannous Fluoride. A Preliminary Investigation, *J. Dent. Hyg., 65,* 289, July-August, 1991.

25. **Walsh,** T.F., Glenwright, H.D., and Huyll, P.L.: Clinical Effects of Pulsed Oral Irrigation with 0.2% Chlorhexidine Digluconate in Patients with Adult Periodontitis, *J. Clin. Periodontol., 19,* 245, April, 1992.

26. **Mazza,** J.E., Newman, M.G., and Sims, T.N.: Clinical and Antimicrobial Effect of Stannous Fluoride on Periodontitis, *J. Clin. Periodontol., 8,* 203, June, 1981.

27. **Boyd,** R.L., Leggott, P., Quinn, R., Buchanan, S., Eakle, W., and Chambers, D.: Effect of Self-administered Daily Irrigation with 0.01% SnF2 on Periodontal Disease Activity, *J. Clin. Periodontol., 12,* 420, July, 1985.

28. **Schmid,** E., Kornman, K.S., and Tinanoff, N.: Changes of Subgingival Total Colony Forming Units and Black Pigmented Bacteroides After a Single Irrigation of Periodontal Pockets with 1.64% SnF2, *J. Periodontol., 56,* 330, June, 1985.

29. **Harper,** D.S., Gordon, J., Fine, J., and Hovliaris, C.: Effect of Subgingival Irrigation with an Antiseptic Mouthrinse on Periodontal Pocket Microflora, *J. Dent. Res., 70,* 324, Abstract No. 474, Special Issue, April, 1991.

30. **Southard,** G.L., Parson, L.G., Thomas, L.G., Woodall, I.R., and Jones, B.J.B.: Effect of Sanguinaria Extract on Development of Plaque and Gingivitis when Supragingivally Delivered as a Manual Rinse or Under Pressure in an Oral Irrigator, *J. Clin. Periodontol., 14,* 377, August, 1987.

31. **Parsons**, L.G., Thomas, L.G., Southard, G.L., Woodall, I.R., and Jones, B.J.B.: Effect of Sanguinaria Extract on Established Plaque and Gingivitis when Supragingivally Delivered as a Manual Rinse or Under Pressure in an Oral Irrigator, *J. Clin. Periodontol., 14,* 381, August, 1987.

32. **Phelps-Sandall**, B.A. and Oxfor, S.J.: Effectiveness of Oral Hygiene Techniques on Plaque and Gingivitis in Patients Placed in Intermaxillary Fixation, *Oral Surg. Oral Med. Oral Pathol., 56,* 487, November, 1983.

33. **Romans**, A.R. and App, G.R.: Bacteremia, a Result from Oral Irrigation in Subjects with Gingivitis, *J. Periodontol., 42,* 757, December, 1971.

34. **Felix**, J.E., Rosen, S., and App, G.R.: Detection of Bacteremia after the Use of an Oral Irrigation Device in Subjects with Periodontitis, *J. Periodontol., 42,* 785, December, 1971.

35. **Pitcher**, G.R., Newman, H.N., and Strahan, J.D.: Access to Subgingival Plaque by Disclosing Agents Using Mouthrinsing and Direct Irrigation, *J. Clin. Periodontol., 7,* 300, August, 1980.

36. **Scopp**, I.W. and Orvieto, L.D.: Gingival Degerming by Povidone-iodine Irrigation: Bacteremia Reduction in Extraction Procedures, *J. Am. Dent. Assoc., 83,* 1294, December, 1971.

37. **Veksler**, A.E., Kayrouz, G.A., and Newman, M.G.: Reduction of Salivary Bacteria by Preprocedural Rinses with Chlorhexidine 0.12%, *J. Periodontol., 62,* 649, November, 1991.

38. **Fine**, D.H., Mendieta, C., Barnett, M.L., Furgang, D., Meyers, R., Olshan, A., and Vincent, J.: Efficacy of Preprocedural Rinsing with an Antiseptic in Reducing Viable Bacteria in Dental Aerosols, *J. Periodontol., 63,* 821, October, 1992.

39. **Newbrun**, E.: Chemical and Mechanical Removal of Plaque, *Compendium, 6,* S110, Supplement No. 6, 1985.

40. **Volpe**, A.R.: Dentifrices and Mouth Rinses, in Stallard, R.E., ed.: *A Textbook of Preventive Dentistry,* 2nd ed. Philadelphia, W.B. Saunders Co., 1982, pp. 170–216.

41. **Ciancio**, S.G.: Nonsurgical Periodontal Treatment, in

Proceedings of the World Workshop in Clinical Periodontics. American Academy of Periodontology, Princeton N.J., 1989, pp. II–2.

42. **American Dental Association,** Council on Dental Therapeutics: *Accepted Dental Therapeutics,* 40th ed. Chicago, American Dental Association, 1984, pp. 322–323.

43. **Weitzman,** S.A., Weitberg, A.B., Stossel, T.P., Schwartz, J., and Shklar, G.: Effects of Hydrogen Peroxide on Oral Carcinogenesis in Hamsters, *J. Periodontol., 57,* 685, November, 1986.

44. **Rees,** T.D. and Orth, C.F.: Oral Ulcerations with Use of Hydrogen Peroxide, *J. Periodontol., 57,* 689, November, 1986.

45. **Mandel,** I.D.: Chemotherapeutic Agents for Controlling Plaque and Gingivitis, *J. Clin. Periodontol., 15,* 488, September, 1988.

46. **Loe,** H. and Schiott, C.R.: The Effect of Mouthrinses and Topical Applications of Chlorhexidine on the Development of Dental Plaque and Gingivitis in Man, *J. Periodontol. Res., 5,* 79, No. 2, 1970.

47. **Segreto,** V.A., Collins, E.M., Beiswanger, B.B., de la Rosa, M., Isaacs, R.L., Lang, N.P., Mallatt, M.E., and Meckel, A.H.: A Comparison of Mouthrinses Containing Two Concentrations of Chlorhexidine, *J. Periodontol. Res., 21,* 23, Supplement No. 2, 1986.

48. **Gisselsson,** H., Birkhed, D., and Bjorn, A.L.: Effect of Professional Flossing with Chlorhexidine Gel on Approximal Caries in 12- to 15-year-old Schoolchildren, *Caries Res., 22,* 187, May-June, 1988.

49. **Tilliss,** T.S.I.: A Closer Look at Tartar Control Dentifrices, *J. Dent. Hyg., 63,* 364, October, 1989.

DENTAL PROSTHESES

10

Care and maintenance of the oral cavity includes care of
any prosthetic device in the mouth. This chapter provides
information on the maintenance of these devices.

TABLE 10.1. Dental Prostheses

Appliance Type	Factors	Maintenance for Oral Health
Orthodontic: fixed, removable, space maintainers	Age: high gingivitis incidence in preteen and teenage years Poor oral hygiene habits Tooth position/access problems Hyperplasia caused by gingival irritation from wires, clasps, rubber bands, plaque, and debris	Customized plaque control instructions Orthodontic brushes Interdental aids Rubber tip, toothpick/holder, floss threaders, proximal brushes, single tuft brushes Fluoride application Dentifrice, brush-on gel, gel trays Oral irrigation (1) Appliance should be kept in water when not in use
Fixed partial dentures: natural teeth supported; implant supported	Should be compatible with (2) the teeth and surrounding periodontium All parts accessible for cleaning Does not interfere with cleaning of natural dentition Does not traumatize oral tissues	Toothbrushing instructions Oral irrigation Floss or yarn with threader Nonabrasive dentifrice with fluoride (Acidulated fluoride contraindicated for composite and porcelain restorations) (3) See Table 9.7

continued

Removable partial dentures	Bacterial plaque accumulates easier and in greater quantities	See Table 10.2, 10.3
	Purposes for cleaning	Power-assisted brush should not be used
Complete dentures, overdentures	Prevent oral tissue irritation (mechanical and chemical)	See Table 10.2, 10.3
	Infection control	
	Prevention of mouth odor	
	Maintain appearance	

TABLE 10.2. Patient Care of Removable Appliances

Rinsing	After every meal, if brushing is not possible, remove appliance and rinse separately from mouth
Brushing	Regular toothbrushes are not recommended; if patient prefers to use a toothbrush on the appliance, a separate brush should be used for the appliance only—not the one used for the natural dentition
	Power-assisted brushes should not be used for the appliance
	Clasp brush: cone-shaped cylinder brushes specifically for clasps
	Denture brush: for smooth surfaces and metal bars
	Caution should be used when cleaning appliances
	Too-firm grasping of the appliance may distort, bend, or fracture the clasps
	Lining the sink with a towel or face cloth or filling the sink partially with water helps prevent accidental breakage if dropped during cleaning
	Thorough cleansing of the appliance is needed to keep the natural teeth and dentition healthy
	Use a nonabrasive, nondiscoloring soap
Immersion	Cleaning and brushing of appliance should be done prior to immersion
	Appliance should be stored in plain water when not in use
	Chemical solutions can be used for cleansing appliances (see Table 10.3)
	Mechanical denture cleansers used with an immersion agent: ultrasonic, sonic, magnetic, and agitating cleansers are commercially available for home use

TABLE 10.3. Care of Complete Dentures (4-7)

Denture cleanser requirements (4)	Ease of patient use
	Reasonably priced
	Effective removal of organic and inorganic deposits without abrasion
	Bactericidal and fungicidal
	Nontoxic
	Harmless to partial or complete denture materials
Chemical solution cleaners (immersion)	Alkaline hypochlorite
	Example: household bleach
	Disadvantage: Odor, tarnish, surface pitting, bleaching effect on soft lining and fiber-containing materials
	Alkaline peroxide
	Example: commercial powders or tablets
	Disadvantage: does not remove heavy stains or calculus
	Dilute acids
	Example: 3–5% hydrochloric acid alone or with phosphoric acid; commercially prepared ultrasonic solutions (not recommended for home use); acetic acid (vinegar)
	Disadvantage: corrosion of metal parts

continued

TABLE 10.3. Care of Complete Dentures (4–7)

	Enzymes
	Incorporated into various immersion-type cleansers
	Disinfectants
	Use of EPA-registered products (8)
	Immersion in full-strength household bleach (sodium hypochlorite) for 5 min (9)
	(thoroughly rinse after 5 min because of bleaching properties)
Abrasive cleansers (brushing)	Denture pastes and powders, toothpastes and powders
	Example: various commercial products
	Disadvantage: can abrade plastic resin base and acrylic teeth
	Household agents
	Salt and bicarbonate of soda—mildly abrasive
	Hand soap—cleanses without much abrasion
	Scouring powders and other abrasives should not be used
Immersion	Rinse thoroughly before and after immersion
	Remove denture adhesive material (brush with light pressure)
	Use a container specific for denture cleansing with a fitted lid; empty and clean the container
	daily and mix fresh solution daily to prevent contamination and growth of
	microorganisms (10)

continued

Use warm water to mix the solution according to manufacturer's instructions

Immersion for commercial preparations is usually 10 to 15 min

Hypochlorite solution

1 tbsp (15 mL) sodium hypochlorite (household bleach)

2 tsp (8 mL) Calgone

4 oz (114 mL) water

Soak dentures for 10–15 min, overnight if there is stain or calculus formation and there are no metal parts that can be corroded

Brushing
See Table 10.2

Whatever type of brush is used, it should access all surfaces of the denture

Precautions

Brushing too vigorously with an abrasive on the impressions surface can alter the fit of the denture

Plastic resin can be abraded, and the roughened surface will collect more debris and calculus

Possible incomplete cleaning of difficult-access areas

Possible uneven pressure when brushing

Possible dropping and breaking when brushing (see Table 10.2)

Additional considerations
Appliances with plastic resin should be immersed in water or cleansing solution when not in mouth

continued

TABLE 10.3. Care of Complete Dentures (4–7)

	Regular professional maintenance should be arranged (not only if the denture accumulates deposits but also to check the appliance fit and oral tissues)
	Residual chemical agents may cause inflammatory or allergic reactions of the mucosa
	Phenolic agents can adversely affect plastic resin
	Temporary soft conditioning lining materials may not be compatible with commercial cleansers. Use cold water and a soft cloth to clean. Outer surfaces can be brushed.
Underlying mucosa	Rinsing
	Each time the denture is removed (warm water or mild salt solution)
	Cleaning
	Edentulous mucosa should be brushed at least once daily using a soft brush with round-ended filaments
	Massage
	Digital—thumb and index finger over the ridge, press and release stroke massage palate with ball of thumb
	Soft toothbrush—use sides of filaments with vibratory action in each area; care should be taken to place the brush and avoid excessive pressure to prevent trauma
	Power-assisted brush—use smooth, even strokes in each area
	Regular maintenance appointments—professional examination of denture and the oral tissues to ensure proper-fitting appliances and detect any oral problems, lesions

TABLE 10.4. Complete Denture-Patient Instruction

Item	Factors to Teach
Food selection	Check each day's diet to fulfill needs for a balanced diet
	Older patients: use foods to prevent diet-induced chronic diseases
	New denture wearers should
	Avoid foods that need incising
	Avoid raw vegetables, fibrous meats, and sticky foods until experience has been gained
	Cut food into small pieces
	Practiced denture wearer
	Select a variety of foods, but do not expect the same efficiency as with the natural teeth
Incision or biting	Use the canine and premolar area. Insert for biting at the angle of the mouth.
	Push back as the food is incised; do not pull or tear the food in a forward direction
Chewing	Take small portions
	Try to chew with some food on each side at the same time to stabilize the denture
	Be patient and practice
Salivary flow	Anticipate an increased flow of saliva when a new denture is worn
Speaking	Speak slowly and quietly
	Practice by reading aloud at home, preferably in front of a mirror
	Repeat and practice words that seem the most difficult

continued

TABLE 10.4. Complete Denture-Patient Instruction

Item	Factors to Teach
Sneezing, coughing, yawning	Anticipate loss of denture retention
	Cover mouth with hand and handkerchief
Denture hygiene	Thoroughly clean dentures twice each day
	Immerse dentures in chemical solution and brush for plaque removal; rinse thoroughly
	Complete denture care is described in Tables 10.2 and 10.3
Mucosa	Tissues need to rest each day; preferable to leave the dentures out while sleeping
	Brush and massage the mucosa to clean away plaque and debris and stimulate circulation
Storage of dentures	After careful cleaning to remove all bacterial plaque, store the dentures in water (or cleaning solution) in a covered container
	Place in a safe place inaccessible to children or house pets
	Change water or cleaning solution daily and wash the container
Over-the-counter products	Never attempt to alter the denture for relief of discomfort
	Do not buy and use self-reline materials, adhesives, or other additives without consulting the dentist.
	They may be harmful to the dentures and/or the oral tissues.
	Consult the dentist for advice about all denture problems

continued

Maintenance	Understand the importance of the dentist's examination of the denture fit, occlusion, and wear, and the condition of the oral mucosa
	First year: expect reline, rebase, or remake of dentures because bone remodeling is greatest during the first year
	Subsequent appointment: an examination each year for most patients, provided the denture hygiene is ideal. Other patients in the cancer-susceptible category need an examination every 3 months.

TABLE 10.5. Implant Maintenance

Basic criteria for implant assessment	Routine, frequent examinations
	No pain or discomfort reported by patient
	No mobility
	No bleeding or increased probing depths on gentle probing
	No bone loss or periimplant radiolucency on radiographs
	No clinical signs of periimplantitis
Maintenance appointments	Review bacterial plaque control and motivational techniques before implant procedures and after, at regularly spaced intervals, based on the patient's home care compliance and abilities to maintain oral health
	Routine review of health history, vital signs, intraoral/extraoral examination
	Selective radiographs (may use special film placement devices) (11, 12)
	Periodontal assessment
	Periimplant tissue—visual examination should show no inflammatory signs
	Probing—plastic probe; very gently
	Mobility determination
	Deposits
	Use of a disclosing agent for bacterial plaque
	Usually calculus is not extensive, hard, or firmly attached to implant abutments or protruding parts

continued

Review bacterial plaque control procedures

Instrumentation

Plastic or wood instruments especially designed for implant maintenance

Prevent damage to implant surfaces and superstructures—severe abrasion can result from the use of an ultrasonic scaler; airbrasives can alter the hydroxylapatite coating on the implant (13, 14)

Stain removal—not routinely included; if stain removal is indicated, use only a nonabrasive agent gently applied with a rubber cup

Professional subgingival irrigation—use after instrumentation when periimplantitis is present; 0.12% chlorhexidine solution is a safe procedure around implants (15)

REFERENCES

1. **Attarzadeh,** F.: Water Irrigating Devices for the Orthodontic Patient, *Int. J. Orthodon.,* 24, 15, Spring, 1986.

2. **Obreschkow,** C.: Oral Hygiene and Periodontal Considerations in Restorative Treatment with Prefabricated Attachments and Precision-milled Prosthetic Devices, *Int. J. Periodont. Restorative Dent.,* 4, 73, No. l, 1985.

3. **American Dental Association,** Council on Dental Materials, Instruments, and Equipment and Council on Dental Therapeutics: Status Report: Effect of Acidulated Fluoride on Porcelain and Composite Restorations, *J. Am. Dent. Assoc.,* 116, January, 1988.

4. **Abelson,** D.C.: Denture Plaque and Denture Cleansers: Review of the Literature, *Gerodontics,* 1, 202, October, 1985.

5. **Budtz-Jorgensen,** E.: Materials and Methods for Cleaning Dentures, *J. Prosthet. Dent.,* 42, 619, December, 1979.

6. **Gallagher,** J.B., Jr.: *Handbook for Complete Dentures,* Boston, Tufts University, School of Dental Medicine, 1981.

7. **American Dental Association,** Council on Dental Materials, Instruments, and Equipment: Denture Cleansers, *J. Am. Dent. Assoc.,* 106, 77, January, 1983.

8. **Cottone,** J.A., Terezhalmy, G.T., and Molinari, J.A.: *Practical Infection Control in Dentistry.* Philadelphia, Lea & Febiger, 1991, p. 190.

9. **Rudd,** R.W., Senia, E.S., McCleskey, F.K., and Adams, E.D.: Sterilization of Complete Dentures with Sodium Hypochlorite, *J. Prosthet. Dent.,* 51, 318, March, 1984.

10. **DePaola,** L.G. and Minah, G.E.: Isolation of Pathogenic Microorganisms from Dentures and Denture-soaking Containers of Myelosuppressed Cancer Patients, *J. Prosthet. Dent.,* 49, 20, January, 1983.

11. **Cox,** J.F. and Pharoah, M.: An Alternative Holder for Radiographic Evaluation of Tissue-integrated Prostheses, *J. Prosthet. Dent.,* 56, 338, September, 1986.

12. **Meijer,** H.J.A., Steen, W.H.W., and Posman, F.:

Standardized Radiographs of the Alveolar Crest Around Implants in the Mandible, *J. Prosthet. Dent., 68,* 318, August, 1992.

13. **Thomson-Neal,** D., Evans, G.H., and Meffert, R.M.: Effects of Various Prophylactic Treatments on Titanium, Sapphire, and Hydroxyapatite-coated Implants: An SEM Study, *Int. J. Periodont. Restorative Dent., 9,* 301, No. 4, 1989.

14. **Rapley,** J.W., Swan, R.H., Hallmon, W.W., and Mills, M.P.: The Surface Characteristics Produced by Various Oral Hygiene Instruments and Materials on Titanium Implant Abutments, *Int. J. Oral Maxillofac. Implants, 5,* 17, Number 1, 1990.

15. **Lavigne,** S.E., Krust, K.S., Gross, K.B., Killoy, W.J., and Theisen, F.: Effects of Subgingival Chlorhexidine Irrigation on Periimplant Tissues, *J. Dent. Res., 71,* 300, AADR Abstract No. 1553, Special Issue, 1992.

DIET AND ORAL HEALTH

11

TABLE 11.1. Diet/Nutrition and Oral Relationships

	Factors
Periodontal tissues (1–3)	*Nutritional deficiencies*
	Nutritionally balanced diet is necessary for healthy periodontal tissue
	Nutritional deficiency does not specifically cause periodontal infections
	Nutritional deficiencies (e.g., protein, ascorbic acid, vitamin B complex) may modify resistance of gingival tissues to plaque microorganisms, causing acceleration and increased intensity of inflammatory conditions
	Periodontal infection effects can alter tissue capacity to utilize nutrients and thereby interfere with healing and repair
	Consistency of food
	Soft, sticky foods encourage accumulation of food and debris, nourishing microorganisms and causing increased bacterial plaque
	Firm, fibrous food may stimulate and improve circulation of the tissues
	Uncooked fruits and vegetables tend to clear away loose debris and give a sensation of cleanliness—they do not remove plaque from the cervical area (4)
	Dietary analysis
	Used as a guide for patient nutritional counseling
	Studies the food habits and patterns of a patient's diet to aid both patient and clinician to focus on modifying behaviors for improving and maintaining oral health

continued

Skin and mucous membrane	*Nutritional deficiencies*
	Severe nutritional deficiencies are rare
	Produce symptoms of mixed clinical entities, infrequently of severe acute disease
	Oral symptoms indicating possible deficiency may in fact indicate multiple nutritional deficiencies
	Effects of deficiency are chronic and of a slow, gradual course
	Clinical manifestations are influenced by trauma, local irritation, or systemic factors that lower tissue resistance
	Oral lesions
	Stomatitis, glossitis, cheilitis, localized ulcerations, areas of atrophic change may indicate underlying nutritional deficiency (5, 6)
	Definitive diagnosis is not really possible, even with histories, diet analysis, and laboratory tests
	Nutrients associated with the health of oral mucosa: iron, ascorbic acid, and various B vitamins
	Extraoral lesions
	Lesions of the skin can indicate deficiencies of nutritional elements (7) (e.g., anorexia nervosa)
Dental caries (8, 9)	Fluoride deficiency during tooth formation years increases dental caries incidence with cariogenic diet exposure
	Dental caries is the result of excess cariogenic food intake rather than a deficiency disease
	Dietary analysis and counseling should be provided for caries-prone individuals and especially those with eating disorders

TABLE 11.2. Dietary Analysis

	Components
Objectives	Aid the individual in objectively recognizing personal dietary habits
	Obtain an overview of food types, preferences, and quantities
	Study food habits: frequency, regularity, and order of food intake
	Obtain baseline data on individual cariogenic food intake for future comparison
	Determine overall consistency of diet, fibrous food intake
	Compare cariogenic exposure frequency with clinical and radiographic findings
	Provide basis for personalized dietary recommendations for oral health
Types	Qualitative: considers the general food groups essential or detrimental to adequate oral health
	Quantitative: done by a nutritionist; provides specific therapeutic diets for physiologic and pathologic conditions (under direction of a physician); does precise mathematic calculations of the chemical constituents of the diet
Food diary	Can be either an oral or written interview for food intake over the last 24 hours or diary kept by the patient for a week or 5 days
	Should be a simple-to-use form (see Figs. 11.1–11.3)

continued

	Patient should indicate
	Portion sizes
	Components of mixed dishes (casseroles, salads, etc.)
	Identify where meals were consumed (home, restaurant, as a guest)
	Vitamins, prescribed medication, water intake
	Is this a normal food intake week?
	Appetite
	Allergies
	Food preferences
	Special diets
	Additions to food: butter, condiments, cream, sauces, etc.
	Types of foods: canned, frozen, fresh, raw, fried, baked, etc.
Summary and analysis	See Fig. 11.3
	Analyze the overall content of the diet
	Note cariogenic food intake and consistency of food intake (frequency, types, times)
	Review dietary analysis with the patient
	Corroborate findings with clinical findings

Food Diary

Example of How Foods Should Be Listed

Breakfast 7:30 A.M.	
Oatmeal	1 cup
with milk	1/2 cup
with brown sugar	2 teasp.
Milk	1-8 oz. glass
Toast - whole wheat bread	2 slices
with butter	generous
Egg - boiled	1
with butter	1/2 teasp.
Prunes - stewed -- with syrup	6 large
Finished 7:45 A.M.	

Between Breakfast and Lunch 10:00 A.M.	
Coffee	1 cup
with cream	1 teasp.
with sugar	2 teasp.
Water (around 11:00)	1 paper cup

Food eaten at lunch and dinner should be listed just as carefully as the breakfast shown above. If sandwiches are eaten, list the contents of the filling, such as egg, beef, lettuce, dressing.

Please show the approximate amounts of every kind of food that you ate. Do not mention any food that is served unless you ate it.

Please record all candy, cough drops, milk shakes, soft drinks, ice cream cones, popcorn, fruit (kinds), or cookies that you ate between meals. Also record vitamin concentrates or medicaments related to diet.

FIGURE 11.1. Food diary cover. On the cover are examples of the way to list foods and indicate household measurements. The blank area on the right is for a summary prepared by the patient during the counseling appointment. Single pages for each day's diary are shown in Figure 11.2.

Name_____

Age_____ Week of_____

Summary

FIGURE 11.1.—*continued.*

Name _____

Day _____ Date _____

The Day's Food Diary

	Amount		Amount
Breakfast_____A.M. Finished_____A.M.		Between Lunch and Dinner _____P.M.	
		Dinner_____P.M.	
Between Breakfast and Lunch _____A.M.			
Lunch_____A.M. Finished_____P.M.		Finished_____P.M.	
		Between Dinner and Retiring_____P.M.	

FIGURE 11.2. Food diary. Example of a form for the patient to use to record the daily diet. A booklet of seven forms can be assembled for a week-long record. The cover for the booklet is shown in Figure 11.1.

Dietary Analysis

Name _____

Age _____ Date _____

FOOD GROUPS		Day 1	2	3	4	5	6	7	Daily average	Recommended Daily Amounts	Adequate	Inadequate
MILK GROUP	Milk									Child Adol. Adult 2–4 4+more 2+more		
	Milk Products											
MEAT GROUP	Meat, Fish Poultry									2–3 servings		
	Eggs, Dry Beans											
VEGETABLE GROUP	Yellow and Dark Green									3–5 servings		
	Other											
	Potato											
FRUIT GROUP	Raw—Citrus									2–4 servings		
	Other											
	Cooked											
BREAD AND CEREALS GROUP										6–11 servings		

FIGURE 11.3. See legend on page 250.

SWEETS											Total	NOTES AND RECOMMENDATIONS
Liquid	With Meal											
	End of Meal											
	Between Meal											
Soft (Sticky Retentive)	With Meal											
	End of Meal											
	Between Meal											
Hard (Sucked-Long-Lasting)	End of Meal											
	Between Meal											

FIGURE 11.3. Dietary analysis recording sheet. From the food diary kept by the patient (Figures 11.1 and 11.2), each item is entered as a check in the space beside the appropriate food group. These are totaled, averaged, and compared with the recommended daily amounts on the right. The lower section provides space to categorize and count cariogenic foods.

TABLE 11.3. Dietary Counseling

Component	Factors
Objectives	Aid the patient in recognizing his/her individual oral health problems and the relationship to current habits
	Explanation of specific changes needed to improve general and oral health
	Dental caries control: substitution of cariogenic foods with healthier food choices, snacking patterns
Planning	Patient attitude: willingness and ability to cooperate
	Identify problems that may interfere with the individual's acceptance of behavior modification recommendations
	Degree of difficulty in change
	Dissatisfaction without usual food
	Lack of appreciation for need to change
	Misconceptions about sugar/energy
	Degree of emphasis—dental disease is not fatal; minor deviations from recommended changes will not produce drastic results
	Social prejudices
	Cultural patterns
	Financial considerations
	Emotional problems
	Parental attitudes

continued

TABLE 11.3. Dietary Counseling

Component	Factors
	Teaching aids
	Patient's record (food diary, radiographs, chartings)
	Visual aids: diagrams, models, charts
	Pamphlets specific to the individual's needs
	Outline of plan with specific recommendations, suggestions
	List of suggested food substitutions, snacks
Setting for counseling	Area should be free from interruptions, background distractions
	Provide comfortable seating
	For children, encourage both parents to be present if possible
	Person who plans and prepares the meals should be present
	Factors related to the treatment plan should be reviewed
Conference considerations	Be prepared and on time
	Keep visual aids simple and few
	Create a congenial atmosphere; use spontaneity during the presentation
	Encourage only the principals to be present during the conference to avoid distractions
	Include everyone present in the discussion
	Use a natural tone of voice
	Adequately discuss all questions
	Avoid notetaking during the session

continued

Presentation	Review purpose of the meeting
	Clarify and be specific about cariogenic foods
	Discuss the relationship between sucrose and dental caries
	Discuss the relationship between frequency of sucrose intake and dental caries
	Discuss the types of foods that are retained in the mouth and can cause dental caries
	Work with the patient in identifying the problems of the current diet; help with food selection substitutes
	Individualize recommendations as much as possible to encourage compliance with habit changes
	Immediate evaluation: the individual's interest and cooperation
Evaluation	3-month follow-up
	5–7-day food diary for analysis
	Review plaque control and make necessary suggestions
	Recommend adherence to restricted diet when indicated
	6-month follow-up
	Examination and clinical procedures
	Comparison of dental caries incidence with previous history
	Dietary recommendations in accord with new assessment
	Overall evaluation
	Consistent reduction in dental caries rate over the years
	Continued maintenance of oral health indicates that learning and behavior modification have occurred

REFERENCES

1. **Carranza,** F.A.: *Glickman's Clinical Periodontology,* 7th ed. Philadelphia, W.B. Saunders Co., 1990, pp. 139–140, 157, 431–443.
2. **Genco,** R.J., Goldman, H.M., and Cohen, D.W., eds.: *Contemporary Periodontics,* St. Louis, The C.V. Mosby Co., 1990, pp. 264–266.
3. **Nizel,** A.E. and Papas, A.: *Nutrition in Clinical Dentistry,* 3rd ed. Philadelphia, W.B. Saunders Co., 1989, pp. 309–338.
4. **Arnim,** S.S.: The Use of Disclosing Agents for Measuring Tooth Cleanliness, *J. Periodontol., 34,* 227, May, 1963.
5. **McCarthy,** P.L. and Shklar, G.: *Diseases of the Oral Mucosa,* 2nd ed. Philadelphia, Lea & Febiger, 1980, pp. 376–388.
6. **Robinson,** H.B.G. and Miller, A.S.: *Color Atlas of Oral Pathology,* 5th ed. Philadelphia, J.B. Lippincott Co., 1990, p. 141.
7. **Miller,** S.J.: Nutritional Deficiency and the Skin, *J. Am. Acad. Dermatol., 21,* 1, July, 1989.
8. **Newbrun,** E.: *Cariology,* 3rd ed. Chicago, Quintessence, 1989, pp. 99–175.
9. **Harris,** N.O. and Madse, K.O.: Nutrition and Plaque Diseases, in Harris, N.O. and Christen, A.G., eds.: *Primary Preventive Dentistry,* 3rd ed. Norwalk, CT, Appleton & Lange, 1991, pp. 347–371.

PREVENTIVE SUPPLEMENTS

12

Fluorides and sealants are covered in this chapter. It should be noted that both are important parts of a total preventive program and should be used in combination with one another as are toothbrushing, flossing, diet, and other preventive measures.

TABLE 12.1. Fluoride Metabolism (1)

Intake absorption	Fluoridated water, supplements, food, and beverages prepared with fluoridated water
	Stomach and small intestine
	Rapidly absorbed
	5% of unabsorbed fluoride is excreted in feces
	Blood stream
	Maximum blood levels within one hour of intake
	Level fluctuates with intake
	Normal plasma level is low (saliva levels lower)
Distribution and retention	Children: Approximately one half of intake deposited in calcifying bones and teeth
	Adults
	Normal bone exchange and maintenance with continuous daily use of fluoridated water
	Accumulates in the skeleton throughout life
	Storage
	95% stored in bone
	Storage amounts vary with intake, time of exposure, age, and development phase of the individual
	Teeth store small amounts (highest levels on tooth surface)

continued

Excretion	Soft tissues
	Some tissues have higher levels than plasma
	Low concentration in human milk
	Most excreted through the kidneys
	Small amount excreted by sweat gland
	5% excreted in feces
	Urine fluoride concentration within 2 hours of intake

TABLE 12.2. Fluoride and Tooth Development

Preeruptive: mineralization stage	Fluoride deposited during the formation of enamel
	Fluoride incorporated as fluorapatite during mineralization
	Fluoride availability to developing teeth via the blood stream to tissues surrounding the tooth buds
	Fluoride ingestion from water, foods, supplements
	Excess fluoride may inhibit ameloblast activity, forming defective enamel matrix and producing dental fluorosis
	Incorporation of fluoride into developing enamel produces fluorapatite that is less soluble than hydroxyapatite and improves mineralized tooth tissue quality
Preeruptive: maturation stage	Fluoride deposition in the surface of enamel continues after completion of mineralization and before tooth eruption
	More fluoride is acquired by the outer surface during this period; fluoride concentration decreases inward from the enamel surface to dentino-enamel junction (2)
	Fluoride introduction within 2 years prior to eruption is beneficial
	Fluoride level is greater in dentin than in enamel (highest concentration is at the pulpal surface) (3)

continued

Posteruptive

Fluoride uptake is rapid during the first years after eruption (especially from supplements)

Continued exposure to fluoride (drinking water, dentifrice, mouthrinses, other surface exposures) inhibits demineralization and facilitates remineralization throughout the life of the teeth

High level of fluoride in cementum; increases with age (3)

Aid maturation of enamel surface

Reduce enamel solubility

Increase enamel resistance

Alter the action of plaque bacteria

TABLE 12.3. Fluoridation Effects and Benefits

	Factors
Appearance	Dental fluorosis with higher than optimum levels (varies from white flecks or bands to brown, mottled enamel) (4); see Table 12.4
Dental caries	Permanent teeth Continuous use of fluoridated water from birth can result in 40–65% fewer carious lesions Anterior teeth (particularly maxillary) receive more protection Benefits teeth erupted prior to fluoride exposure (5–7) Caries rate is slowed (8) Primary teeth Caries incidence reduced up to 50% in primary teeth with fluoridation from birth (5, 9) Root caries Incidence is approximately 50% less in lifelong residents of a fluoridated community (10, 11)
Prenatal	Can pass through the placental barrier and become incorporated in the fetal calcifying tissues Fluoride ingested *after* birth has greater influence on primary teeth
Tooth loss	Primary and permanent tooth loss is greater in teeth without fluoride (9)
Malocclusion	Fewer extractions (especially premature loss of primary molars); lower incidence of malocclusion from local causes (12)

continued

Adulthood	Lifelong residence in fluoridated areas gives significantly lower caries incidence (13)
	Edentulous statistics are much lower in individuals with lifelong fluoridation (14)
Bone	Important to maintenance of normal bone
	Improves calcium metabolism
	Fewer bone fractures
Periodontal disease	Indirect favorable effects
	May have effect on bone resorption, resistance to local factors
	Reduction of tooth loss, dental caries, and malocclusion affect periodontal factors
Defluoridation	System used in areas with excessive fluoride in the water supply (14)
	Significant reduction in objectionable dental fluorosis (15, 16)
Cost	After installation of system, can be as low as 15 cents per person per year (17)
	Reduces the total cost of restorative dentistry and time lost from work and school by millions of dollars per year

TABLE 12.4.   Descriptive Criteria and Scoring System for the Tooth Surface Index of Fluorosis (TSIF)

Numerical Score	Descriptive Criteria
0	Enamel shows no evidence of fluorosis.
1	Enamel shows definite evidence of fluorosis, namely areas with parchment-white color that total less than one-third of the visible enamel surface. This category includes fluorosis confined only to incisal edges of anterior teeth and cusp tips of posterior teeth ("snowcapping").
2	Parchment-white fluorosis totals at least one-third of the visible surface, but less than two-thirds.
3	Parchment-white fluorosis totals at least two-thirds of the visible surface.
4	Enamel shows staining in conjunction with any of the preceding levels of fluorosis. Staining is defined as an area of definite discoloration that may range from light to very dark brown.
5	Discrete pitting of the enamel exists, unaccompanied by evidence of staining of intact enamel. A pit is defined as a definite physical defect in the enamel surface with a rough floor that is surrounded by a wall of intact enamel. The pitted area is usually stained or differs in color from the surrounding enamel.
6	Both discrete pitting and staining of the intact enamel exist.
7	Confluent pitting of the enamel surface exists. Large areas of enamel may be missing, and the anatomy of the tooth may be altered. Dark-brown stain is usually present.

Reprinted with permission from Horowitz, H.S., Driscoll, W.S., Meyers, R.J., Heifetz, S.B., and Kingman, A.K.: A New Method for Assessing the Prevalence of Dental Fluorosis—the Tooth Surface Index of Fluorosis. *J. Am. Dent. Assoc., 109*, 37, July, 1984.

TABLE 12.5. Dietary Fluoride

Types	Factors
Foods	Do not contain enough for caries prevention
	Tea and fish have larger amounts than meat, eggs, vegetables, cereals, fruits
Salt	Fluoridated salt reduces dental caries incidence but is not comparable to fluoridated water
Supplements	Determine need for supplements (see Table 12.6)
	Limit amount of prescriptions to 264 mg of sodium (below toxic or lethal doses)
	Need to adjust amount/dose for nonfluoridated or partially fluoridated water supplies (18)
	Breast-fed infants
	If totally breast-fed after 6 months, need daily supplement
	In fluoridated areas, if receiving other sources of liquid with fluoride, no supplement is needed
	Vitamins with fluoride factors
	Difficult to adjust the prescribed fluoride to amount already received in water supply
	Contains a fixed amount of fluoride
	No evidence that vitamins enhance the effect of fluoride
	Expense of vitamins is not needed or prescribed

TABLE 12.6. Use of Fluoride Supplements

Criteria	For individuals using a private water supply without natural fluoride or one that is not practical to fluoridate
	When water fluoride level is less than optimum
	For those in communities with nonfluoridated water supplies
	For children too old to receive the full benefits from fluoridation at the start of a fluoridation program (fluoride applications and other methods)
	Fluoride dentifrices as a supplement to fluoridation
Determination of need	Review patient history to make sure other fluoride supplements are not being used
	Refer to list of fluoridated water supply areas (available from state or local health departments)
	Request water analysis when private water source fluoride level has not been determined

TABLE 12.7. Fluoride Supplements Dosage Schedule in mg F/Day[a]

Age of Child (Years)	Water Fluoride Concentration (ppm)		
	Less Than 0.3	Between 0.3–0.6	Greater Than 0.6
Birth–6 mos	0	0	0
6 mos–3 yrs	0.25 mg	0[b]	0[b]
3–6 yrs	0.50 mg	0.25 mg	0
6–16 yrs	1.0 mg	0.50 mg	0

Recommendations from the American Dental Association, Chicago, IL

[a] 2.2 mg sodium fluoride provide 1 mg fluoride ions.

[b] Infants receiving their total diet from breast-feeding need a 0.25-mg supplement.

TABLE 12.8. Comparison of Topical Fluoride Agents for Professional Application

	NaF	APF	SnF$_2$
Concentration	Solution 2%	Gel, foam, or solution 1.23%	Solution 8%
Fluoride ion %	0.91%	1.23%	1.95%
ppm fluoride	9,040 ppm	12,300 ppm	19,360 ppm
Mg F/mL	9.04	12.0	19.36
Efficacy	29%	28%	32%
Application frequency	4/year at ages 3, 7, 10, 13	1 or 2/year	1 or 2/year
Taste	Bland	Bitter without flavoring	Astringent
Tooth discoloration	None	None	Brown
Gingival reaction	None	None	Occasional

Modified from Ripa, L.W.: Professionally (Operator) Applied Topical Fluoride Therapy: A Critique, *Int. Dent. J., 31*, 105, June, 1981.

TABLE 12.9. Procedures to Reduce Fluoride Ingestion During Topical Gel-Tray Application

Patient	Seat upright
	Instruct not to swallow
	Tilt head forward with trays; tilt away from side with cotton-roll holder
Trays	Custom-made or appropriate size with absorptive liners; post-dam; border rim
	Use minimum amount of gel; 2 mL per tray, less for small tray; no more than total of 5 mL for large trays
Isolation	Use saliva ejector with maximum efficiency suction
	Cotton-roll holder technique: position for security, stability; place saliva absorber in cheek
Attention	Do not leave patient unattended
Timing	Use a timer; do not estimate
Completion	Tilt head forward for removal of tray or cotton-roll holder
	Request patient to expectorate for several minutes; do not allow swallowing
	Wipe excess gel from teeth with gauze sponge
	Use high-power suction to draw out saliva and gel
	Instruct patient not to rinse, eat, drink, or brush teeth for at least 30 minutes

Recommendations based on Oral Health Policies for Children: Protocol for Fluoride Therapy, American Academy of Pediatric Dentistry, 211 E. Chicago Avenue, Chicago, IL 60611.

TABLE 12.10. Self-Applied Fluorides

Method	Indications for Use	Precautions
Mouth tray (19) (custom or disposable)	Rampant enamel or root caries Xerostomia Radiation therapy Caries prevention under an overdenture Root surface hypersensitivity	Do not use acidulated preparations on porcelain (20), titanium restorations Do not swallow during procedure Expectorate several times after tray removal
Mouthrinses (low-potency/high frequency, high-potency/low frequency, oral rinse supplements) (21)	General prevention of dental caries High-risk preteen and adolescent years Individuals with demineralization areas Root exposure Moderate to rampant dental caries Individuals with plaque-retentive appliances Xerostomia Root surface hypersensitivity	Not for use by children under the age of 6 years or individuals unable to rinse and expectorate Low-potency products can be purchased OTC, (over-the-counter); all others are by prescription Commercial preparations containing alcohol should not be used by children or recovering alcoholic individuals *continued*

Dentifrices	Dental caries prevention Caries-risk individuals Desensitization	ADA-approved dentifrice ensures clinical and laboratory efficacy Children should not use more than a small pea-sized amount on brush Children should not swallow dentifrice Container should be kept out of the reach of children
Brush-on gel	Adjunct to daily fluoride dentifrice use Supplement to professional applications Regular use helps control demineralization around orthodontic appliances (24) Provides protection against postirradiation caries in conjunction with other fluoride applications (25)	Limited and conflicting research of efficacy (22, 23) Toothbrushing and flossing precede application (gel is not used as a dentifrice) APF gels not for use on porcelain or composite (20)

TABLE 12.11. Fluoride Safety

	Factors
Fluoride management	Use and recommend only approved fluoride preparations (FDA and ADA)
	Use only researched and recommended amounts and methods
	Know potential toxicity of products used
	Be prepared to treat emergencies in case of accidental toxic responses
	Instruct patient in proper use and care of fluoride products
	Prescription of less than toxic or lethal doses
	Large quantities not stored in home
	Emphasize parental supervision of brushing, fluoride administration
	Child-proof containers, stored out of reach of children and others unable to understand hazards
Acute toxicity	Rapid intake of excess dose over a short time
	Acute fluoride poisoning is rare (26)
	Certainly lethal dose (CLD) (27)—amount of drug likely to cause death if not intercepted by antidotal therapy (see Table 12.12)
	Safely tolerated dose (STD)—one fourth of the CLD
	Children 12 years old and under: 1 g (1000 mg) may be fatal
	½ g (500 mg) exceed the STD for all ages
	500 mg lethal to children under 6 years of age (27)

continued

Signs and symptoms of acute toxic dose
Symptoms begin within 30 minutes of ingestion and may persist up to 24 hours
Nausea, vomiting, diarrhea
Abdominal pain
Increased salivation, thirst
Symptoms of hypocalcemia
Hyperreflexia, convulsions, paresthesias
Cardiovascular and respiratory depression (may lead to death within a few hours if not treated)
Emergency treatment
Induce vomiting: digital stimulation or Ipecac syrup
Have second person call emergency service
Administer fluoride binding liquid when patient is not vomiting (milk, lime water (CaOH2 solution 0.15%))
Support respiration, circulation

continued

TABLE 12.11. Fluoride Safety

	Factors
	Emergency room therapy
	Calcium gluconate for muscle tremors or tetany
	Gastric lavage
	Cardiac monitoring
	Endotracheal intubation
	Blood monitoring: calcium, magnesium, potassium, pH
	IV for restoration of blood volume, calcium
Chronic toxicity	Skeletal fluorosis—isolated instances of osteosclerosis after 20 or more years' use of 10–25 ppm fluoridated water or industrial exposure (26)
	Dental fluorosis—ingestion of excess fluoride during crown development years (birth until 8 or 9 years of age)
	Mild fluorosis—no esthetic or health problem; inadvertent ingestion of excess fluoride during topical procedures (self-applied or professional); see Table 12.12, Fig. 12.1 (27–29)

TABLE 12.12. Lethal and Safe Doses of Fluoride

A. Lethal and Safe Dosages of Fluoride for a 70-kg Adult

Certainly Lethal Dose (CLD)

5–10 g NaF

or

32–64 mg F/kg

Safely Tolerated Dose (STD) = ¼ CLD

1.25–2.5 g NaF

or

8–16 mg F/kg

B. CLDs and STDs of Fluoride for Selected Ages

Age (years)	Weight (lbs)	CLD (mg)	STD (mg)
2	22	320	80
4	29	422	106
6	37	538	135
8	45	655	164
10	53	771	193
12	64	931	233
14	83	1,206	301
16	92	1,338	334
18	95	1,382	346

Reprinted with permission from Heifetz, S.B. and Horowitz, H.S.: The Amounts of Fluoride in Current Fluoride Therapies: Safety Considerations for Children, *ASDC J. Dent. Child., 51,* 257, July-August, 1984.

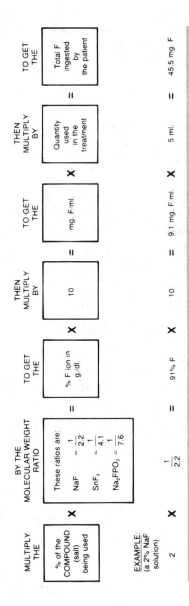

FIGURE 12.1. Fluoride calculation. The flowchart shows the steps in the calculation of the amount of fluoride in a compound used in treatment. The example shows that 5 mL of a 2% solution of NaF contains 45.5 mgF, an amount slightly greater than half of the safely tolerated dose (STD) for a 2-year old child (Table 12.12). (Reprinted with permission from Heifetz, S.B. and Horowitz, H.S.: The Amounts of Fluoride in Current Fluoride Therapies: Safety Considerations for Children, *ASDC J. Dent. Child.*, 51, 257, July-August, 1984.)

TABLE 12.13. Sealants

	Factors
Definition and action	Organic polymer that bonds to the enamel surface, mainly by mechanical retention
	Physical barrier to prevent bacteria and other materials from penetrating within a pit or fissure
Types	Filled, unfilled, fluoride-releasing filled
	Chemical cured (autopolymerization or visible light-cured (photopolymerization))
Tooth selection	Primary and permanent teeth that have pits and fissures including buccal pits, palatal pits, cigulum pits
	Deep, narrow pits and fissures
	Application as soon as possible after eruption
	Previous history of dental caries
	Not indicated when proximal caries in the same tooth require restoration
	Incipient pit and fissure caries are arrested by sealant placement (30–32)
	Age as a factor: caries-free teeth may benefit from sealant placement (teen years, pregnancy, change of habits)
Retention	Preparation of tooth surface can be accomplished by acid etch alone, bristle brush and water (33–35), or traditional rubber cup or bristle brush with plain pumice
	Retention should be tested with explorer immediately after placement
	Adjust occlusion if needed (unfilled sealants may wear down readily; filled sealants are more resistant because of the viscosity and flow) (36, 37)

continued

TABLE 12.13. Sealants

	Factors
	Sealant in pits and fissures and microspaces of enamel remain and provide protection even though surface sealant may be lost (38)
	Improper technique is a major cause of early sealant loss
	Any contamination of the etched enamel prior to application of sealant decreases the effectiveness of the sealant
	Sealants should be examined at each maintenance appointment
Replacement	Same tooth preparation as initial placement
	Retained sealant areas do not need removal in order to replace lost sealant areas
	Re-etching is necessary with each replacement
Topical fluoride application	Advised for promotion of remineralization of surfaces etched but not covered with sealant

REFERENCES

1. **Murray,** J.J., Rugg-Gunn, A.J., and Jenkins, G.N.: *Fluorides in Caries Prevention,* 3rd ed. Oxford, Wright, Butterworth-Heinemann, 1991, pp. 262–271.

2. **Brudevold,** F., Gardner, D.E., and Smith, F.A.: The Distribution of Fluoride in Human Enamel, *J. Dent. Res., 35,* 420, June, 1956.

3. **Ekstrand,** J., Fejerskov, O., and Silverstone, L.M., eds.: *Fluoride in Dentistry.* Copenhagen, Munksgaard, 1988, pp. 44–50.

4. **Dean,** H.T., Arnold, F.A., Jr., and Elvove, E.: Domestic Water and Dental Caries. V. Additional Studies of the Relation of Fluoride Domestic Waters to Dental Caries Experience in 4424 White Children, Aged 12 to 14 Years, of 13 Cities in 4 States, *Public Health Rep., 57,* 1155, August, 7, 1942.

5. **Arnold,** F.A., Dean, H.T., Jay, P., and Knutson, J.W.: Effect of Fluoridated Public Water Supplies on Dental Caries Prevalence. Tenth Year of the Grand Rapids Muskegon Study, *Public Health Rep., 71,* 652, July, 1956.

6. **Hayes,** R.L., Littleton, N.W., and White, C.L.: Posteruptive Effects of Fluoridation on First Permanent Molars of Children in Grand Rapids, Michigan, *Am. J. Public Health, 47,* 192, February, 1957.

7. **Russell,** A.L. and Hamilton, P.M.: Dental Caries in Permanent First Molars After Eight Years of Fluoridation, *Arch. Oral Biol., 6,* 50, July, 1961.

8. **Backer Dirks,** O., Houwink, B., and Kwant, G.W.: Some Special Features of the Caries Preventive Effect of Water Fluoridation, *Arch. Oral Biol., 4,* 187, August, 1961.

9. **Ast,** D.B. and Fitzgerald, B.: Effectiveness of Water Fluoridation, *J. Am. Dent. Assoc., 65,* 581, November, 1962.

10. **Burt,** B.A., Ismail, A.I., and Eklund, S.A.: Root Caries in an Optimally Fluoridated and a High Fluoride Community, *J. Dent. Res., 65,* 1154, September, 1986.

11. **Stamm,** J.W., Banting, D.W., and Imrey, P.B.: Adult Root Caries Survey of Two Similar Communities with Contrasting Natural Water Fluoride Levels, *J. Am. Dent. Assoc., 120,* 143, February, 1990.

12. **Salzmann,** J.A.: The Effects of Fluoride in the Prevalence of Malocclusion, *J. Am. Coll. Dent., 35,* 82, January, 1968.

13. **Russell,** A.L. and Elvove, E.: Domestic Water and Dental Caries. VII. A Study of the Fluoride-Dental Caries Relationship in an Adult Population, *Public Health Rep., 66,* 1389, October 26, 1951.

14. **Englander,** H.R. and Wallace, D.A.: Effects of Naturally Fluoridated Water on Dental Caries in Adults, *Public Health Rep., 77,* 887, October, 1962.

15. **Murray,** J.J., Rugg-Gunn, A.J., and Jenkins, G.N.: *Fluorides in Caries Prevention,* 3rd ed. Oxford, Wright, Butterworth-Heinemann, 1991, pp. 94–99.

16. **Horowitz,** H.S., Maier, F.J., and Law, F.E.: Partial Defluoridation of a Water Supply on Dental Fluorosis—Final Result in Bartlett, Texas, after 17 Years, *Am. J. Public Health Rep., 82,* 965, November, 1967.

17. **Ripa,** L.W.: A Half-century of Community Water Fluoridation in the United States: Review and Commentary, *J. Public Health Dent., 53,* 17, Winter, 1993.

18. **American Dental Association,** Council on Dental Therapeutics. Chicago, American Dental Association, 1994.

19. **American Dental Association:** A Guide to the Use of Fluorides for the Prevention of Dental Caries, 2nd ed., *J. Am. Dent. Assoc., 113,* 558, September, 1986.

20. **American Dental Association,** Council on Dental Materials, Instruments, and Equipment and Council on Dental Therapeutics: Status Report: Effect of Acidulated Phosphate Fluoride on Porcelain and Composite Restorations, *J. Am. Dent. Assoc., 116,* 115, January, 1988.

21. **Ripa,** L.W.: Fluoride Rinsing: What Dentists Should Know, *J. Am. Dent. Assoc., 102,* 477, April, 1981.

22. **Tolle,** S.L., Bauman, D.B., and Allen, D.S.: Effects of Fluoride Gels on Plaque and Gingival Health, *Dent. Hyg., 61,* 280, June, 1987.

23. **Naleway,** C.A.: Laboratory Methods of Assessing Fluoride Dentifrices and Other Topical Fluoride Agents,

in Wei, S.H.Y., ed.: *Clinical Uses of Fluorides.*
Philadelphia, Lea & Febiger, 1985, pp. 144–146.

24. **Strateman,** M.W. and Shannon, I.L.: Control of
    Decalcification in Orthodontic Patients by Daily Self-
    administrated Application of a Water-free 0.4-Percent
    Stannous Fluoride Gel, *Am. J. Orthodon., 66,* 273,
    September, 1974.

25. **Wescott,** W.B., Starcke, E.N., and Shannon, I.L.:
    Chemical Protection Against Postirradiation Dental
    Caries, *Oral. Surg. Oral Med. Oral Pathol., 40,* 709,
    December, 1975.

26. **Hodge,** H.C. and Smith, F.A.: Fluoride Toxicology, in
    Newbrun, E., ed.: *Fluorides and Dental Caries,* 3rd ed.
    Springfield, IL, Charles D. Thomas, 1986, pp. 199–220.

27. **Heifetz,** S.B. and Horowitz, H.S.: The Amounts of
    Fluoride in Current Fluoride Therapies: Safety
    Considerations for Children, *ASDC J. Dent. Child.,
    51,* 257, July-August, 1984.

28. **Bayless,** J.M. and Tinanoff, N.: Diagnosis and
    Treatment of Acute Fluoride Toxicity, *J. Am. Dent.
    Assoc., 110,* 209, February, 1985.

29. **Lyon,** T.C.: Topical Fluorides: How Much Are You
    Using? *Dent. Hyg., 59,* 58, February, 1985.

30. **Swift,** E.K.: The Effect of Sealants on Dental Caries:
    A Review, *J. Am. Dent. Assoc., 116,* 700, May, 1988.

31. **Handelman,** S.L.: Therapeutic Use of Sealants for
    Incipient or Early Carious Lesions in Children and
    Young Adults, *Proc. Finn. Dent. Soc., 87,* 463, No.
    4, 1991.

32. **Weerheijm,** K.L., de Soet, J.J., van Amerongen, W.E.,
    and de Graaff, J.: Sealing of Occlusal Hidden Caries
    Lesions: An Alternative for Curative Treatment? *ASDC
    J. Dent. Child., 59,* 263, July-August, 1992.

33. **Mertz-Fairhurst,** E.J., Fairhurst, C.W., Williams, J.E.,
    Della-Giustina, V.E., and Brooks, J.D.: A Comparative
    Clinical Study of Two Pit and Fissure Sealants: 7-year
    Results in Augusta, GA, *J. Am. Dent. Assoc., 109,* 252,
    August, 1984.

34. **Simonsen,** R.J.: The Clinical Effectiveness of a Colored
    Pit and Fissure Sealant at 36 Months, *J. Am. Dent.
    Assoc., 102,* 323, March, 1981.

35. **Simonsen,** R.J.: Retention and Effectiveness of Dental Sealant after 15 Years, *J. Am. Dent. Assoc., 122,* 34, October, 1991.

36. **Tilliss,** T.S.I., Stach, D.J., Hatch, R.A., and Cross-Poline, G.N.: Occlusal Discrepancies after Sealant Therapy, *J. Prosthet. Dent., 68,* 223, August, 1992.

37. **Stach,** D.J., Hatch, R.A., Tilliss, T.S., and Cross-Poline, G.N.: Change in Occlusal Height Resulting from Placement of Pit and Fissure Sealants, *J. Prosthet. Dent., 68,* 750, November, 1992.

38. **Buonocore,** M.G.: Pit and Fissure Sealing, *Dent. Clin. North Am., 19,* 367, April, 1975.

PRACTICE APPLICATIONS/ ADJUNCTIVE TREATMENTS

13

This chapter provides information on a variety of practice procedures. The topics range from ultrasonics and instrument sharpening to treating hypersensitive teeth.

Treatment of periodontal infection has shifted to include modalities other than the traditional use of manual instruments. The emphasis is on creating conditions that will promote the healing of periodontal tissue and infection. The development of ultrasonic tips designed for accessing periodontal pockets and furcations expands the parameters of periodontal treatment beyond a focus on only root smoothness. Adjunctive treatment with antimicrobials, oral irrigation, and local and systemic antibiotic therapies are part of nonsurgical periodontal therapy (1).

TABLE 13.1. Ultrasonic/Sonic Scalers

Type	Mechanism	Cycles/Second (Vibrations)	Tip Motion/Activation
Ultrasonic: magnetostrictive	Magnetostrictive stacks or rods Converts high-frequency electrical current into rapid mechanical vibrations	20,000–42,000	Elliptical or rotational 360° around tip
Ultrasonic: piezoelectric	Crystal converts electrical energy into ultrasonic vibrations	29,000–50,000	Linear Two sides of the tip
Sonic	Air pressure handpiece on dental unit	2,500–7,000	Elliptical or orbital 360° around tip

TABLE 13.2. Ultrasonic/Sonic Scaling Indications, Precautions, Contraindications

Indications	Precautions, Contraindications
Supragingival calculus removal	Patients with known communicable diseases transmitted by aerosols
Periodontal debridement	Immunosuppressed individuals
Initial debridement for acute necrotizing ulcerative gingivitis (ANUG)	Pulmonary/respiratory risk individuals (2)
Oral surgery preparation	Patients with swallowing and/or gagging problems
Orthodontic cement removal, debonding (3)	Individuals with cardiac pacemakers—consult cardiologist
Removal of overhangs	Children
	Teeth: demineralized areas; exposed cemental surfaces; sensitivity areas
	Restorative materials: porcelain crowns (4); composite resins; laminate veneers (5); amalgam surfaces and margins (6); titanium implants (7, 8)

TABLE 13.3. Ultrasonic Procedure Factors (9, 10)

Preparation	Minimize water contamination (11)
	Tune according to manufacturer's specification
	Review histories, radiographs, treatment plan
	Make sure antibiotic premedication has been taken if indicated by history (12)
	Explain procedure: sounds, vibrations, water spray (individuals with hearing aids should be instructed to turn them off)
	Have patient rinse with antimicrobial mouthrinse prior to commencement of procedure
	Both clinician and patient should have protective coverings over clothing and eyes (patient should remove contact lenses)
Instrumentation	Patient in supine position
	Use high-volume evacuation (dental assistant); adaptors are available to convert high-volume evacuation to a saliva ejector; devices are also available that attach to the ultrasonic handpiece for fluid removal
	Keep the tip in motion at all times
	Use sweeping, overlapping strokes
	Tapping strokes against the cervical edge of a deposit (the opposite of manual instrumentation) (13)
	Very light pressure is used; heavier pressure decreases the effectiveness and can cause damage to root surfaces
	New tips designed for periodontal pocket access and debridement are changing the manner in which scaling and root planing are used for periodontal treatment

continued

Postoperative	Plaque control procedures as recommended
	Use of fluoride dentifrice and mouthrinse for newly exposed tooth surfaces
	Advise on tooth sensitivity to temperature, which may persist for a few days
	Warm saline rinses for gingival sensitivity
Advantages (14)	Periodontal inserts: improved subgingival access; instrumentation efficiency; emphasis on soft tissue healing; cementum conservation; minimal damage
	Reduced instrumentation time
	Increased patient comfort
	Reduced operator fatigue

TABLE 13.4. Types of Sharpening Stones

Type	Characteristics
Natural abrasive stones	Quarried from mineral deposits (e.g., Arkansas stone)
Artificial materials	Hard, nonmetallic substances impregnated with aluminum oxide, silicon carbide, or diamond particles
	Larger and coarser than particles of Arkansas stone (e.g., ruby stone, carborundum stones, diamond hone)
	Ceramic aluminum oxide
	Steel alloys (e.g., tungsten carbide steel [Neivert whittler])
Unmounted (manual)	Stationary flat stones
	Hand stones
	Other types (sharpening devices)
Mandrel mounted (power-driven)	Cylindrical (straight or tapered) small stones
	Various diameters, designed for variously sized instruments

FIGURE 13.1. Selection of cutting edge to sharpen. Both cutting edges and the rounded toe are sharpened for a universal curet (*left*). An area-specific curet is sharpened on the longer cutting edge and the rounded toe. A scaler is sharpened on the two sides, and the tip is brought to a point.

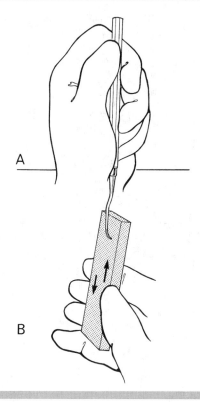

FIGURE 13.2.   Stationary instrument—moving stone technique. **A.** Grasp the instrument with the nondominant hand. Stabilize the hand on the edge of a stationary table or bench and put good light on the instrument. **B.** The stone is angled with the face of the instrument at 100–110° (Fig. 13.3) to maintain the internal angle of the blade at 70–80°.

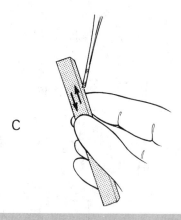

FIGURE 13.2—*continued.* **C.** The stone is reversed to sharpen the opposite cutting edge of a universal curet.

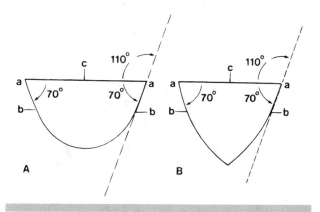

FIGURE 13.3. Angulation for sharpening. Cross sections of a curet (**A**) and a sickle scaler (**B**) show correct angulation of the face of the blade with the flat sharpening stone (*broken line*) to reproduce the internal angle of the instrument at 70°. Note the cutting edges (*a*) and the lateral surfaces (*b*).

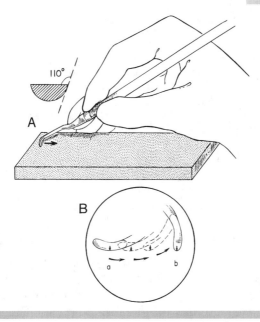

FIGURE 13.4. Stationary stone—moving instrument technique. **A.** The stone is placed flat with the blade in position at the beginning of the sharpening stroke. With the finger rest stabilized on the edge of the stone, the cutting edge is maintained at the proper angulation (110°) as the instrument is drawn along the stone with an even, moderate pressure. **B.** The movement of the blade is shown by the arrows, which indicate each portion of the cutting edge as the blade is turned on the stone from the beginning (a) to the completion (b) of the stroke at the center of the round toe of the curet. For a universal curet, the instrument is turned over, and the opposite cutting edge is sharpened.

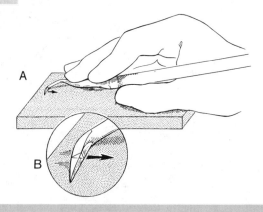

FIGURE 13.5. Stationary stone technique for a scaler. **A.** With a modified pen grasp and a finger rest established on the side of the stone, the scaler is positioned for sharpening. **B.** The portion of the cutting edge nearest the lower shank is applied first with an angle of 100–110° between the face and the stone. The instrument is turned continuously to follow the arc-like shape of the blade. The cutting edges are sharpened to the pointed tip.

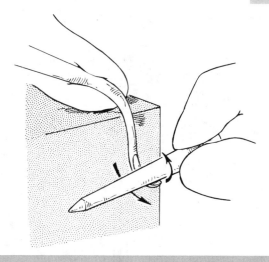

FIGURE 13.6.   Sharpening cone. A cylindrical Arkansas stone is applied to the face of a curet. The instrument is stabilized over a firm block, and the stone is positioned to fit the curvature of the surface to be sharpened. An even pressure is applied across the face of the instrument so that both cutting edges will be sharpened on the same plane.

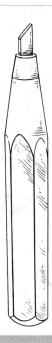

FIGURE 13.7. The Neivert whittler. The working end is made of tungsten carbide steel and the handle is made of stainless steel.

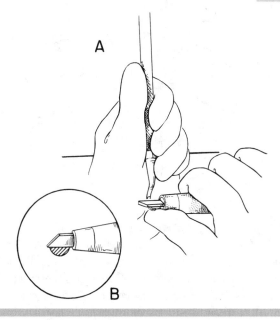

FIGURE 13.8. Sharpening with a Neivert whittler. **A.** The instrument is stabilized in the nondominant hand, and the whittler is held in a palm grasp with the thumb rest close to the instrument to be sharpened. **B.** Close-up shows position of the blade of the sharpener across the face of the curet.

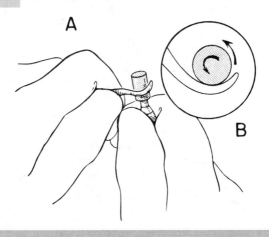

FIGURE 13.9.   Mandrel mounted sharpening stone. **A.** A mounted stone with a diameter appropriate for the curved blade to be sharpened is positioned across the face for even sharpening of the cutting edges. The hands and arms are stabilized for precision and control. **B.** With low speed to minimize heat production, the rotating stone is passed along the face of the instrument. Near the toe, the stone is moved upward to prevent flattening of the instrument.

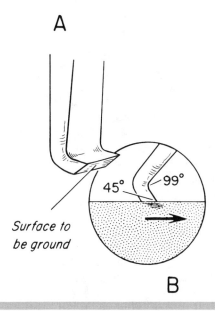

A

B

45°   99°

*Surface to
be ground*

FIGURE 13.10.   Sharpening a hoe scaler. **A.** The surface to be ground. **B.** The hoe is adapted to the surface of a stationary flat stone at the proper angle to maintain the original bevel of 45°. The arrow indicates the direction of the sharpening stroke leading into the cutting edge.

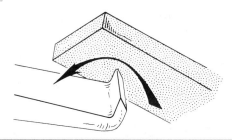

FIGURE 13.11. Rounding a hoe scaler. To round the sharp corners of the hoe scaler, a flat stone is rubbed over the instrument with a gentle rolling motion.

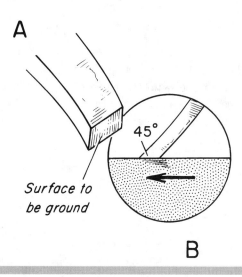

FIGURE 13.12. Sharpening a chisel scaler. **A.** The surface to be ground. **B.** The chisel is adapted to the surface of a stationary flat stone at the proper angle to maintain the original bevel of 45°. The arrow indicates the direction of the sharpening stroke leading into the cutting edge.

TABLE 13.5. Gingival Curettage Objectives

Overall	Specific	Technique
Treatment component to restore gingival health	Abate inflammation by edema drainage	Removal of diseased pocket lining epithelium and underlying inflamed connective tissue
Reduction or elimination of inflammation	Shrinkage of free gingiva (pocket depth)	
Reduction or eradication of gingival or periodontal pockets	Removal of diseased soft tissue to deter disease redevelopment	Removal of tissue debris and chronic granulation tissue
	Promotion of fibrosis and healing	Removal of calcified debris remaining after irrigation and suction post scaling and root planing
	Allow replacement of diseased pocket lining with new connective tissue and sulcular epithelium	
	Aid in return of normal gingival contour	Removal of microorganisms embedded within tissue

TABLE 13.6. Selection of Treatment Areas for Gingival Curettage

Indications for Definitive Curettage	Contraindications	Indications for Nondefinitive Curettage
Gingival tissue soft, spongy consistency with other signs of inflammation	Firm, fibrous gingival tissue	Preparation for surgical pocket elimination
Shallow (4–5 mm) suprabony pockets	Thin, fragile pocket walls	Maintenance therapy (recurrent infection control)
Persistent hyperemia, edema, and pocket depth after complete scaling and root planing	Acute periodontal inflammatory lesions	
	Conditions that require specific surgical treatment	
	Deep and/or infrabony pockets	
	Areas of narrow attached gingiva or mucogingival involvement	
	Furcation involvement	

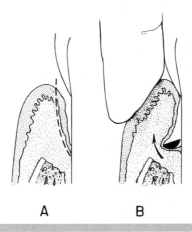

A   **B**

FIGURE 13.13.   Gingival curettage. **A.** The broken line shows pocket tissue to be removed during gingival curettage, namely the pocket epithelium and the underlying inflamed connective tissue. **B.** The curet positioned at the bottom of the pocket with the cutting edge toward the gingival tissue wall. Pressure applied with a finger on the outside of the pocket provides support for the pressure of the curet as it is activated. The curet is angled for a vertical stroke, as shown by the cross section of the blade and the arrow.

TABLE 13.7.   Effect of Instrumentation on Pocket Micro-flora

Periodontal Infection Before Treatment	Periodontal Health After Treatment
Predominant flora is	Predominant flora is
Anaerobic	Aerobic
Gram-negative	Gram-positive
Motile	Nonmotile
Spirochetes, motile rods; pathogenic	Coccoid forms; nonpathogenic
Very high total count of all types of microorganisms	Much lower total counts of all types of microorganisms
Many leukocytes	Lower leukocyte counts

TABLE 13.8. Professional Subgingival Irrigation

Delivery Methods	Recommendations for Use	Special Considerations
Disposable hand syringe Specially designed jet irrigator Air-driven irrigation handpiece Some ultrasonic devices	Proprocedural delivery: antimicrobial agents can reduce microorganisms in aerosol contamination Preanesthesia application: reduction of microorganisms prior to topical anesthetic application and administration of local anesthetic Procedural: irrigation with antimicrobial during ultrasonic use Maintenance phase: postprocedural Irrigation: 　Tissue sites unresponsive to traditional periodontal treatment 　Gingivitis superimposed on periodontitis 　Areas inaccessible to mechanical instrumentation and in which open scaling and root planing or surgical intervention is not an option	Variety of antimicrobial agents, saline, water, and products such as chlorhexidine gluconate and stannous fluoride can be used for irrigation (15–18) Antibiotic premedication needed for patients susceptible to effects of bacteremia Use caution with irrigation pressure used with disposable hand syringes

TABLE 13.9. Acute Gingival Conditions

	Predisposing Factors	Etiology	Treatment
Necrotizing ulcerative gingivitis/ periodontitis (NUG/NUP)	Local Preexisting gingivitis and/or periodontitis Inadequate personal oral care Tobacco use Factors related to retention of plaque and deposits Stress factors: anxiety, emotional stress Systemic: disease-resistance factors Inadequate diet, nutrition Illness, disease Side effects of chemotherapy and radiation Fatigue, insufficient sleep	Fusiospirochetal complex of microbes that develops and increases in association with predisposing factors that have lowered body's immune system response (19–22)	Relief of acute symptoms Debridement of teeth and gingiva Subgingival scaling and root planing Chlorhexidine 0.12% rinse twice daily Personal care instructions Dietary, health counseling (23) Multivitamin supplement recommendation Possible systemic antibiotic therapy Several appointments may be necessary to resolve the acute phase *continued*

TABLE 13.9. Acute Gingival Conditions

	Predisposing Factors	Etiology	Treatment
			Successive treatment
			Evaluation and complete assessment
			Treatment of gingival and bony craters
Periodontal abscess	Existing periodontal disease	Polymorphonuclear leukocytes and other defense cells mixed with cell and tissue debris, forming pus	Relief of acute symptoms
	Trauma from foreign objects impacted in sulcus or instrumentation (24)		Relieve pain
			Establish drainage
	Incomplete instrumentation of pocket depth (25)		Determine need for systemic antibiotic
			Hot saline rinses every 2 hours
			Follow-up appointment in 24 to 48 hrs
			Initiation of plaque control instruction
			Scaling and root planing
			Definitive therapy for elimination of pocket

TABLE 13.10. Hypersensitive Teeth

Contributing factors	Exposure of cementum and dentin
	Gingival recession (26, 27)
	Periodontal infection with attachment loss
	Trauma: hard toothbrush; overly vigorous brushing; use of abrasive dentifrice; bruxing; malocclusion
	Periodontal surgery
	Anatomy of cementoenamel junction: dentin zone between enamel and cementum (28)
	Loss of cementum: abrasion; erosion; dental caries; scaling; root planing; polishing with abrasive agent or airbrasive instrument
	Loss of enamel: dietary erosion; fractures; toothbrush abrasion; occlusal wear; parafunctional habits
	Dental factors: cracked tooth syndrome; dental caries; defective restorations (margin leakage, fractures); fractured or chipped teeth
Types of pain stimuli (29)	Mechanical (tactile)
	Toothbrush filaments or bristles
	Eating utensils
	Periodontal and dental instruments
	Friction from denture clasps or other appliances
	Habits (toothpicks, fingernails, etc.)

continued

TABLE 13.10. Hypersensitive Teeth

	Chemical
	Acids produced by bacterial plaque
	Citrus fruits
	Condiments
	Thermal
	Hot or cold food or beverages
	Air
	Osmotic
	Concentrated solutions (sugar, salt) induce fluid movement in dentin
Untreated: spontaneous remission	Formation of reparative and/or secondary dentin
	Deposition of fluoride, minerals (diet, fluoridated water, dentifrice) at opening of tubules
	Calculus formation over sensitive area
	Control intake of pain-causing factors
Treatment: desensitizing agents	Modes of action
	Surface coating of tubule entrance
	Intratubular mineralization or precipitation
	Irritation and stimulation to encourage secondary dentin formation
	Criteria for acceptable desensitizing agent (30)
	Rapid action
	Ease of application

continued

Biologic acceptance by body tissues
Long-lasting or permanent effects
No side effects
No pain during application
Consistent effectiveness
Desensitizing agents (shown effective for certain patients)
Silver nitrate (30)
Formalin (30)
Glycerine (31)
Strontium chloride (32, 33)
Potassium nitrate (34–36)
Fluorides
Sodium fluoride (39–41)
Stannous fluoride (42, 43)
Sodium citrate (44)
Potassium oxalate (45)
Calcium compounds
Dicalcium phosphate (37)
Calcium hydroxide (35, 38)
Cyanoacrylate (46)
Resin (47)

continued

TABLE 13.10. Hypersensitive Teeth

Professional applications	Methods available are not consistently effective for all patients. Few patients respond to a single form of treatment. Effective home-care plaque control influences the success rate with professional applications.
	Sealing dentinal tubules with albumin precipitants
	Cavity varnishes; thin mixes of crown and bridge cement; zinc oxide and eugenol; Gottlieb's solution for thermal shock
	Composite resin precede with acid etch (47)
	Laser (48)
	Hypnosis (49)
	Sodium fluoride desensitizing (40)
	33% sodium fluoride, 33% kaolin, 33% glycerin
	Clean and isolate area; wipe with 2% sodium fluoride solution, dry area, apply paste mixture with wood point and gently burnish for 3 minutes
	Iontophoresis (50, 51)
	Impregnation of tissue with ions from dissolved salts with aid of an electric current. Promotes ionic transport of fluoride onto a tooth surface. Follow manufacturer's directions for equipment use.
Patient self-care	Consistent vigorous plaque control; special care in cervical areas
	Fluoride dentifrice, desensitizing dentifrice, or combination daily
	Self-applied fluoride: tray/gel; brushing with gel; rinses
	Identify foods, beverages that cause sensitivity (food diary)

REFERENCES

1. **Young,** N.A.: Periodontal Debridement: Re-examining Non-surgical Instrumentation, Part I: A New Perspective on the Objectives of Instrumentation, *Seminars In Dental Hygiene, Vol. 4, No. 4, November, 1994.*

2. **Krell,** K.V., Courey, J.M., and Bishara, S.E.: Orthodontic Bracket Removal Using Conventional and Ultrasonic Debonding Techniques, Enamel Loss, and Time Requirements, *Am. J. Orthod. Dentofacial Orthop., 103, 258,* March, 1993.

3. **Suzuki,** J.B. and Delisle, A.L.: Pulmonary Actinomycosis of Periodontal Origin, *J. Periodontol., 55, 581,* October, 1984.

4. **American Dental Association,** Council on Dental Materials, Instruments, and Equipment: *Dentist's Desk Reference: Materials, Instruments, and Equipment,* 2nd ed. Chicago, American Dental Association, 1983, pp. 361–362.

5. **Carr,** E.H.: Laminate Veneers. Restoration Alternative Means Special Care, *RDH, 2,* 11, July-August, 1982.

6. **Rajstein,** J. and Tal, M.: The Effect of Ultrasonic Scaling on the Surface of Class V Amalgam Restorations—A Scanning Electron Microscopy Study, *J. Oral Rehabil., 11, 299,* May, 1984.

7. **Thomson-Neal,** D., Evans, G.H., and Meffert, R.M.: Effects of Various Prophylactic Treatments on Titanium, Sapphire and Hydroxy-coated Implants, *Int. J. Periodontics Restorative Dent., 9, 301,* No. 4, 1989.

8. **Rapley,** J.W., Swan, R.H., Hallmon, W.W., and Mills, M.P.P.: The Surface Characteristics Produced by Various Oral Hygiene Instruments and Materials on Titanium Implant Abutments, *Int. J. Oral Maxillofac. Implants, 5, 47,* No. 1, 1990.

9. **Holbrook,** T.E. and Low, S.B.: Power-driven Scaling and Polishing Instruments, in Hardin, J.F., ed.: *Clark's Clinical Dentistry,* Revised edition—1989. Philadelphia, J.B. Lippincott Co., 1989, Section 5A, pp. 1–24.

10. **Clark,** S.M.: A Compact Guide to Ultrasonic Instrumentation, *Compendium, 12, 760,* October, 1991.

11. **Larato,** D.C., Ruskin, P.F., and Martin, A.: Effect of an Ultrasonic Scaler on Bacterial Counts in Air,

J. Periodontol., 38, 550, November-December (Part I), 1967.

12. **Bandt,** C.L., Korn, N.A., and Schaffer, E.M.: Bacteremias from Ultrasonic and Hand Instrumentation, *J. Periodontol., 35,* 214, May-June, 1964.

13. **American Dental Hygienists' Association:** Periodontal Debridement Therapy, Audio Cassette Course, Chicago, Copyright, 1983.

14. **Bray,** K.K.: Innovations in Periodontal Debridement: Re-examining the Role of Power-Driven Scaling, *Dental Hygiene Connection, Vol. No. l, Issue No. 1,* Dentsply Cavitron, 1995.

15. **Southard,** S.R., Drisko, C.L., Killoy, W.J., Cobb, C.M., and Tira, D.E.: The Effect of 2% Chlorhexidine Digluconate Irrigation on Clinical Parameters and the Level of *Bacteroides gingivalis* in Periodontal Pockets, *J. Periodontol., 60,* 302, June, 1989.

16. **Schmid,** E., Kornman, K.S., and Tinanoff, N.: Changes of Subgingival Total Colony Forming Units and Black Pigmented Bacteroides after a Single Irrigation of Periodontal Pockets with 1.64% SnF2, *J. Periodontol., 56,* 330, June, 1985.

17. **Mazza,** J.E., Newman, M.G., and Sims, T.N.: Clinical and Antimicrobial Effect of Stannous Fluoride on Periodontitis, *J. Clin. Periodontol., 8,* 203, June, 1981.

18. **Schlagenhauf,** U., Stellwag, P., and Fiedler, A.: Subgingival Irrigation in the Maintenance Phase of Periodontal Therapy, *J. Clin. Periodontol., 17,* 650, October, 1990.

19. **Loesche,** W.J., Syed, S.A., Laughon, B.E., and Stoll, J.: The Bacteriology of Acute Necrotizing Ulcerative Gingivitis, *J. Periodontol., 53,* 223, April, 1982.

20. **Falkler,** W.A., Martin, S.A., Vincent, J.W., Tall, B.D., Nauman, R.K., and Suzuki, J.B.: A Clinical, Demographic and Microbiologic Study of ANUG Patients in an Urban Dental School, *J. Clin. Periodontol., 14,* 307, July, 1987.

21. **Dennison,** D.K., Smith, B., and Newland, J.R.: Immune Responsiveness and ANUG, *J. Dent. Res., 64,* 197, Abstract 204, March, 1985.

22. **Rowland,** R.W., Mestecky, J., Gunsolley, J.C., and Cogen, R.B.: Serum IgG and IgM Levels to Bacterial Antigens in Necrotizing Ulcerative Gingivitis, *J. Periodontol., 64,* 195, March, 1993.

23. **Nizel,** A.E.: *Nutrition in Preventive Dentistry: Science and Practice,* 2nd ed. Philadelphia, W.B. Saunders Co., 1981, pp. 485–488.

24. **Armitage,** G.C.: *Biologic Basis of Periodontal Maintenance Therapy.* Berkeley, CA, Praxis Publishing Co., 1980, pp. 154–159.

25. **Gillette,** W.B. and Van House, R.L.: Ill Effects of Improper Oral Hygiene Procedures, *J. Am. Dent. Assoc., 101,* 476, September, 1980.

26. **Grant,** D.A., Stern, I.B., and Listgarten, M.A., eds.: *Periodontics,* 6th ed. St. Louis, The C.V. Mosby Co., 1988, pp. 460–467.

27. **Carranza,** F.A.: *Glickman's Clinical Periodontology,* 7th ed. Philadelphia, W.B. Saunders Co., 1990, pp. 118–122.

28. **Bhaskar,** S.M., ed.: *Orban's Oral Histology and Embryology,* 11th ed. St. Louis, The C.V. Mosby Co., 1991, p. 192.

29. **Grant,** D.A., Stern, I.B., and Listgarten, M.A., eds.: *Periodontics,* 6th ed. St. Louis, The C.V. Mosby Co., 1988, pp 638–641.

30. **Grossman,** L.I.: A Systematic Method for the Treatment of Hypersensitive Dentin, *J. Am. Dent. Assoc., 22,* 592, April, 1935.

31. **Colaneri,** J.N.: A Simple Treatment of Hypersensitive Cervical Dentin, *Oral Surg. Oral Med. Oral Pathol., 5,* 276, March, 1952.

32. **Meffert,** R.M. and Hoskins, S.W.: Effect of a Strontium Chloride Dentifrice in Relieving Dental Hypersensitivity, *J. Periodontol., 35,* 232, May-June, 1964.

33. **Minkoff,** S. and Axelrod, S.: Efficacy of Strontium Chloride in Dental Hypersensitivity, *J. Periodontol., 58,* 470, July, 1987.

34. **Hodosh,** M.: A Superior Desensitizer—Potassium Nitrate, *J. Am. Dent. Assoc., 88,* 831, April, 1974.

35. **Green,** B.L., Breen, M.L., and McFall, W.T.: Calcium

Hydroxide and Potassium Nitrate as Desensitizing Agents for Hypersensitive Root Surfaces, *J. Periodontol., 48,* 667, October, 1977.

36. **Tarbet,** W.J., Silverman, G., Stolman, J.M., and Fratarcangelo, P.A.: Clinical Evaluation of a New Treatment for Dentinal Hypersensitivity, *J. Periodontol., 51,* 535, September, 1980.

37. **Hiatt,** W.H. and Johansen, E.: Root Preparation. I. Obturation of Dentinal Tubules in Treatment of Root Hypersensitivity, *J. Periodontol., 43,* 373, June, 1972.

38. **Pashley,** D.H., Kalathoor, S., and Burnham, D.: The Effects of Calcium Hydroxide on Dentin Permeability, *J. Dent. Res., 65,* 417, March, 1986.

39. **Lukomsky,** E.H.: Fluorine Therapy for Exposed Dentin and Alveolar Atrophy, *J. Dent. Res., 20,* 649, December, 1941.

40. **Hoyt,** W.H. and Bibby, B.G.: Use of Sodium Fluoride for Desensitizing Dentin, *J. Am. Dent. Assoc., 30,* 1372, September 1, 1943.

41. **Minkov,** B., Marmari, I., Gedalia, I., and Garfinkel, A.: The Effectiveness of Sodium Fluoride Treatment with and without Iontophoresis on the Reduction of Hypersensitive Dentin, *J. Periodontol., 46,* 246, April, 1975.

42. **Miller,** J.T., Sannon, I.L., Kilgore, W.G., and Bookman, J.E.: Use of a Water-free Stannous Fluoride-containing Gel in the Control of Dental Hypersensitivity, *J. Periodontol., 40,* 490, August, 1969.

43. **Blong,** M.A., Volding, B., Thrash, W.J., and Jones, D.L.: Effects of a Gel Containing 0.4-Percent Stannous Fluoride on Dentinal Hypersensitivity, *Dent. Hyg., 59,* 489, November, 1985.

44. **Zinner,** D.D., Duany, L.F., and Lutz, H.J.: A New Desensitizing Dentifrice: Preliminary Report, *J. Am. Dent. Assoc., 95,* 982, November, 1977.

45. **Muzzin,** K.B. and Johnson, R.: Effects of Potassium Oxalate on Dentin Hypersensitivity In Vivo, *J. Periodontol., 60,* 515, March, 1989.

46. **Javid,** B., Barkhordar, R.A., and Bhinda, S.V.: Cyanoacrylate—A New Treatment for Hypersensitive

Dentin and Cementum, *J. Am. Dent. Assoc., 114,* 486, April, 1987.

47. **Brannstrom,** M., Johnson, G., and Nordenvall, K.J.: Transmission and Control of Dentinal Pain: Resin Impregnation for the Desensitization of Dentin, *J. Am. Dent. Assoc., 99,* 612, October, 1979.

48. **Renton-Harper,** P. and Midda, M.: NdYag Laser Treatment of Dentinal Hypersensitivity, *Br. Dent. J., 172,* 13, January 11, 1992.

49. **Starr,** C.B., Mayhew, R.B., and Pierson, W.P.: The Efficacy of Hypnosis in the Treatment of Dentin Hypersensitivity, *Gen. Dent. 37,* 13, January-February, 1989.

50. **Gillam,** D.G. and Newman, H.N.: Iontophoresis in the Treatment of Cervical Dentinal Sensitivity—A Review, *J. West. Soc. Periodont./Periodont. Abstr., 38,* 129, No. 4, 1990.

51. **McBride,** M.A., Gilpatrick, R.O., and Fowler, W.L.: The Effectiveness of Sodium Fluoride Iontophoresis in Patients with Sensitive Teeth, *Quintessence Int., 22,* 637, August, 1991.

TREATMENT FACTORS FOR SPECIAL NEEDS

14

This chapter provides information on patients with special needs or conditions as well as factors to consider when rendering treatment. It should be noted that every patient has special needs and conditions of which we must be aware. Cultural, ethnic, and socioeconomic factors also play an important part in influencing oral healthcare treatment.

TABLE 14.1. Pregnancy and Treatment (See Table 14.2)

Oral Hygiene Care	Precautions/Contraindications
Oral hygiene/plaque control education on the gingival problems that may arise as a result of poor oral hygiene: Generalized gingival enlargement (pregnancy gingivitis) (7–9) Isolated gingival enlargement ("pregnancy tumor," epulis gravidarum, pregnancy granuloma (10), pyogenic granuloma (11)) Scaling and root planing to promote gingival health Dietary counseling: Promote adequate nutrition, increased daily allowances (5, 6) Counteract effects of morning sickness Counseling on oral care for infant (see Table 14.4)	Consult with patient's physician concerning dental treatment (1) Second trimester is the safest period for treatment (2) Radiographs only if necessary Monitor vital signs Extensive periodontal or dental treatment other than emergencies or to correct obvious disease problems should be postponed Exercise caution in recommending or prescribing any drugs because of the teratogenic effects (3, 4) See Table 14.3. Morning sickness with vomiting over an extended period may cause enamel erosion

TABLE 14.2. Appointment Adaptations for the Prenatal Patient

Characteristics	Dental Hygiene Implication
Fatigues easily, may even fall asleep	Short appointments; several in series, as needed Work with an assistant to accomplish more at each appointment
Discomfort of remaining in one position too long	Interrupt in middle of appointment to change chair position Assistance with evacuation during intraoral instrumentation can shorten appointment time
Backache	Adjust chair appropriately for comfort
Frequent urination	Allow sufficient appointment time for interruptions Suggest at beginning of appointment that patient mention need for interruption
General awkwardness because of new shape and weight gain	Attend to details, such as gently lowering and straightening chair for patient Make sure rinsing facilities are convenient; or, preferably, an assistant attends to evacuation
Dyspnea (aggravated by supine chair position)	Adapt chair for patient comfort
Faintness and dizziness	Be prepared for emergency Place the patient on her *side* and not in supine or Trendelenburg position because pressure from the *continued*

TABLE 14.2. Appointment Adaptations for the Prenatal Patient

Characteristics	Dental Hygiene Implication
	enlarged uterus and the abdominal organs on the inferior vena cava can interfere with venous return; placental separation could result
Nausea and vomiting (first trimester) Unpleasant taste in mouth Gagging	Suggest toothbrushing or rinsing at frequent intervals Recommend a small toothbrush Turn head down over sink while brushing; helps to relax throat and allow saliva to flow out Take care in instrument and radiographic film placement
Exaggerated reactions to odors and flavors of medicaments and other office materials	Determine particularly obnoxious odors for an individual patient and remove them Pay attention to cleanliness of cuspidor
Physician's recommendations for alleviation of symptoms: frequent eating of small amounts of foods	Encourage use of noncariogenic foods
Unusual food cravings	If cravings are for sweets, clearly define relationship of frequent nibbling of cariogenic foods to dental caries Provide list of nutritious noncariogenic snacks

TABLE 14.3. Drugs Contraindicated During Pregnancy and Breastfeeding

Classification	Drugs Prescribed for Treatment	Possible Adverse Effects on Fetus and Infant
Anticoagulant	Warfarin (Coumadin) (D)[a] Dicumarol (D)	Hemorrhagic; fetal death Birth malformations
Anticonvulsant	Barbiturates (phenobarbital) (D) Phenytoin sodium (D) Trimethadione (D) Valproate sodium (D)	Congenital malformations Developmental delays Fetal phenobarbital syndrome Fetal hydantoin syndrome Fetal trimethadione syndrome Fetal valproate syndrome
Antimicrobial	Streptomycin (B) Tetracycline (D)	Toxic action on ear: 8th cranial nerve damage Bone growth inhibition; intrinsic dental stain
Antineoplastic	Cyclophosphamide (Cytoxan) (D) Mercaptopurine (D) Methotrexate (D)	Multiple anomalies; fetal death

continued

TABLE 14.3. Drugs Contraindicated During Pregnancy and Breastfeeding

Classification	Drugs Prescribed for Treatment	Possible Adverse Effects on Fetus and Infant
Hormones	Clomiphene (Clomid) (X) Estrogenic substances (X) Diethylstilbestrol (X) Prednisone (C) Progesterone (X)	Increased anomalies; neural tube defects Cancer of the vagina and cervix; genital tract anomalies; congenital heart defects
Psychotrophic	Antianxiety Chlordiazepoxide (Librium) (D) Diazepam (Valium) (D) Meprobamate (Miltown) (D) Antimanic Lithium carbonate (D)	Low heart rate, muscle tone, respiration, poor sucking reflex Birth defects Lethargy, cyanosis, teratogenic (dose related)
Drugs of Abuse	*Alcohol*	Fetal alcohol syndrome Spontaneous abortion; low birth rate Mental retardation

continued

Cocaine	
Prenatal exposure	Decreased birth weight; prematurity
	Fetal growth retardation; microcephaly
	Teratogenic effects
Inhale free-base vapors (postpartum)	Increased rate of seizures
Narcotics	
Heroin	Decreased birth weight
	Withdrawal symptoms
Methadone	Convulsions; sudden infant death
Tobacco	
Cigarette smoking	Low birth weight; prematurity; miscarriage; still birth; infant mortality
	Sudden infant death syndrome
Involuntary smoking	Children: increased respiratory infections and symptoms
Environmental	Deficiencies in physical growth, intellectual development
Second-hand	Higher incidence in mortality rate of infant and child

[a] United States Food and Drug Administration (FDA) categorizes drugs and their relation to pregnancy as **A.** No risk demonstrated to fetus in any trimester. **B.** No adverse effects in animals; no human studies available. **C.** Only given after risks to fetus are considered; animal studies have shown no adverse reactions; no human studies available. **D.** Definite fetal risks; may be given in spite of risks if needed in life-threatening conditions. **X.** Absolute fetal abnormalities; not to be used at any time in pregnancy.

TABLE 14.4. Infants and Toddlers

Area of Concern	Birth to 6 Months	6 to 12 Months	18 Months
Developmental milestone	Eruption of first tooth Pattern of eruption	Pattern of eruption Expected new teeth	Check tooth contacts Close contacts; teach to floss
Nutrition and feeding	Appropriate use of nursing bottle Use of only tap water Causes of nursing caries Discourage parent sleeping with child	Discontinue bottle feeding Use Tippy Cup Discuss sugar use, sugar retention, and caries initiation	Nutrition, snacking based on child's diet Snacking safety (aspiration)
Oral hygiene and caries prevention	Clean teeth after each feeding (wash cloth, soft brush)	Use of brush Position of infant for brushing	Disclose for bacterial plaque Review brushing
Fluoride information	Need for fluoride (F) Provide systemic F Check water supply for existing F Prescribe supplements when deficient	Review fluoride used Discuss compliance Review manner of storage	Update fluoride status Use of pea-size fluoride dentifrice on brush

continued

Trauma prevention		Trauma-proofing Confirm emergency access to dental provider	Discuss oral electrical burns and child-proofing home
Habits/function behaviors	Discuss teething, nonnutritive sucking, and *Streptococcus mutans* transmission	Discuss oral signs of child abuse	Home preparation for dental hygiene visit
Dental/dental hygiene visit	What happens at baby's dental visit	First visit within 6 months of eruption first tooth	Frequency depends on parent compliance with home preventive measures

Adapted from Casamassimo, P.S., Griffiths, P., and Nowak, A.: Anticipatory Guidance in Dentistry. *Dentalhygienistnews, 5*, 19, Fall, 1992.

TABLE 14.5. Cleft Lip or Palate

General physical characteristics	Higher incidence of other congenital anomalies (13)
	Other facial deformities
	Predisposition to upper respiratory and middle ear infections
	Higher incidence of hearing loss
	Speech difficulties (anatomic, hearing loss, psychologic)
	Possible undernourishment
Oral characteristics	Higher incidence of missing, supernumerary, abnormalities of teeth
	Frequent malocclusion requiring orthodontic treatment
	Possible lack of muscle coordination of lips, tongue, cheeks, floor of mouth, or throat, causing compensatory habits for speech
	Gingival disturbances from bacterial plaque accumulation caused by physical problems associated with condition
	Early periodontal disease with bone and attachment loss common in adolescents (14)
	No difference in caries incidence; physically related problems may make bacterial plaque control more difficult
	Surgical correction suture lines may be evident
	Patient may have prosthesis, obturator, or speech aid

continued

TABLE 14.5. Cleft Lip or Palate

Dental hygiene care	Treatment to correct the condition has usually been provided by a team of specialists with progress closely monitored at each age period (15, 16)
	Consultation with attending physician
	Frequent maintenance appointments (3 to 4 months)
	Appointment considerations
	Alleviate stress factors as much as possible
	Treat patient with same consideration as other patients
	If patient has speech difficulties, provide pencil and paper or have attending parent or caregiver present for interpretation
	Open fissure lines increase susceptibility to infection (prevent debris from entering or being retained in the clefts)
	Cleaning of prosthesis or speech aid same as for removable denture
	Bacterial plaque control instructions adapted for special needs, care for prosthesis (include caregiver)
	Dietary counseling
	Presurgery care: caution because of infection susceptibility See Table 14.15
	Postsurgery care
	Careful rinsing after each feeding
	Careful brushing (usually by caregiver) to avoid damage to healing suture lines
	Toothbrush with suction attachment may be used

TABLE 14.6. Adolescence (17, 18)

General Characteristics	Oral Factors

Hormonal changes, development of sex organs
Growth spurt (irregular, uneven stages of growth may result in poor coordination and awkwardness)
Nutrition requirements
  Male: highest of lifetime
  Female:
    Exceeded only during pregnancy
    Iron-deficiency anemia not uncommon in teenage girls
Skin disorders
Personal factors: increased self-interest, growing independence, concern over physical characteristics
	Higher incidence in communities without fluoridation
	Periodontal infections
	  All categories
	  "Puberty" gingivitis (exaggerated response to local irritants may be related to hormonal changes) (19, 20)
	  Early-onset periodontitis (loss of periodontal attachment, bone) (21–25)
	  Juvenile periodontitis (26) localized (LJP), generalized (GJP)
	  Necrotizing ulcerative gingivitis/periodontitis highest frequency in older adolescents and young adults
	Other possible oral health problems: (27)
	  Oral manifestations of sexually transmitted infections (STI)
	  Effects of tobacco use
	  Potential effects of oral contraceptives (28)
	  Anorexia nervosa, bulimia
	  Traumatic injuries to teeth and oral, facial structures

Dental hygiene care: Bacterial plaque control instruction, instrumentation, fluoride treatment program, dietary analysis and/or counseling, regular maintenance, evaluation

TABLE 14.7.	Menopause and Climacteric
Definitions	Climacteric: female period of transition from reproductive to nonreproductive stage of life (through menopause and after when body adjusts to endocrine and other changes)
	Menopause: cessation of menstruation
Oral factors	Oral disturbances relatively uncommon
	Control of local factors (bacterial plaque) through oral hygiene care lessens any exaggerated tissue response to hormonal changes
	Menopausal gingivostomatitis is rare (29)—also may occur after ovary removal or radiation therapy to ovaries
	Mucous membranes and tongue
	Possible dryness with burning or unusual taste
	Epithelium may become thin, atrophic; decreased keratinization; less tolerance for removable prostheses
	Inadequate diet and eating habits may contribute to adverse changes (frequently resemble vitamin deficiency symptoms, especially B vitamins), dental caries
	Decreased salivary output, xerostomia
Dental hygiene care	Professional maintenance appointments
	Emphasis on daily plaque control
	Recommendation of saliva substitute if needed
	Emphasis on relationship between general and oral health
	Dietary analysis and counseling
	Fluoride therapy: dentifrice and brush-on gel before retiring recommended

TABLE 14.8. Oral Factors and the Geriodontic Patient[a]

Soft tissues

Lips

Loss of elasticity, dehydration within tissues

Angular Cheilitis (30, 31): not specifically age-related but frequently seen in the elderly (related to reduced vertical dimension or inadequate support of the lips, moisture from drooling; secondarily: riboflavin deficiency or infection (*Candida albicans* or other organisms)

Oral mucosa

Decreased secretion of salivary and mucous glands affect surface texture

Xerostomia associated with certain diseases and medications

Atrophic changes: thinner, less vascular, elastic tissue; thinning of epithelium

Hyperkeratosis: result of irritation

Capillary fragility: facial bruises and petechiae of the mucosa are common

Tongue

Atrophic glossitis (burning tongue): appears smooth, shiny, bald, atrophied papillae (related to iron deficiency anemia or other combinations of deficiencies), not age specific but nutritional

Taste sensations: reduced or abnormal taste reactions may occur but not normally in healthy elderly individuals (primarily with disease condition) (32)

Sublingual varicosities: occurs frequently, not necessarily in relationship to systemic conditions

continued

	Xerostomia
	Normal salivary flow in healthy individuals (33)
	Usually in conjunction with pathologic states, drug-induced changes, or radiation-induced salivary gland degeneration
Teeth	Color: changes from long-term habits (tobacco, food), dental restorations
	Attrition: frequently shows signs of wear—long-term effects of diet, occupational factors, or bruxism
	May have chipping, seem brittle
	Abrasion: at neck of tooth from long-term use of hard toothbrush, horizontal brushing with abrasive dentifrice
	Dental caries
	Root caries: result of root exposure, not age (periodontal therapy and maintenance can prevent increased incidence) (34)
	Rampant caries ["retirement caries" (35)]: influencing factors include: xerostomia, impaired masticatory abilities, lifestyle changes (snacking, irregular mealtimes, poor food selections)
	Dental pulp (36)
	Questionable if changes are related to aging
	Changes seen more frequently in older persons
	Narrowing of pulp chambers and root canals
	Increased deposition of secondary dentin
	Progressive deposition of calcified masses (pulp stones or denticles)

continued

TABLE 14.8. Oral Factors and the Geriodontic Patient[a]

Periodontium	Bone
	Osteoporosis may be present (nutrition and hormone related)
	Depressed vascularity, reduced metabolism, reduced healing ability
	Cementum
	Increased thickness (37)
	Gingiva
	Most gingival changes from effects of infection or anatomic factors
	Predisposing factors may be insufficient attached gingiva or malpositioned teeth
	Predisposing factors may include inappropriate toothbrushing, laceration, inflammation, dental treatment
Personal factors	Possible factors that may affect the elderly patient:
	Insecurity (economic status, self-respect, feeling of being needed, inability to work, reduced activity [physical limitations, family overprotection], family rejection, health anxiety)
	Depression: limited or declining physical abilities, physical appearance changes, loneliness
	Inability to adjust to change (tendency to develop fixed habits and ideas)
	Slowing of voluntary responses
	Tendency to introspection (narrowing of interests, living in the past)

continued

Dental hygiene care	See Tables 14.9–14.12
	Awareness of reasons elderly individuals may not seek regular professional care:
	Lack of perceived need, physical or mental disabilities, chronic disease, physical barriers (transportation, access)
	Professional maintenance appointments
	Review of medical history, taking of vital signs, intraoral and extraoral examination (should be routinely for any age)
	Instruction in daily bacterial plaque control, dental caries control, control of xerostomia, diet concerns
	Dietary counseling
	Fluoride therapy as needed

[a]Changes related to aging must be separated from the long-term effects of chronic diseases.

TABLE 14.9. Adaptation in Treatment Procedures for the Geriodontic Patient

Appointment Factors	Characteristics	Dental Hygiene Implication
Medical history review	Many forms of chronic diseases	Poor medical prognosis may limit extent of total treatment
	Variety of medications used	Need for antibiotic premedication for decreased immune response
Appointment planning	Low stress tolerance	Morning appointments
	Tires more easily than a younger patient	Shorter appointments
		Need for frequent maintenance appointments to provide high-level preventive care
		Appreciation of the real effort patient has made to get there
	Slower voluntary responses	Do not rush
	Sensitivity about shortcomings of lack of motor control	Do not make the patient feel old by obvious physical assistance

continued

	Lowered tolerance to extremes of heat and cold; less body cooling through perspiration	Adjust room temperature
	Impaired hearing: difficulty in hearing when there are distractions	Speak clearly and slowly; provide written memorandum of date and time of each appointment
		Eliminate background noises and music
Instrumentation	Loss of elasticity of lips and oral mucosa	Difficulty in retraction may provide patient discomfort
	Slowing of voluntary responses	Do not demand quick response to request for change of position of head, rinsing
	Cannot adjust to sudden muscular demands	
	Pulp recession; variable pain threshold	Ask patient before administering anesthesia; the patient may not need it
	Reduction in growth and repair processes	Provide as little trauma to gingiva as possible during instrumentation
	Decreased resistance to infection	
	Healing slowed	Suggest postoperative care procedures to promote healing
	Inability to recover readily from stresses and strains	At completion of appointment, straighten chair back slowly and let patient sit up for short time before dismissing; assist out of chair
	Unsteadiness; tendency to postural hypotension	

TABLE 14.10. Characteristics Affecting Instruction for the Geriodontic Patient

Characteristics	Suggested Relation to Patient Instruction
Tendency for introspection; desire for attention	Patience needed in taking time to listen to complaints and accounts of past experiences
Feelings of insecurity Deprivation of physical capabilities Touchy sensitiveness, exaggerated imaginary or real pains, or attitudes of suspicion	Sympathetic understanding needed Build up self-confidence
Resistance to change; tendency to maintain fixed habits	Should not attempt to change all lifelong habits, only detrimental habits
Vision impaired	For the patient who wears prescription eyeglasses, make sure the glasses are worn while instruction is being given Recommend that eyeglasses be worn at home while performing plaque control procedures

continued

Hearing impaired; loss of sensitivity to higher tones	Speak distinctly in normal voice; look directly at patient while speaking—many are lip readers
Slowing of voluntary responses Slowing of speed of thought associations Difficulty in timing sequential events; skills become separate movements, as by a child Least comfortable when must respond quickly to demanding sequential stimuli Rate of learning changed, ability to learn not changed Changes in speed of vocalization	Make suggestions gradually, over a series of appointments Do not demand learning a completely new procedure; adapt procedure already used Guide patient's demonstration of toothbrushing to prevent embarrassment Do not expect perfection; go slowly, anticipate difficulties, give cues, clues Distinguish between slowness of learning and inability to learn
Memory shortened, mainly the result of lack of attention, lack of interest, or more selection of what patient wants to remember	Use motivating factors carefully; provide written instructions; spoken instructions may be forgotten or misunderstood
Need for personal achievement	Help patient gain sense of accomplishment; commend for any success, however minor Never compare the patient's condition with that of other patients

TABLE 14.11. Effects of Medications

Effect of Medication Adjust Procedure	Drug Classes Involved
Abnormal hemostasis	Aspirin Warfarin (Coumadin) Dipyridamole
Need to minimize vasoconstrictor use	Antiarrhythmics Cardiac glycosides Sublingual and systemic nitrates Tricyclic antidepressants
Decreased tolerance for stress	Beta-blockers Calcium-channel blockers Cardiac glycosides Sublingual and systemic nitrates
Altered host resistance	Long-term antibiotics Insulin Oral hypoglycemics Systemic corticosteroids
Xerostomia	Antianxiety agents Anticholinergics Antidepressants Antihistamines/decongestants Antihypertensives Antiparkinsons Antipsychotics Chemotherapy agents Diuretics
Movement disorders	Antipsychotics Levodopa Lithium
Gingival overgrowth	Phenytoin Nifedipine Cyclosporine

Adapted from Levy, S.M., Baker, K.A., Semla, T.P., and Kohout, F.J.: Use of Medications with Dental Significance by a Noninstitutionalized Elderly Population, *Gerodontics, 4,* 119, June, 1988.

TABLE 14.12.   Common Impairments Associated with Alzheimer's Disease

Early stage
Forgetfulness
Personality changes
Employment performance
   difficulty
Social withdrawal
Apathy
Errors in judgment
Inattentiveness
Personal hygiene neglect

Middle stage
Disorientation
Loss of coordination
Restlessness/anxiety
Language difficulty
Sleep pattern disturbance
Progressive memory loss
Catastrophic reactions
Pacing

Advanced stage
Profound comprehension
   difficulty
Gait disturbances
Bladder and bowel incontinence
Hyperoralia
Inability to recognize family
   members
Seizures
Aggression
Lack of insight into deficits

Terminal stage
Physical immobility
Contractures
Dysphagia
Emaciation
Mutism
Pathologic reflexes
Unawareness of environment
Total helplessness

Reprinted with permission from Fabiszewski, K.J.: Caring for the Alzheimer's Patient, *Gerodontology, 6,* 53, Summer, 1987, © Beech Hill Enterprises, Inc.

TABLE 14.13. Edentulous Patient Care and Factors (See Tables 10.2–10.4)

Bone	Residual ridges remodel continuously after teeth extraction Alveolar bone undergoes resorption (varies with individual) Major bony changes occur during first year after extraction, but continuation of change occurs throughout life Mandibular bone loss is greater than maxilla (38)
Mucous membrane	Support (cushioning) effect for the denture depends on the makeup of the submucosa and differs in various parts of the mouth
New dentures counseling	Clearly outline procedures and treatment Follow through initial postinsertion appointment (instruction on denture care, tissue management, maintenance/examination appointment [at least annually]) Occasionally dentures must be constructed for children to replace primary teeth or permanent teeth (congenital conditions, rampant decay, trauma), the parent or caregiver must take part in the counseling sessions
Postinsertion care	Immediate denture: leave in place 24 to 48 hours; upon return to facility, denture is removed, mouth is rinsed, and instructions are given for future care New dentures over healed ridges: series of adjustment appointments, first appointment within 48 hours after insertion, review care instructions over several periods (39); See Table 10.4

continued

Denture-related oral changes	Alveolar ridge remodeling (40): residual ridge size reduction may cause loss of denture support, facial height, and lip support, increased chin prominence, temporomandibular joint manifestation, and occlusal disharmony
	Patient adaption to bone changes by compensating adjustments in denture wear and management or through commercial products (adhesives, self-reline), which may be detrimental and cause further damage (41)
	Dentures need relining, rebasing, or reconstruction periodically
	Oral mucosa
	Tissue reactions vary among individuals
	Influencing factors: systemic conditions that alter host response; aging; denture and tissue hygiene; constant denture wearing; xerostomia; fit and occlusion of denture
	Xerostomia: influences denture retention and tissue lubrication, reduces resistance of oral mucosa to trauma and infection
	Sensory changes: may decrease tactile sensitivity to small objects, alteration of taste (plaque retention on denture can alter taste also)
Denture-induced oral lesions	Thorough intraoral examination should be done whether or not the patient presents with any symptoms
	Principal causes of lesions under dentures: infection, trauma, ill fit, inadequate oral hygiene, constant denture wear (no tissue relief; should be removed for part of every 24 hours)

continued

TABLE 14.13. Edentulous Patient Care and Factors (See Tables 10.2–10.4)

Inflammatory lesions:

Localized (sore spots): isolated red inflamed area, sometimes ulcerated, trauma from ill fit, rough spot on denture, tongue bite

Generalized: "denture sore mouth," "denture stomatitis"

Generalized redness over denture-supporting tissues; pain or burning sensation may be present (more frequent in maxilla)

Contributing factors: trauma from fit, occlusion, or parafunction habits; inadequate denture hygiene and mucosa care; chemotoxic effect from residual cleansing paste or solution, allergy to denture base (rare); constant denture wear without relief for tissues; self-treatment with commercial products for relining; systemic influence on tissue tolerance to trauma and lowered infection resistance; *Candida albicans* infection (42)

Ulcerative lesions: usually related to overextended denture border, should be biopsied if persists longer than expected healing time

Papillary hyperplasia: palatal vault, rarely outside the bony ridge confines, group of closely arranged, pebble-shaped, red, edematous projections; unknown cause, associated with poor denture hygiene, ill-fitting dentures, possible *Candida albicans* infection

continued

	Denture irritation hyperplasia (epulis fissuratum): chronic inflammatory tissues in single or multiple elongated folds related to ill-fitting denture border
	Angular cheilitis (30, 31) See Table 14.8
Prevention and maintenance	Develop good attitude and understanding in patient
	Daily preventive measures: denture hygiene; massage and clean oral mucosa; rest for tissue, nutrition, and dietary care; xerostomia relief (saliva substitute if needed); dental caries control of overdenture wearers
	Professional supervision: adjustment appointments, relining, rebasing, remake within the first year, annual appointments thereafter—high-risk patients more frequently
	Maintenance appointment: review history, vital signs; intraoral and extraoral examination, examine and clean dentures; review care instructions as needed, examine oral tissues and fit of denture, treat as needed
	Denture marking for identification (required by law in most states in the U.S. and in some countries) (43)

TABLE 14.14. Categories of Oral and Maxillofacial Treatment

Dentoalveolar surgery
  Exodontics
  Impacted tooth removal
  Alveolar bone surgery: alveoloplasty
Infections
  Abscesses
  Osteomyelitis
Traumatic injury
  Fractures of jaws, zygoma
  Fracture of teeth, alveolar bone
Neoplasms
  Cysts
  Tumors
Dental implant placement
Preprosthetic reconstruction
  Maxillofacial prosthetics
Orthognathic surgery
  Prognathism correction
  Facial esthetics
Cleft lip/palate
Temporomandibular disorders (TMD)
Salivary gland obstruction

TABLE 14.15. Oral and Maxillofacial Surgery

Patient preparation: dental hygiene objectives	Reduce oral bacterial count: promotes aseptic field, reduces postoperative infection
	Reduce gingival inflammation, improve tissue tone: less local bleeding during surgery, promotes postoperative healing
	Calculus removal: removes plaque retention sources, prevents interference of surgical instrument placement, prevents calculus pieces from breaking off during surgery (may be inhaled or contaminate surgical site or socket)
	Instruction on preoperative personal oral care procedures
	Nutrition and dietary counseling
	Explanation of preoperative preparation directions
	Patient motivation
Possible patient personal factors	Apprehension and fear
	Impatience: difficulty understanding need for oral hygiene procedures prior to surgery
	Shame (appearance, neglect)
	Resignation (inevitability, lack of appreciation of natural teeth)
	Discouragement
	Resentment (work time loss, financial aspects, inconvenience, discomfort)

continued

TABLE 14.15. Oral and Maxillofacial Surgery

Dental hygiene care: preoperative	Review histories, treatment plan
	Instruction and counseling; bacterial plaque control, nutrition, and diet (44)
	Instrumentation
	Scaling
	Stain removal: contraindicated for enlarged, inflamed, sensitive gingiva; deep pockets, profuse hemorrhage
	Postprocedure rinsing: saline or antimicrobial
	Follow-up evaluation of tissue response pre- and post-surgery
	Preoperative instructions (45, 46)
	Explanation of general procedures of anesthesia and surgery
	Provide printed instructions
	Food and liquid intake
	Alcohol and medication restrictions
	Transport to and from the appointment
	Procedures for the night before surgery
	Personal items: clothing, care of contact lenses, prostheses

continued

Postoperative care   Immediate instructions: printed

Bleeding control

gauze sponge over surgical site for ½ hr

at home: gauze sponge or cold wet teabag for ½ hr

Rinsing: no rinsing for 24 hrs after surgery; warm salt water after tooth brushing and every 2 hrs thereafter

Plaque control: thorough brushing, avoid surgical site

Rest: avoidance of strenuous exercise for 24 hrs; keep mouth from excessive movement; 8 to 10 hrs of sleep nightly

Diet: high protein, liquid or soft; plenty of water and fruit juices; avoid excess chewing

Pain: follow oral surgeon's directions

Swelling: apply icepack 15 min on, 15 or 30 min off as directed by oral surgeon

Complications

provide telephone numbers

complications may include: uncontrollable pain, excessive bleeding, temperature rise, difficulty in opening mouth, unusual swelling a few days after surgery

Dental hygiene participation: suture removal; irrigation of sockets; personal care instructions; diet supervision

TABLE 14.16. Intermaxillary Fixation Dental Hygiene Care

Problems	Development of gingivitis or periodontal complications
	Gingivitis can develop in 9 to 19 days (47)
	Lack of normal stimulation to periodontium circulation
	Reduction of cleansing effects of tongue, lips, and facial muscle actions
	Difficult plaque control due to tender, sensitive gingiva
	Dental caries: limited cariogenic foods for liquid or soft diet make diet planning difficult
	Loss of appetite: monotonous liquid or soft diet can lead to weight loss and lowered physical resistance, which may result in secondary infections
	Mouth opening difficulty: compromises effectiveness of toothbrushing, muscular trismus after appliance removal
Instrumentation	Preoperative: removal of gross calculus if possible before wiring or placement of splints, trauma may prevent access
	During treatment: limited access, facial aspects only; need to use continuous suction during procedure
	After appliance removal: plaque control procedures initiated; complete scaling and planing
Diet	Nutritional needs: promote tissue building and repair (44)
	All essential food elements
	Emphasis on protein, vitamins (especially A and C), minerals (especially calcium and phosphorus)

continued

Usual caloric requirements for patient's age with consideration to the amount of physical exercise and loss of appetite while recuperating

Feeding methods: straw, spoon, nasogastric tube

Liquid diet indications

All patients with jaws wired together

Patients with mouth opening difficulties that hinder insertion of food or manipulation of food in the mouth

Soft solids diet indications

No appliance or single-jaw appliance

After appliance removal for several days to 1 wk

Nonhospitalized patient

Give instruction sheets with specific meal plans

Express nutritional needs in quantities or servings

Show methods of varying the diet

Give recommendations on limiting cariogenic foods

continued

TABLE 14.16. Intermaxillary Fixation Dental Hygiene Care

Personal oral care procedures	Dependent on the appliance: condition of the lips, tongue, and other oral tissues; extent of trauma; cooperation of the patient
	Toothbrushing, however limited, as soon as possible (patient or caregiver)
	Irrigation
	First few days after surgical procedure, adjunct to toothbrushing
	Mouthrinse selection: consult oral surgeon (saline, chlorhexidine gluconate, fluoride)
	Early postsurgical cleansing
	Premoistened swab or toothette
	Very soft toothbrush with suction
	Customized bacterial plaque control instruction using toothbrushes adapted for conditions present and other aids (limited because of access [48]); irrigation techniques
	After appliance removal
	Bacterial plaque control instruction
	Daily self-applied fluoride in addition to fluoride dentifrice

TABLE 14.17. General Surgery Dental Hygiene Care

Prevention	Complete periodontal and dental treatment prior to elective or planned surgery
	Protection against complications related to broken restoration or appliances or tooth or gingival problems
Risk status patients	Infection-susceptible patients Prosthetic heart valves Joint replacements Organ transplant recipients Chemotherapy patients Users of immunosuppressant drugs
	Education/instruction in bacterial plaque control; completion of oral care treatments prior to surgery
Mouth preparation prior to general inhalation anesthesia	Reduces the oral bacterial count
	Possible inhalation of debris and fluids during anesthetic administration or coughing
Long convalescence	Lessened postoperative oral care problems in healthy mouth

---

TABLE 14.18. Oral Cancer

Incidence	Oral soft tissue neoplasm: more than 90% are malignant squamous cell carcinomas (spread by local extension and the lymphatic system)
	Approximately 3% in men, 2% in women
	Most common location of oral tumors: tongue and floor of mouth (48)
	Highest numbers of lip and tongue cancers: men, between ages of 40 and 65 years
	Approximately 2.2% of cancer-related deaths
Predisposing factors (49)	Weakened immunity
	History of syphilis and other infections
	History of herpes simplex and other viruses
	Diet (particularly in colon cancer)
	Long-term exposure to sun's rays
	Tobacco use (50)
	Chronic alcoholism
Preparation of mouth prior to cancer treatment	Restoration of mouth to optimal health prior to surgery, radiation, or chemotherapy
	Condition of the teeth and soft tissues prior to cancer therapy affect the extent and severity of the after effects of the therapy

continued

Reduce oral microbial count, improve environment for surgical procedures, and enhance healing conditions

Preventive bacterial plaque control program

Fluoride therapy

Removal of nonrestorable teeth

Surgical procedures: removal of residual root tips and other subsurface pathologic areas in edentulous areas

Endodontic therapy (essential abutment teeth, prosthetic replacement treatment planning)

Periodontal therapy: scaling, root planing, surgical procedures (time permitting), occlusal adjustment

Restoration of carious lesions

Indications for surgery (51)

Nonradiosensitive neoplasms; neoplasms that cannot be treated by radiotherapy alone

Recurrence of neoplasm in area of previous radiotherapy

Side effects of radiation more severe than healed surgical defects

Neoplasms involving bone, lymph nodes, and salivary glands

continued

TABLE 14.18. Oral Cancer

Radiation therapy[a]

May be the sole treatment or in conjunction with surgery (51, 52)

Effects of radiation therapy (53, 54)

Effects appear during treatment and continue for weeks to months after therapy; other effects may not become evident until months or years after irradiation

Taste alteration (55)

Loss of appetite

Mucosa: mucositis

Most severe in patients with susceptible tissues secondary to alcoholism and/or heavy smoking

Inflammation, edema, ulceration, necrotization with sloughing, fibrosis develops later

May appear as early as 1 wk after the start of radiation therapy

Sensitivity to temperature extremes, pressure

May develop swallowing and speaking problems (55)

Greatest risk: lips, buccal mucosa, soft palate, borders of tongue, floor of mouth (55)

Symptoms disappear a few weeks after radiation is stopped (epithelium will remain thin and more fragile than normal)

Salivary glands: Gland tissue does not recover from radiation damage (55)

Xerostomia: third or fourth day after start of radiation reduction of saliva volume (may be 50–100%) (55)

continued

Saliva changes: mucinous, acidic, less well distributed in the mouth (55)

Mucosal changes: may be prone to cracks and bleeding

Difficulty in speaking, swallowing, wearing prostheses; increased dental caries

Bone

Change in growth potential, lowered resistance to infection; bone changes are not reversible, children may experience altered craniofacial growth (55)

Osteoradionecrosis (ORN):

more frequent in mandible

spontaneous or trauma-caused (tooth extraction, invasive periodontal therapy, intraoral prosthetic appliances) (55)

pain, trismus, exposed bone, sequestration, pathologic fracture, suppuration, halitosis

prevention: lowered incidence with correct pre- and postradiation procedures, maintenance of oral cleanliness and health

Teeth

"Radiation caries"

exposed root surfaces are more susceptible

redisposing factors (xerostomia, plaque control, diet, soreness, changes in oral flora) are the cause, not radiation directly

prevention: aggressive plaque control, fluoride application therapy, fluoride-containing saliva substitutes

continued

TABLE 14.18. Oral Cancer

	Tooth development: affects odontogenic cells in children; tooth bud can be destroyed if irradiated before mineralization has started
	Tooth sensitivity: all teeth may react to temperature extremes, particularly those with obvious decay
	Trismus: may occur 3 to 6 months after completion of therapy
Chemotherapy (56, 57)	Side effects
	Immunosuppressive: inhibits antibody response, induces leukopenia
	Myelosuppressive: depresses bone marrow activity, resulting in leukopenia and thrombocytopenia
	Appetite loss, nausea, vomiting, diarrhea
	Oral complications (58, 59):
	Fewer side effects with optimum oral health maintenance (60)
	Oral complications, most commonly ulceration, in patients with malignancies unrelated to the head and neck (adult—40%; children—90%) (61)
	Cytotoxicity: ulcerations, loss of surface characteristics, higher incidence in younger patients, complicated by nutrition loss factors
	Hemorrhage
	Spontaneous gingival bleeding

continued

Thrombocytopenia

Presence of petechiae

Frequency/severity of bleeding related to presence of mucositis and/or periodontitis, radiation therapy

Infection

Chronic infection: increase in severity, become acute

Oral microflora changes, predominance of Gram-negative microorganisms and fungi (candidiasis most frequent)

Viral infections infrequent; herpes simplex may be reactivated

Patient factors: fear, anxiety, depression; concerns about: treatment, deformity/disfigurement, pain, finances, hospitalization

Explanation to allay fear

Empathy, positive attitude, instill trust, caring

Counsel/assist with changing detrimental habits; refer to support and/or professional groups

Bacterial plaque control

Nutrition and diet counseling

Instruction on care of dental prostheses

Instrumentation

Ideally, complete periodontal treatment prior to cancer treatment; excessive tissue manipulation a few days prior to surgery is contraindicated

Dental hygiene care

continued

TABLE 14.18. Oral Cancer

Scaling and root planing
Removal of rough and overhanging margins, all restorations finished
Fluoride
Daily use of fluoride dentifrice
Daily use of fluoride gel (custom tray; brush-on after regular brushing) (55)
Saliva substitute: no restriction on use frequency; contraindicated for patients on low-sodium diet
Maintenance
Emphasis on daily oral hygiene home care
Daily examination of oral mucosa, supervision of gingival and dental health during therapy,
    weekly after completion of therapy, then monthly as conditions warrant
Consult with patient's physician/oncologist concerning premedication if on immunosuppressive
    drugs, scaling and root planing completion, probing[a]
Review of fluoride procedures
Extraoral/intraoral soft tissue examination
Gingival examination and evaluation
Evaluation of home bacterial plaque control

[a]Consultation with the patient's physician and/or oncologist must be done prior to any dental hygiene or dental treatment.

TABLE 14.19. Characteristics of Benign and Malignant Neoplasms

Characteristics	Benign	Malignant
Cell characteristics	Cells resemble normal cells of the tissue from which the tumor originated	Cells often bear little resemblance to the normal cells of the tissue from which they arose; there is both anaplasia and pleomorphism
Mode of growth	Tumor grows by expansion and does not infiltrate the surrounding tissues; encapsulated	Tumor grows at the periphery and sends out processes that infiltrate and destroy the surrounding tissues
Rate of growth	Rate of growth is usually slow	Rate of growth is usually relatively rapid and is dependent on level of differentiation; the more anaplastic the tumor, the more rapid the rate of growth
Metastasis	Does not spread by metastasis	Gains access to the blood and lymph channels and metastasizes to other areas of the body *continued*

TABLE 14.19. Characteristics of Benign and Malignant Neoplasms

Characteristics	Benign	Malignant
Recurrence	Does not recur when removed	Tends to recur when removed
General effects	Is usually a localized phenomenon that does not cause generalized effects unless by location it interferes with vital functions	Often causes generalized effects, such as anemia, weakness, and weight loss
Destruction of tissue	Does not usually cause tissue damage unless location interferes with blood flow	Often causes extensive tissue damage as the tumor outgrows its blood supply or encroaches on blood flow to the area; may also produce substances that cause cell damage
Ability to cause death	Does not usually cause death unless its location interferes with vital functions	Usually causes death unless growth can be controlled

Reprinted with permission from Porth, C.: *Pathophysiology: Concepts of Altered Health States*, 2nd ed. Philadelphia, J.B. Lippincott Co., 1986.

TABLE 14.20. Vocabulary Terms Used with Patients with Disabilities

Accessibility standards: the ADA prohibits discrimination on the basis of a disability and requires places of public accommodation and commercial facilities to meet requirements of accessibility by removing architectural, transportation, and communication barriers.

ADA: Americans with Disabilities Act (U.S.A. 1991).

Barrier-free: area that is freely accessible to all without discrimination on the basis of a disability; obstacles to passage or communication have been removed.

Behavior modification: an approach to correction of undesirable conduct that focuses on changing observable actions; modification of behavior is accomplished through systematic manipulation of the environmental and behavioral variables related to the specific behavior to be changed.

Behavior therapy: an approach in which the focus is on the patient's observable behavior, rather than on conflicts and unconscious processes presumed to underlie the maladaptive behavior; accomplished through systematic manipulation of the environmental and behavioral variables related to the specific behavior to be modified.

Deinstitutionalization: returning patients to home and community as quickly as possible after treatment rather than housing them permanently or for long periods in custodial institutions; the elimination of mental health institutions, for example, has been made possible (1) by the use of new medications that control the symptoms of illness and (2) by community health centers that serve as support.

continued

TABLE 14.20. Vocabulary Terms Used with Patients with Disabilities

Desensitization: the treatment of phobias and related disorders by intentionally exposing the patient, in imagination or real life, to emotionally distressing stimuli; desensitization of a fearful patient to accept dental treatment might consist, for example, of short exposures to the dental chair, instruments, air syringe, and the sound of a handpiece along with building trust in the dental team members.

Developmental disability: a substantial handicap of indefinite duration with onset before the age of 18 years, attributable to mental retardation, autism, cerebral palsy, epilepsy, or other incurable neuropathy.

Disability: any restriction or lack of ability (resulting from an impairment) to perform an activity in the manner or within the range considered normal for a human being of the same age, sex, and background.

Handicap: a disadvantage for an individual, resulting from an impairment or a disability, that limits or prevents fulfillment of a role that is within the normal range for a human of the same age, sex, and social and cultural factors as the affected individual.

Impairment: any loss or abnormality of psychologic, physiologic, or anatomic structure or function.

Mainstreaming: integration of people with disabilities into their community through programs of rehabilitation; process by which persons with special needs (educational, physical, psychologic) are included within the mainstream of society rather than segregated.

Normalization: making available to all individuals patterns and conditions of everyday life that are as close as possible to the norms and patterns of the mainstream of society.

TABLE 14.21. Impairments, Disabilities, and Handicaps

Impairments	Disabilities	Handicaps
Intellectual impairments	Behavior disabilities	Orientation handicap
Mental retardation	Awareness	To surroundings
Memory, thinking	Motivation	Relates to behavior and communication
Psychologic impairments	Communication disabilities	disability
Consciousness	Speaking	Physical independence handicap
Perception	Listening	Dependence on others
Language impairments	Personal care disabilities	Mobility handicap
Communication	Personal hygiene	Reduced mobility
Voice function	Dressing	Dwelling restriction
Aural impairments	Locomotor disabilities	Occupation handicap
Hearing impairment	Ambulation	Adjusted occupation
Auditory sensitivity	Transport	Restricted because of disability

continued

TABLE 14.21. Impairments, Disabilities, and Handicaps

Impairments	Disabilities	Handicaps
Ocular impairments	Body disposition disabilities	Social integration handicap
Visual acuity	Subsistence	Restricted participation
Blindness	Dexterity disabilities	Socially isolated
Visceral impairments	Daily activity	Economic self-sufficiency handicap
Internal organs	Grasping	Fully self-sufficient
Impaired mastication, swallowing	Situational disabilities	Impoverished
Skeletal impairments	Environmental temperature	
Mechanical and motor	Dependence	
Deficiency of parts	Endurance	
Paralysis	Particular skill disability	
Disfiguring impairments	Task fulfillment	
Structural deformity	Learning ability	
Generalized, sensory impairment	Dexterity	
Susceptible to trauma		

Reprinted with permission from World Health Organization: *International Classification of Impairments, Disabilities and Handicaps*, Geneva, 1980.

TABLE 14.22. Dental Hygiene Care of Patients with Disabilities

Objectives	Motivate patient and/or caregiver
	Contribute to general health
	Prevent need for extensive dental and periodontal treatment
	Aid improvement of appearance
	Make appointments pleasant and comfortable experiences
Pretreatment planning	Preliminary information:
	Medical, dental history
	Information relative to the disability
	Specific information about disabling condition
	Medications
	Muscular capabilities
	Communication capabilities
	Mental capacities
	Degree of independence
	Special needs/requirements needed to treat (portable headrest [63], chair padding, restraints, wheelchair transfer, etc.)

continued

TABLE 14.22. Dental Hygiene Care of Patients with Disabilities

	Consent forms
	Physician/specialist consultation
	Discussion with parent and/or caregiver
	Appointment scheduling
	Special requirements may determine scheduling time, length of appointment
	Transportation requirements
	Allow sufficient time for procedures
	Follow-up appointments according to need, ability
Oral manifestations	Oral diseases are not different from those of nondisabled persons
	Dental hygiene and dental treatment is the same with adjustments for the disability
	Congenital conditions
	Cleft lip or palate; see Table 14.5
	Other craniofacial anomalies
	Tooth defects
	Increased incidence with developmental disabilities
	Variation in number and structure of teeth
	Dentinogenesis imperfecta, amelogenesis imperfecta, enamel hyperplasia, and other anomalies

continued

Oral injuries
   Attrition: common among individuals with cerebral palsy or mental retardation caused by
      bruxism
   Trauma: teeth and soft tissues from accidents related to instability, falling, self-abuse, seizure
Facial weakness or paralysis
Malocclusion: frequent among individuals with developmental disabilities
Dental caries: varied findings cannot support generalization of caries incidence in person with
      disabilities, dependent on the oral health care or lack thereof (64)
Gingival and periodontal diseases (65)
   Increased incidence in individuals with mental retardation or physical disabilities that prevent
      daily self-care
   Individuals with Down's syndrome have a higher incidence of severe periodontal disease with
      earlier bone loss than those with other types of mental retardation
Therapy-related
   Phenytoin-induced gingival overgrowth
   Chemotherapy
   Radiation therapy

continued

TABLE 14.22. Dental Hygiene Care of Patients with Disabilities

Functioning levels	Refers to daily living skills (bathing, dressing, etc.) that individuals can accomplish by themselves, with assistance, or dependent on others for complete care
	Classified as *high, moderate, or low*; also referred to as *self-care, partial care, or total care* (66)
	Other terminology: *supervised, supervised/assistance,* and *maintenance (by others)* (67)
	High functioning, self-care level: able to toothbrush and floss on their own
	Moderate functioning, partial-care level: able to perform part of their oral hygiene needs but need training, assistance, direct supervision
	Low functioning, total-care level: unable to provide their own care; dependent
Dental hygiene care (68)	Parent or caregiver included in all educational/counseling sessions
	Bacterial plaque control
	Adaption of toothbrushing and interdental cleaning techniques and aids
	See Figures 14.1–14.3
	Fluoride
	Daily self-applied fluoride
	Periodic professional application
	Fluoridated water
	Fluoride supplement as needed
	Dentifrice, if able to use

continued

Pit and fissure sealants

Artificial saliva for xerostomia

Nutrition and diet counseling

Instrumentation

 Premedication as needed: antibiotic, sedatives

 Adaption of techniques: external finger and hand rests may be safer for the clinician in some
 instances (69)

 Stabilization: may need to use mouth prop (use precaution)

 Ultrasonic scaler contraindicated for aspiration-risk patients

 Single-end instruments preferrable in case of sudden involuntary patient movement

Regular maintenance appointments

See Figures 14.1, 14.2

Self-care aids

Floss holder handles can be adapted like toothbrush handles

Additional handle adaptions

 Insert handle into foam rubber hair roller

 Quick-cure acrylic grip made from wax impression of patient's hand grasp

Lengthening

 Wood cylinder with handle cemented inside (70)

 Remove head from old brush and affix to new brush handle

continued

TABLE 14.22. Dental Hygiene Care of Patients with Disabilities

Tongue depressors
 commercially available metal extenders with wing nut and bolt (71)
 bicycle spoke, coat hanger fixed with acrylic resin handle (72, 73)
Specially designed toothbrushes that reach multiple surfaces with each stroke (74)
Head movements instead of hand movements to brush
Power-assisted brushes
 Advantages
  Thicker handle and weight make them easier to grasp
  Can be mounted for stationary use
  Can be used with Velcro cuff around the hand
 Disadvantages
  On/off mechanism may be difficult to manage if finger coordination or strength is poor
  Vibration of instrument cannot be tolerated by some patients
  Weight can be a problem in patients with limited arm strength
Removable dental prostheses (70, 76); see Figure 14.4, Tables 10.2, 10.3
 Use handle adaption techniques for toothbrush
 Fingernail or denture brush with suction cups (71)

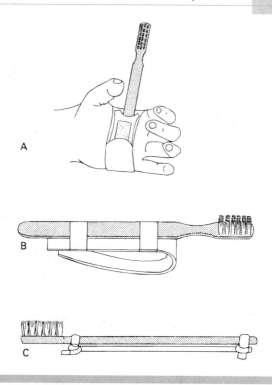

FIGURE 14.1. Aids for patients who cannot grasp and hold. **A.** Adjustable Velcro strap around hand has a pocket designed to hold the toothbrush handle. **B.** Handle of a fingernail brush attached to a toothbrush by adhesive tape. **C.** Rubber tubing attached firmly to a toothbrush handle enables the patient to hold the brush across the palm of the hand. A floss holder may also be held by these methods.

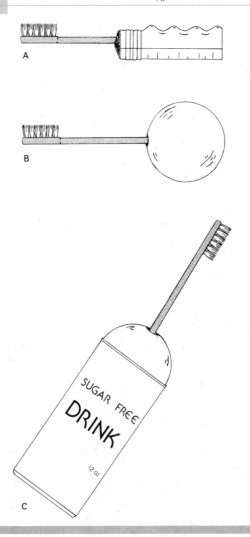

FIGURE 14.2. Aids for patients with limited grasp. **A.** Toothbrush inserted into a bicycle handle grip. **B.** Toothbrush inserted into a soft rubber ball. **C.** Toothbrush in a soft rubber ball inserted into a juice or soda pop can provides a handle of appropriate diameter for patients with limited hand closure.

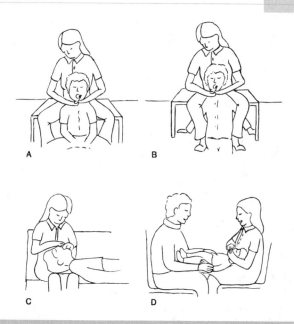

FIGURE 14.3.   Positions for child or disabled patient during bacterial plaque removal. **A.** Patient seated on the floor with the head turned back into the lap of a caregiver. **B.** Patient's arms restrained by the legs of a caregiver. **C.** Patient reclining on a couch with the head in the lap of a caregiver. **D.** Two people participating with a small child in between. One holds the patient for stabilization while the other holds the head for toothbrushing and flossing.

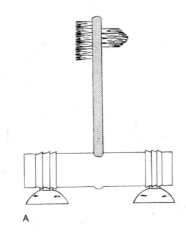

A

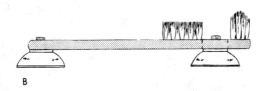

B

FIGURE 14.4. Denture brushes with suction cups. **A.** Denture brush in a commercially available mounting. **B.** Suction cups attached directly to a denture brush. Either brush may be positioned in a sink to aid the person who has one hand or who needs to grasp the denture with two hands to prevent accidental dropping and breakage.

TABLE 14.23. Group In-service Education

Preparation	Customize presentation materials to the audience
	Interesting, appropriate visual aids and content
	Knowledge of functioning levels of clientele
	Assess current oral care procedures of the facility
	Preworkshop visit for observation, review of clinic records; collect baseline data (gingival/plaque index) if possible
Program content	Participants' own plaque control
	Facts about cause and prevention
	Oral examination
	Oral mucosa
	Tongue
	Gingiva
	Bacterial plaque
	Denture-supporting mucosa
	Dentures
	Denture marking procedures
	Mouth care/disease control techniques
	Staff trained to work in pairs (77)
	Plaque control
	Fluoride application
	Denture care
	Saliva substitute
	Record keeping
	Question and answer period
Follow-up and continuing education	Question and answer period
	Review/comparison of gingival/plaque index
	New employee orientation
	Periodic in-service sessions for continuing education

TABLE 14.24. Homebound and Bedridden, Unconscious Patient

Preparation	Consideration of characteristics related to the illness or disease
	Consideration of age-related special problems
	Review of medical, dental history
	Consultation with patient's physician, dentist
	Equipment
	Sterile equipment, instruments
	Disposable items
	Protective barriers: including patient drape, towels to cover pillows
	Instruction materials
	Emesis basin
	Lighting: use portable lighting or adapted available household lighting
	Wheelchair headrest
	Container for prostheses
	Schedule appointments with consideration of patient's daily care routines
Dental hygiene care	Adapt to working with the environment
	Assessment
	Vital signs
	Extraoral/intraoral examination
	Periodontal assessment
	Dental examination
	Personal care instructions to patient and caregiver
	Instrumentation: adaption of patient and clinician positions as needed
	Fluoride: customized to fit special circumstances
	Nutrition and diet counseling in collaboration with patient's physician
	Recommendations for home care; adaptions to toothbrush; interdental care
	Schedule regular maintenance appointments

continued

TABLE 14.24.   Homebound and Bedridden, Unconscious Patient

Care of unconscious or helpless patient	Instruction of caregivers is essential
	Objectives
	Prevent mouth debris from being aspirated
	Minimize oral infection possibility
	Clean mouth, provide patient comfort
	Denture care
	Removal of dentures if patient is unconscious
	Clean and store covered container with water
	Daily change of water or cleansing solution to prevent bacterial growth (78)
	General mouth cleaning
	At least three times daily (prevents dryness and sordes)
	Toothbrushing and flossing if possible; swabs and gauze sponges are not as effective (79)
	Use of power-assisted brush, mouth prop, or toothbrush with suction attachment (80, 81); see Fig. 14.5
	Xerostomia relief
	Frequent swabbing of oral mucosa with saliva substitute or swabs prepared with saliva substitute (82)
	Alcohol- or glycerin-containing products dry the oral tissues and should not be used (83, 84)
Sources for suction toothbrushes	Ora Genics
	5699 S.E. International Way, Unit D.
	Milwaukie, OR 97222
	(*Vac-U-Brush*)
	Trademark Corp.
	1053 Headquarters Park
	Fenton, MO 63026-2033
	(*Plak-Vac*)

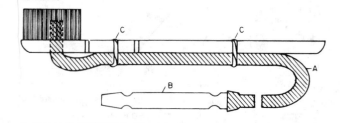

FIGURE 14.5. Suction toothbrush. **A.** Plastic tubing. **B.** Adapter for attachment of the tubing to an aspirator or suction outlet. **C.** Small rubber bands attach the tubing to the brush handle. The plastic tube is inserted through a hole in the head of the brush and extended to a level slightly below the brushing plane.

TABLE 14.25. Physically Impaired Patient (Also See Tables 14.22, 14.24)

Condition	Factors Pertaining to Condition	Dental Hygiene Care Factors
Spinal cord dysfunctions	Signs and symptoms depend on the nature and level of the injury site	Wheelchair considerations
	Impairment or no sensation or motor function below level of lesion	Dental chair positioning to accommodate appliances, prevent hypotension (85)
	Other possible effects	Prevention of pressure sore: change body position of patient at intervals; use padding
	Impairment of voluntary bladder and bowel control	Dental assistant needed for all procedures
	Sexual function impairment	Care of removable appliances includes oral orthosis (mouth-held appliances) (86)
	Impairment of vasomotor and body temperature mechanisms	Disease control: complete preventive program
	Possible secondary complications (85, 86)	Caregiver instruction
	Respiratory difficulties	Consultation with patient's physician before any treatment
	Decubitus ulcer (pressure sore)	Antibiotic premedication for patients with shunt
	Spasticity	Check patient medications; seizures may be controlled with phenytoin, which can result in gingival overgrowth
	Body temperature regulation	
	Infection vulnerability	
	Autonomic dysreflexia (hyperreflexia)—life-threatening sharp increase in blood pressure	

continued

TABLE 14.25. Physically Impaired Patient (Also See Tables 14.22, 14.24)

Condition	Factors Pertaining to Condition	Dental Hygiene Care Factors
	Major causes	
	Trauma	
	Neoplasms	
	Viral or bacterial infections	
	Progressive degenerative disorders	
	Vascular accidents	
	Arthritic spur compression	
	Congenital anomalies or deformities	
Cerebrovascular accident (stroke)	Two-thirds of survivors have some degree of permanent disability	Elective treatment not advised until 6 mo or longer after stroke
	Affected side of face and body is opposite that of brain injury	Consult with patient's physician concerning medical release, medications
	Third leading cause of death in U.S.	Regular appointments may need to be of shorter duration
	Common signs and symptoms	Complete scaling and root planing; bacterial
	Paralysis: hemiplegia or partial paralysis	plaque control instruction (with adaptions);
	Speech difficulty	daily fluoride application
	Difficulty in saliva control, swallowing	

continued

	Sensory: superficial anesthesia or increased sensitivity to pain or touch Mental function: may be unaffected or show slowness, poor memory, loss of initiative Personal factors: personality changes, anxiety, depression	Caregiver instructions
Muscular dystrophies (87)	Progressive severe weakness; loss of use of muscle groups Generally limited to skeletal muscles; rarely involves heart muscle Range from mild to severe types: Becker: mild, later onset Duchenne (pseudohypertrophic) Primarily males, transmitted by female carriers Present at birth, apparent before age of 10 yrs Severe disablement by puberty Rarely survive past 30 yrs	See Table 14.22 Walking assistance: may do better without help—ask patient Watch patient balance whether standing or sitting Facial muscle weakness may interfere with self-cleansing mechanisms, rinsing Oral tissues: the gaping lips effect is similar to mouth breathing Arm and shoulder weakness: power-assisted or adapted handle toothbrushes Caregiver instructions Consult with patient's physical or occupational therapist for advice or assistance

continued

TABLE 14.25. Physically Impaired Patient (Also See Tables 14.22, 14.24)

Condition	Factors Pertaining to Condition	Dental Hygiene Care Factors
	Facioscapulohumeral Male and female equally Onset: average 13 years, after puberty; mild symptoms may appear at later age Facial muscle involvement, particularly obicularis oris Shoulder muscle weakness Slower progression than Duchenne, normal life span Incapacitation later in life	
Myasthenia gravis (88)	Autoimmune neuromuscular disease Weakness and fatigue of symmetrical voluntary muscles Early involvement of cranial nerves affecting facial and oral areas Onset Early peak: age 20, women twice more frequently than men	Short appointment duration early in day in conjunction with medication schedule Weakness increases with activity Frequent maintenance appointments to control and eliminate oral infection Be prepared for respiratory emergency Dental assistant to monitor vital signs, provide suction

continued

Late adult: more males than females

Precipitating factors affecting severity of muscular
  involvement
  Emotional excitement
  Surgical procedures
  Sleep loss
  Alcoholic intake
  Infection

Check patient medication and if taken on
  schedule

Stress reduction procedures

Types of crises (88)
  Myasthenic: undermedication, increased
    severity of symptoms
  Sudden onset: inability to speak, swallow, or
    maintain airway
  Emergency care: suction, provide a patent
    airway, obtain medical assistance
  Cholinergic: overmedication
  Onset: within 30—60 min after taking
    medication
  Increased muscle weakness, excessive
    pulmonary secretion, cramps, diarrhea
  Emergency care:
    Maintain airway, ventilation
    Prompt medical assistance

continued

TABLE 14.25. Physically Impaired Patient (Also See Tables 14.22, 14.24)

Condition	Factors Pertaining to Condition	Dental Hygiene Care Factors
Multiple sclerosis (disseminated sclerosis) (89, 90)	Chronic demyelinating disease of the central nervous system	See Table 14.22
	Progressive disability	Keep patient mentally and physically relaxed
	Nerve impulse transmission interference	Atmosphere should be warm, quiet, comfortable
	Frequent involvement of spinal cord and optic nerves	Frequent short-duration appointments
	Onset	Plaque control with needed adaptations
	Between 20 and 40 yrs of age	Giving patient instructions: patient may respond slowly; may have visual disturbances
	Rare before 15 yrs or after 55 yrs	
	More prevalent in temperate climates	
	Relapses and remissions	
	Precipitating factors	
	Infection	
	Stress and emotional trauma	
	Injury	
	Heavy exercise and fatigue	
	Pregnancy	

continued

	Physical symptoms	Possible oral characteristics
Cerebral palsy	Involuntary motion of eyes	Disturbances of facial musculature
Injury to area of brain affecting motor control	Speech disorders	Malocclusion
Results in paralysis or disruption of motor parts	Muscular coordination and gait changes, spasms, loss of balance	Attrition
Injury can occur prenatally, natally, or postnatally	Paralysis of one or more extremities, occasionally of the face	Fractured teeth
Variety of causes from pregnancy conditions to disease/infection to trauma	Autonomic function difficulty	
	Infection susceptibility, especially upper respiratory	

continued

TABLE 14.25. Physically Impaired Patient (Also See Tables 14.22, 14.24)

Condition	Factors Pertaining to Condition	Dental Hygiene Care Factors
	Characteristics classified by motor activity, area of brain damaged differs for each type (91, 92):	Dental caries may be slightly higher due to predisposing factors of the condition
	Spasticity—motor area of cerebral cortex	Periodontal disease (high percentage)
	Athetosis—basal ganglia	Phenytoin-induced gingival overgrowth
	Ataxia—cerebellum	Difficulty with plaque control procedures, mouth breathing, disrupted self-cleansing mechanisms
	Rigidity	
	Tremor	
	Flaccidity	Special adaptations for plaque control
	Mixed—combinations of the six types	Inability to communicate does not mean lack of comprehension
	Other conditions that may occur	Severe management patients may need general anesthesia in a hospital setting for dental treatment
	Mental retardation—50%	
	Learning disabilities	
	Seizures	Caution during instrumentation because sudden movements can injure both clinician and patient
	Sensory disorders	

continued

Bell's palsy	Paralysis of the facial muscles innervated by the facial or seventh cranial nerve	Dental assistant needed during procedures
		Premedication, sedation, restraining procedures may be needed
	Occurrence:	Caregivers can give suggestions for management of patient
	Relatively rare; incidence increases with each decade of life	Instruction and frequent appointments to supplement home care for damaged side
	Before age 50: frequency more female	Caution when anesthesia used for opposite side (sensory responses are still intact if only the seventh cranial nerve is involved)
	After age 50: frequency more male	Protective eyewear for patient because of compromised ability to close lid
	Cause unknown, possible agents implicated:	
	Bacterial and viral infections	
	Trauma from tooth extraction	
	Surgery of the parotid gland area	

continued

TABLE 14.25. Physically Impaired Patient (Also See Tables 14.22, 14.24)

Condition	Factors Pertaining to Condition	Dental Hygiene Care Factors
	Characteristics (93):	
	Abrupt weakness or paralysis of facial muscles on one side	
	Usually without preceding pain	
	Corner of mouth droops, uncontrollable salivation, drooling	
	Cannot close eyelid, watering of eye	
	Speech and mastication difficulties	
	Return to normal function within a month, often a spontaneous recovery; some may have residual effects or permanent paralysis	
Parkinson's disease (paralysis agitans, Parkinson's syndrome, Parkinsonism)	Progressive disorder of central nervous system	Facial and oral characteristics
	Occurrence: primarily middle-aged and older individuals, higher incidence in males	Fixed, mask-like expression with diminished eye blinking
	Cause unknown	Lips, tongue, neck tremor
	Degeneration of neurons in substantia nigra of basal ganglia controlling posture, support	Difficulty in swallowing
		Excess salivation and drooling

continued

and voluntary motion; severe deficiency of dopamine

Characteristics

Bent body posture, head; general stiffness

Motion, responses slowed

Difficulty keeping balance

Slow, shuffling gait

Tremor in one or both hands

Intellect seldom affected except in advanced cases

Special adaptations for plaque control

See Tables 14.8, 14.22

Arthritis

Joint inflammation, acute or chronic, localized or generalized

Polyarthritis—many joints involved

Rheumatoid arthritis (94):

Chronic, immunologic systemic disease

Inflammation of joints occurs in exacerbations and remissions

Onset: usually between ages 20 and 40, may occur at any age; more women are affected

Presence of joint prostheses requires antibiotic premedication (95)

Temporomandibular joint may be involved and require adaptations for treatment

Check on medications, over the counter as well as prescription, which may cause excess bleeding during treatment

Adaptations for plaque control devices

continued

TABLE 14.25. Physically Impaired Patient (Also See Tables 14.22, 14.24)

Condition	Factors Pertaining to Condition	Dental Hygiene Care Factors
	Juvenile rheumatoid arthritis	
	Children under 16 yrs of age	
	Onset more acute; prolonged fever, enlargement of spleen, and lymph nodes	
	Inflammation of many joints may appear after a few weeks	
	May have complete remission, increasing disability, or have mild symptoms persisting for years	
	Degenerative joint diseases (DJD)	
	Also called osteoarthritis	
	Affects weight-bearing joints	
	Inflammation is not the basic joint problem	
	Onset between 50 and 70 yrs of age	
	Up to 85% of individuals over age 70 have evidence of DJD	

continued

Scleroderma (progressive, systemic sclerosis)	Autoimmune disease of connective tissue Overproduction of collagen Onset usually between ages 30 and 50 but can affect any age group, including infants 2 to 5 times more common in females **General characteristics** May be localized, involving only the skin or generalized, involving all body organs Joints: pain, swelling, stiffness of fingers and knee joints Polyarthritis, similar to rheumatoid Skin: immobility and rigidity; hard and fixed; ivory-white, yellow, or gray, may have brown pigmentation in late stages Face: When affected is mask-like and expressionless	**Oral characteristics (96):** Lips: thin, rigid, with oral stricture, difficulty opening and closing Mucosa: thin, pale, tender, rigid; poor healing capacity Gingiva: pale, unusually firm Tooth mobility is common Marked widening of periodontal ligament spaces (sometimes considered pathognomonic for scleroderma) Mastication is difficult Limited movement of temporomandibular joint Tongue may be immobile Speech is difficult Oral treatment and self-care are difficult to perform Patients are sensitive to cold, dampness, stress, undue emotional tension, fatigue Major efforts should be made to preserve health of teeth and gingiva to prevent need for extensive treatment

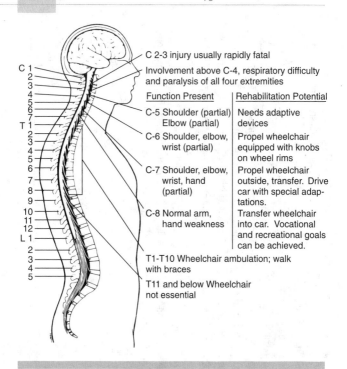

C 2-3 injury usually rapidly fatal

Involvement above C-4, respiratory difficulty and paralysis of all four extremities

Function Present	Rehabilitation Potential
C-5 Shoulder (partial) Elbow (partial)	Needs adaptive devices
C-6 Shoulder, elbow, wrist (partial)	Propel wheelchair equipped with knobs on wheel rims
C-7 Shoulder, elbow, wrist, hand (partial)	Propel wheelchair outside, transfer. Drive car with special adaptations.
C-8 Normal arm, hand weakness	Transfer wheelchair into car. Vocational and recreational goals can be achieved.

T1-T10 Wheelchair ambulation; walk with braces

T11 and below Wheelchair not essential

FIGURE 14.6. Levels of spinal cord injury. On the left, the vertebrae are designated as C (cervical), T (thoracic), and L (lumbar). The effects of spinal cord injury depend on the level of injury, as shown by the information under Function Present at the specific level. The most severely disabled patient has a lesion above level C6. (Reprinted with permission from Smeltzer, S.C. and Bare, B.G.: *Brunner and Suddarth's Textbook of Medical-Surgical Nursing*, 7th ed. Philadelphia, J.B. Lippincott Co., 1992, p. 1739.)

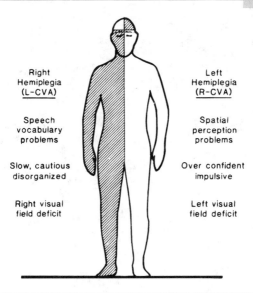

FIGURE 14.7. Cerebrovascular accident (stroke). Right hemiplegia is the result of left-side brain damage; left hemiplegia results from right-side brain damage.

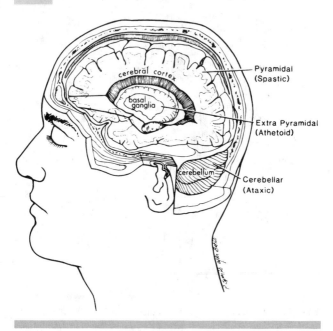

FIGURE 14.8. Cerebral palsy. Shown are the major parts of the brain involved in each of the three major types of cerebral palsy—spastic, athetoid, and ataxic. (Reprinted with permission from Bleck, E.E. and Nagel, D.A.: *Physically Handicapped Children. A Medical Atlas for Teachers.* New York, Grune & Stratton, 1975.)

TABLE 14.26. Sensory Disability and Dental Hygiene Care

Disability	Dental Hygiene Factors

Visual impairment	Totally blind
	  No unique characteristics except inability to see
	  Patient relies on other senses to compensate for sight loss
	  Speak before touching patient
	  Verbal communication and tone of voice convey information
	  Explanation of each procedure in detail using other sensory descriptive terms: taste, feel, sound
	  Allow patient to handle instruments that are not hazardous
	  Tell patient when you will be using power-driven instruments, air syringes
	  Guide dogs: do not distract by speaking or touching it
	  Give clear and concise instructions for plaque control using the patient's mouth for demonstration
	Partially sighted
	  Can use same techniques as with totally blind
	  Positioned patient for best vision when giving plaque control instruction
	  Avoid glare of light into eyes
	  Chair positioned too far back may cause discomfort for a patient with glaucoma
	  Do not expect patient to see fine detail

Hearing impairment	Modes of communication (97):
	  Sign language
	  Finger spelling
	  Oral communication: combination of speech, residual hearing, speech, reading
	  Speech reading (lip reading)

continued

TABLE 14.26. Sensory Disability and Dental Hygiene Care

Disability	Dental Hygiene Factors
	Writing on paper or slate may be method of choice for communication or the use of caregiver or sign language interpreter
	Hearing aid
	Do not touch when the device is operating; some devices react with a high-pitched sound if too near
	Ask patient to turn off device when power-driven instruments are used, especially an ultrasonic scaler
	Partial hearing ability
	Speak clearly, distinctly
	Eliminate interfering noises as much as possible
	Speech Reader
	Face patient directly
	Speak in normal tone; do not raise voice; pause more frequently
	Use alternate words if not understood
	Write proper names or unusual words if not understood
	Sign language: use same techniques as speech reader
	General suggestions
	Use clipboard with large paper, clear writing for written communication
	Do not startle patient by tapping to gain attention
	Plan in advance for a signal patient can use to convey reaction or discomfort
	Teach by demonstration
	Written appointment card
	Use judgement in prolonging conversation; some tire easily, others enjoy communicating

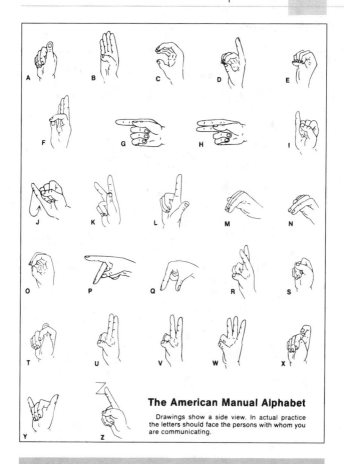

The American Manual Alphabet

Drawings show a side view. In actual practice the letters should face the persons with whom you are communicating.

FIGURE 14.9.   American manual alphabet. Fingerspelling is used in combination with signs and lip reading. (Reprinted with permission from Riekehof, L.L.: *The Joy of Signing,* Second Edition, Gospel Publishing House, Springfield, Missouri. Copyright 1987.)

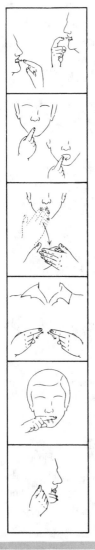

TEETH

Run the tip of the bent index finger across the teeth.
Usage: strong white *teeth*.

TONGUE

Touch the tip of the tongue with the index finger.
Usage: A look at your *tongue* tells the doctor something.

MOUTH

Point to the mouth.
Usage: The dentist looked into my *mouth*.

LIPS

Trace the lips with the index finger.
Usage: Your *lips* are easy to read.

GOOD, WELL

Touch the lips with the fingers of the right hand and
then move the right hand forward placing it palm up in
the palm of the left hand.
Origin: It has been tasted and smelled and offered as
acceptable.
Usage: *good* food; doing *well* at work.

PAIN, ACHE, HURT

The index fingers are jabbed toward each other several
times.
Note: This sign is generally made in front of the body
but may be placed at the location of the pain, as:
headache, toothache, heartache, etc.
Usage: suffered *pain* after the accident; *aching* all over;
    my knee *hurts*; have an *earache*.

TOOTHBRUSH

Using the index finger as a brush, imitate the motion of
brushing the teeth.
Usage: *brushing teeth* twice a day.

DAILY, EVERY DAY

Place the side of the "A" hand on the cheek and rub it
toward the chin several times.
Origin: Indicating several tomorrows.
Usage: *daily* bread.
    drive to work *every day*.

FIGURE 14.10. Examples of signing. Selected words that
may be used during a patient's dental appointment. (Reprinted with
permission from Riekehof, L.L.: *The Joy of Signing*, Second Edition,
Gospel Publishing House, Springfield, Missouri. Copyright 1987.)

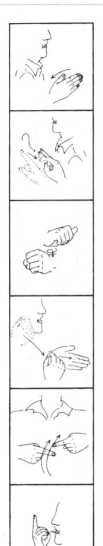

ASK, REQUEST

Place the open hands palm to palm and draw them toward the body.
Origin: Hands held as in prayer.
Usage: *Ask* for help. What is your *request?*

QUESTION

Draw a question mark in the air with the index finger; draw it back and direct it forward as if placing the dot below the question mark.
Usage: That *question* is hard to answer.

ENGAGEMENT, APPOINTMENT, RESERVATION

Make a small circle with the right "A" hand and then place the wrist on the wrist of the left "S" which is facing right.
Origin: Indicating one is bound.
Usage: a dinner *engagement* tonight.
       a 4 o'clock *appointment.*
       a plane *reservation.*

SECRETARY

Take an imaginary pencil from the ear, write into the left hand and make the "PERSON" ending.
Origin: A person who takes notes.
Usage: Teri is my good *secretary.*

COME

Index fingers rotating once around each other move toward the body. Or, use the open hand in a beckoning motion.
Origin: Using the hands in a natural motion.
Usage: When can you *come* to my home?
       Come, I'm waiting for you. (Use second description.)

DENTIST

Place the right "D" at the teeth.
Origin: The initial sign at the teeth.
Usage: Let the *dentist* check your teeth.

FIGURE 14.10.   *(continued)*

TABLE 14.27. Epilepsy and Dental Hygiene Care (See Tables 14.28, 14.29)

Description (99–101)	Term used to describe a symptom or group of symptoms of disordered function of the central nervous system
	Seizure is a convulsive disorder that results from a transient, uncontrolled alteration in brain function, abrupt onset of symptoms that may be of a motor, sensory, or psychic nature
Seizure emergencies (101)	Most likely caused by
	Epilepsy, hypoglycemia, anoxia/hypoxia secondary to syncope
	Local anesthetic overdose
	Precaution and preparation when treating patient with epileptic/seizure history
	Emergency materials/equipment conveniently located
	Have patient remove any appliance or denture during duration of appointment
	Have dental personnel available for assistance in an emergency
	Provide calm, reassuring atmosphere
	Emergency procedure
	Terminate procedure; call for assistance; place medical emergency call
	Position patient: lower chair, tilt to supine and slightly elevate legs
	Move obstacles aside (trays, equipment)
	Loosen belt, tie, collar, necktie
	DO NOT PLACE OR FORCE ANYTHING BETWEEN THE TEETH
	Establish airway, check for breathing obstruction, and provide basic life support if indicated

continued

continued

	Monitor vital signs
	Protect patient from injury
	Postictal phase
	Allow patient to rest
	Reassure patient
	Check oral cavity for trauma
	Complete emergency record
	Discharge patient to hospital, physician, or home
	Follow-up phone check several hours after incident
Precipitating factors	Psychologic stress, apprehension
	Fatigue, sleep deprivation
	Sensory stimuli (flashing lights, noises, peculiar odors)
	Alcohol use: withdrawal from alcohol, other substances
	Aura—warning before seizure
Oral factors	Epilepsy itself produces no oral changes
	Phenytoin-induced gingival overgrowth occurs in 25–50% of individuals using phenytoin for treatment
	(Dilantin hyperplasia, Dilantin-induced hyperplasia, diphenylhydantoin-induced hyperplasia, diphenylhydantoin gingival hyperplasia, Dilantin-induced gingival fibrosis, phenytoin-induced hyperplasia)
	Anterior gingiva affected more than posterior
	Maxillary more than mandibular

TABLE 14.27. Epilepsy and Dental Hygiene Care (See Tables 14.28, 14.29)

	Facial and proximal areas usually larger than lingual and palatal areas
	Rare in edentulous areas, usually associated with sources such as trauma, irritation, or presence of dental implant, retained roots, or unerupted teeth (102, 103)
	Complicating factors: plaque and gingivitis, mouth breathing, defective restorations, large carious lesions, calculus, other plaque-retaining factors
	Effects of accidents during seizures: scarring of lips and tongue, fractured teeth
Dental hygiene treatment	Patient history: include types and doses of medications; history of seizures, type, frequency, severity, duration, precipitating factors; other drugs used to treat epilepsy such as valproic acid may factor in blood coagulation defects (bleeding and bruising) (104); others cause drowsiness
	Treatment of phenytoin-induced gingival overgrowth
	Plaque control instituted prior to phenytoin treatment or decrease gingival overgrowth (105–108)
	Antiplaque agents (stannous fluoride [108], chlorhexidine [109]) can be effective in decreasing bacterial plaque formation and gingival overgrowth
	Scaling—if tissue is fibrotic, shrinkage will not occur
	Consult with patient's physician about possible medication change (other drugs do not induce gingival enlargement)
	Surgical removal of excess tissue (tissue may return to overgrowth stage)
	Aggressive patient bacterial plaque control program

TABLE 14.28. International Classification of Seizures

Partial seizures (seizures beginning locally)
A. Simple partial seizures (without loss of consciousness)
1. With motor signs
2. With somatosensory or special sensory symptoms
3. With autonomic symptoms
4. With psychic symptoms
B. Complex partial seizures
1. Simple partial onset followed by impairment of consciousness
2. With impairment of consciousness at onset
C. Partial seizures evolving to generalized tonic-clonic convulsions (secondarily generalized)
Generalized seizures (bilaterally symmetrical, without local onset)
A. Nonconvulsive seizures
1. Absence seizures
2. Atypical absence seizures
3. Myoclonic seizures
4. Atonic seizures
B. Convulsive seizures
1. Tonic-clonic seizures
2. Tonic seizures
3. Clonic seizures
Unclassified epileptic seizures

Reprinted with permission from International League Against Epilepsy, Commission on Classification and Terminology: Proposal for Revised Clinical and Electroencephalographic Classification of Epileptic Seizures, *Epilepsia, 22,* 489, August, 1981.

TABLE 14.29. Key Words: Seizures

Absence: a generalized seizure of sudden onset characterized by a brief period of unconsciousness; formerly called **petit mal**

Ataxia (ah-tak′sē-ah): failure of muscular coordination; irregularity of muscular action

Atonic: relaxed; without normal tone or tension

Aura (aw′rah): warning sensation felt by some people immediately preceding a seizure; may be flashes of light, dizziness, peculiar taste, or a sensation of prickling or tingling

Automatism (aw-tōm′ah-tizm): involuntary motor activity, such as lip smacking or repeated swallowing

Autonomic symptoms: pallor, flushing, sweating, pupillary dilation, cardiac arrhythmia, incontinence

Clonic: alternate contraction and relaxation of muscle; **clonic phase** is the convulsion phase of a seizure

Consciousness: degree of awareness and/or responsiveness of a person to externally applied stimuli

Convulsion: violent spasm

Cryptogenic (krĭp′tō-jen′ik): a disorder for which the cause is hidden or occult

Electroencephalography (e-lek′trō-en-sef′ah-log′rah -fē): the recording of changes in electric potentials in various areas of the brain by means of electrodes placed on the scalp or on/in the brain itself and connected to a vacuum-tube radio amplifier that amplifies the impulses more than a million times, the impulses move an electromagnetic pen that records the brain waves; a clinical test used for partial diagnosis of epilepsy

Grand mal (grahn mahl): former name for a generalized or major seizure as contrasted with **petit mal** (pĕ-tē′mahl), a minor or relatively mild seizure

Ictal (ik′tal): pertaining to or resulting from a stroke of an acute epileptic seizure

Myoclonus (mi′ōk-lō′-nus): isolated or repetitive shock-like contractions of a muscle or group of muscles; *adj.* myoclonic

continued

TABLE 14.29.   Key Words: Seizures

Paresthesia (par′es-thē′zē-ah): an abnormal sensation, such as burning, prickling, or tingling

Paroxysm (par′ok-sizm): sharp spasm or convulsion, sudden recurrence or intensification of symptoms

Prodrome (prō′drōm): a premonitory symptom; a symptom indicating the onset of a disease or condition; *adj.* prodromal

Psychic (sī′kik): pertaining to the mind or psyche

Seizure (sē′zhur): paroxysmal spell of transitory alteration in consciousness, motor activity, or sensory phenomenon; convulsion

Spasm (spazm): sudden involuntary contraction of a muscle or group of muscles; may be tonic or clonic; may vary from small twitches to severe convulsions

Status epilepticus (sta′tus ĕp′ĭ-lĕp′tĭ cus): rapid succession of epileptic spasms without intervals of consciousness; life threatening; emergency care urgent

Tonic (ton′ik): state of continuous, unremitting action of muscular contraction; patient appears stiff

Tonic-clonic: in a seizure, a sudden sharp tonic contraction of muscles followed by clonic convulsive movements

TABLE 14.30. Mental Retardation and Dental Health (see Tables 14.31, 14.32)

Condition	Factors Pertaining to Condition	Oral/Dental Hygiene Factors
Mental retardation	Significant subaverage general intellectual functioning existing concurrently with deficits in adaptive behavior One of several developmental disorders Mild retardation IQ: 50–55 to 70, third to sixth grade level Can learn practical skills, maintain personal hygiene Moderate retardation IQ: 35–40 to 50–55, can be trained in personal care and hygiene, not completely capable of self-maintenance Severe retardation IQ: 20–25 to 35–40 Some personal care with supervision Profound retardation IQ: below 20 or 25 Nursing care needed	Higher incidence of oral developmental malformations, some specific to particular syndromes or conditions Lips: thicker Teeth: may have imperfect formation, delayed or irregular eruption Periodontal conditions (110, 111): Gingivitis, periodontitis common; more severe in Down's syndrome Greater incidence in institutionalized individuals (112) Habits: increased incidence of clenching, bruxing, tongue thrust Dental caries (110, 111): Preventive factors are the same Higher incidence in noninstitutionalized individuals (110) Severe and profound retardation groups experience significantly higher dental caries rate (110) Basic periodontal therapy: intensive daily plaque control, scaling, frequent maintenance supervision

continued

| Down's syndrome (trisomy 21 syndrome) | Chromosomal abnormality
Incidence in U.S.: 1 in 800 live and stillbirths (113)
Relatively constant combination of characteristic abnormalities
IQ generally under 70; long-term institutionalized individuals may show lower IQ scores
Susceptibility to infection, hepatitis B (116, 117)
Adults age prematurely—many develop Alzheimer's-like dementia with pathologic brain changes similar to those of Alzheimer's disease (119) | Adaptive techniques for both personal and professional care
Mouth may be habitually open with tongue protruding
Lips may be thickened, cracked, and dry
Tongue appears large, generally fissured
Narrow jaw; short and narrow palate
Greater incidence of cleft lip, palate, uvula than general population (114)
Delayed, irregular sequence of tooth eruption
Possible anomalies: microdontia, congenitally missing teeth, fused teeth, peg lateral incisors
Angle's class III, posterior crossbite common
Periodontal disease (115):
Increased susceptibility to plaque and bacterial products
Bone loss, other effects of periodontal disease at early ages
Altered immune system relates to the severity of periodontal infection (leukocyte function) (116)
NUG superimposed, over gingivitis and periodontitis is more prevalent than in other types of mental retardation
continued |

TABLE 14.30. Mental Retardation and Dental Health (see Tables 14.31, 14.32)

Condition	Factors Pertaining to Condition	Oral/Dental Hygiene Factors
Autistic disorder (other names that have been used: Kanner's syndrome, early infantile autism, primary autism, infantile or childhood autism, childhood psychosis)	Pervasive behavioral developmental disorder manifested by limited ability to understand and communicate Appears during first 36 months of life There may be an associated diagnosis of mental retardation with an IQ below 70 Three to four times more frequent in males than in females Normal life span See Table 14.32	May be difficult to treat; some may need sedation, general anesthesia, or soft physical restraints (120, 121) Dental care may have been neglected because of problems associated with the condition (122, 123) No specific oral manifestations Staff preparation and orientation prior to appointments to review and discuss treatment, procedures, and information gathered from history and other persons involved in the patient's care Same dental personnel should be involved at each appointment Provide predictable and consistent experiences Environment free from sensory stimuli Use parent or caregiver to assist with experience, teaching, conditioning Use patience, firmness, repetition

TABLE 14.31.   Developmental Disorders[a]

Mental retardation
 Mild, moderate, severe, profound
Learning disorders
 Reading
 Mathematics
 Written expression
Motor skills disorders
 Coordination
Pervasive developmental disorder
 Autistic disorder
Disruptive behavior disorders
 Overaggressiveness, hostility, hyperactivity, inattention,
  impulsiveness
 Poor attention span
 Conduct disorder; delinquency
 Use of alcohol; stealing; destructive acts
Anxiety disorders
 Chronic anxiety, timid, inhibited
 Unrealistic fears of the unfamiliar
 Fear of separation
 Overanxious
Feeding disorders
 Failure to eat adequately
 Pica
 Rumination disorder
Tic disorders
 Tourette's syndrome
 Chronic motor or vocal tic disorder
Speech and language disorders
 Expressive language
 Voice disorder (pitch, tone)
 Stuttering
 Elective mutism

[a]Disorders usually first diagnosed during infancy, childhood, or adolescence.

TABLE 14.32. Characteristics of Autism

A. **Impairment in Social Interaction**
  1. Impaired awareness of others; unable to relate
  2. Lack of social or emotional reciprocity
  3. Rarely seeks comfort or affection even at times of distress
  4. Failure to develop peer relationships appropriate to developmental level
  5. Absent or impaired imitation

B. **Impairment in Communication**
  1. A delay or total absence of spoken language with markedly abnormal nonverbal communication
  2. Abnormal pitch, intonation, rate, rhythm, or stress of speech
  3. Stereotyped and repetitive use of language or idiosyncratic language
  4. Failure to use social or emotional cues to regulate communication
  5. Absent or impaired imaginative play

C. **Restricted Patterns of Behavior**
  1. Insistence on sameness (resistance to change)
  2. Persistent preoccupation with parts of objects
  3. Stereotyped body movements
  4. Markedly restricted range of interests

D. **Abnormal Development Prior to Age 3**
  1. Delays or abnormal functioning in social development
  2. Delays in language used in social communication or play

TABLE 14.33.   Mental Disorders and Dental Hygiene Treatment (See Table 14.34)

Disorder	Oral/Dental Hygiene Factors
Schizophrenia see Table 14.35 (124–127)	Elective dental hygiene and dental treatment is not done during acute exacerbation
	Decompensation during treatment requires immediate referral
	Side effects from medication may persist after dosages are lowered or discontinued
	Patient may have overall degeneration of health factors
	Patient may have concurrent alcohol and/or drug abuse, smoking
	Xerostomia with related problems
	Review medical history/consult with physician and/or psychiatrist
	Decrease stimulation during appointment; keep routine simple and consistent each appointment
Major depressive disorder see Table 14.37 (128, 129)	Patient may lack interest in self-care, omit general health habits
	Side effects of medications include xerostomia, photosensitivity
	Possible loss of taste perception
	Monitor medical history and medication; consult with patient's physician and/or psychiatrist
	Local anesthesia for scaling and root planing, very sensitive, need profound anesthesia
	Use no more than .05 mg local anesthesia with epinephrine (1/100,000) (3 cartridges) (128–130)
	If patient has a suicidal history, keep sharp instruments out of view
	Use care to prevent postural hypotension

continued

TABLE 14.33. Mental Disorders and Dental Hygiene Treatment (See Table 14.34)

Disorder	Oral/Dental Hygiene Factors
Bipolar disorder see Table 14.38	Depressive phase of bipolar disorder has the same characteristics as major depressive order (see Table 14.37) (131) Oral hygiene needs are often unmet Reporting of injuries or illness by patient unlikely Gingival tissues may appear abraded and lacerated Xerostomia may require saliva substitute, daily fluoride therapy, diet modifications Metallic taste may be reported (lithium side effect) Simplify appointment surroundings; do not rush patient (131, 132) Patient may have short attention span (131, 132)
Postpartum mood disturbances (133)	Puerperium (6-week period after childbirth) Degrees of emotional reactions: postpartum blues to psychosis (major psychiatric emergency)
Anxiety disorders	See Tables 14.39, 14.40 Medications: antianxiety (frequently benzodiazepines), antidepressants (134–136) Hypersensitivity of teeth Xerostomia related to medications Oral cleanliness may not be present or may be excessive

continued

continued

Eating disorders

Appointments (137, 138):

Help patient feel in control, explain each step, give short breaks during procedures

Use effective pain control (local anesthesia)

Morning appointments are best; adjust length of appointment; avoid unnecessary waiting

Anorexia Nervosa: see Table 14.41

Patient may be preoccupied with food, weight loss; may exercise excessively

Depression may be apparent

Frequently a high achiever, scholastically motivated, socially isolated, withdrawn, shy

Xerostomia—enamel, cervical cemental dental caries

Perimyolysis, other findings as in bulimia

Medical history review; diet analysis; use of laxatives, diuretics

Record vital signs

Bulimia nervosa: see Table 14.42

Psychiatric compulsive disorder; recurrent episodes of uncontrollable binge eating

Tendency to be socially extroverted; pursues perfection (especially physically through body shape and weight); aware of abnormal eating habits, so may have low self-esteem, guilt feelings (139–141)

TABLE 14.33. Mental Disorders and Dental Hygiene Treatment (See Table 14.34)

Disorder	Oral/Dental Hygiene Factors
	Oral (142, 143):
	Perimylolysis: earliest evidence on smooth palatal surfaces, later on occlusal, incisal surfaces
	Enamel erosion around restoration margins
	Increase in dental caries, particularly cervical caries
	Saliva decrease in quantity, quality, pH (limitation of buffering, lubrication properties)
	Dehydration of oral soft tissues
	Xerostomia
	Hypersensitive teeth
	Oral trauma from implements used to induce vomiting; pharyngeal trauma from swallowing and regurgitating food bolus; possible scarring of fingers or knuckles from vomit inducement
	Parotid gland enlargement may occur 2 to 6 days after binge (related to malnutrition)
	Bruxism
	Taste perception impairment
	Appointments (140, 142):
	Patient instruction in cause and prevention of conditions related to disorder
	Do not brush after vomiting (may abrade demineralized areas)

continued

	Use alkaline rinse of sodium bicarbonate or magnesium hydroxide solution to neutralize acid
	.05% sodium fluoride rinse also used
	Fluoride therapy to reduce hypersensitivity, caries
	Xerostomia: saliva substitutes with fluoride, sugarless gum, or mints
	Advise use of sugarless foods, fluoride dentifrice, rinses
Psychiatric emergencies	Rare in dental facilities
	Most common: panic attack, atypical drug reaction, schizophrenic or manic decompensation (144)
	Be prepared
	Complete medical history, consult with physician
	Be alert to risks, characteristics of disorder
	Stress management techniques
	Knowledge of patient's medications and any that can be used during a possible emergency
	Ready reference of names, numbers of persons responsible for patient's care: case worker, psychiatrist, caregiver/family member
	Know facility emergency procedures
	Management of panic attack patient
	Stay with patient; request staff person to contact person responsible for patient
	Remain calm, firm
	Move patient to quieter surroundings
	Assist with medication when indicated

TABLE 14.34. Primary Mental Disorders: Classification

Cognitive impairment disorders
  Delirium
  Dementia (HIV, Alzheimer's,
    Parkinson's)
  Amnestic disorders
Substance-related disorders
  Drugs of abuse
  Alcoholism
Schizophrenia
Mood disorders
  Depressive disorder
  Bipolar disorder
Anxiety disorders
  Panic disorder with and
    without agoraphobia
  Phobias
  Obsessive-compulsive disorder
  Posttraumatic stress disorder
  Generalized anxiety disorder
Somatoform disorders
  Conversion disorder
  Hypochondriasis
  Body dysmorphic disorder
  Pain disorder
	Factitious disorders
	  Physical symptoms
	  Psychologic symptoms
	Dissociative disorders
	  Dissociative amnesia
	  Dissociative fugue
	  Multiple personality disorder
	  Depersonalization disorder
	Sexual disorders
	  Sexual dysfunctions
	  Paraphilias
	Eating disorders
	  Anorexia nervosa
	  Bulimia nervosa
	Sleep disorders
	Impulse control disorders
	  Kleptomania
	  Pyromania
	  Pathologic gambling
	Personality disorders
	  Paranoia
	  Narcissism

Adapted from American Psychiatric Association, DSM-IV Options Book, 1991, pp. B:2–B:10.

TABLE 14.35. Symptoms of Schizophrenia

Prodromal and Residual Symptoms	Active-Phase Symptoms
Marked social isolation or withdrawal	Positive symptoms
Marked impairment in role functioning (as wage earner, student, homemaker)	Delusions
	Hallucinations
	Disorganized speech
Markedly peculiar behavior	Catatonia
Marked impairment in personal hygiene	Disorganized or bizarre behavior
Blunted or inappropriate affect	Negative symptoms
Digressive, vague speech or lack of speech	Flat affect
	Lack of voluntary action
Odd beliefs or magical thinking	Speechlessness
Unusual perceptual experiences	No pleasure from events that usually give pleasure
Marked lack of initiative, interests, or energy	

Adapted from American Psychiatric Association: *DSM-IV Options Book,* 1991, pp. F2–F5.

TABLE 14.36. Effects of Antipsychotic Medication

Side Effects[a]	Implications for Appointment
Dystonia	Laryngeal spasm; coughing
Muscle contractions	Unable to turn head
Dysarthria	Communication problems
Difficult speech	
Parkinson-like syndrome	Difficult to gain cooperation
Shuffling gait	Patient positioning
Muscular rigidity	Instrument positioning; retraction
Resting tremor (pill rolling)	
Facial grimacing	

continued

TABLE 14.36. Effects of Antipsychotic Medication

Side Effects[a]	Implications for Appointment
Akathisia Restlessness Pacing	Plan short appointments

Akinesia
  Loss of voluntary movement
  Lethargy, fatigue feelings
	Adjust patient position

Tardive dyskinesia
  Involuntary mouth
    movements
	Difficulty in instrumentation
	Wearing dentures difficult or
	  impossible
	Muscle fatigue; may need
	  mouth prop

Anticholinergic effects
  Xerostomia
  Blurred vision
	Dental caries prevention
	Fluoride dentifrice; saliva
	  substitute
	Seeing visual aids

Cardiovascular
  Postural hypotension
  Tachycardia, palpitations
	Have patient sit up slowly and
	  wait before standing
	Monitor vital signs

Sedation
  Drowsiness
	Interfere with patient's daily
	  routine
	Patient may be late; needs
	  reminders

Blood
  Reduced leukocytes
  Agranulocytosis
	Increased susceptibility to
	  infection
	  Oral candidiasis may be
	  present

[a]For additional side effects, see Kaplan, H.I. and Sadock, B.J.: *Pocket Handbook of Clinical Psychiatry,* Baltimore, WIlliams & Wilkins, 1990, pp. 240–251.

TABLE 14.37. Characteristics of Major Depression

- Depressed mood
- Markedly diminished interest or pleasure in all or almost all activities
- Marked weight loss or gain, or decrease or increase in appetite
- Insomnia or hypersomnia
- Psychomotor agitation or retardation
- Fatigue or loss of energy
- Feelings of worthlessness or excessive guilt
- Diminished ability to think or concentrate or indecisiveness
- Recurrent thoughts of death or suicide
- Feelings of hopelessness

Adapted from Potter, W.Z., Rudorfer, M.V., and Manji, H.: The Pharmacologic Treatment of Depression, *N. Engl. J. Med., 325,* 633, August, 1991.

TABLE 14.38. Characteristics of Manic Episode

- Inflated self-esteem or grandiosity
- Decreased need for sleep
- More talkative than usual or pressure to keep talking
- Flight of ideas or subjective experience that thoughts are racing
- Distractibility (that is, attention easily drawn to unimportant or irrelevant external stimuli)
- Increase in goal-directed activity (socially, at work or school, or sexually) or psychomotor agitation
- Excessive involvement in pleasurable activities that have a high potential for painful consequences (for example, engages in unrestrained buying sprees, sexual indiscretions, or foolish business investments)

Adapted from American Psychiatric Association: DSM-IV Options Book, 1991.

TABLE 14.39. Anxiety Disorders

- Panic disorder without agoraphobia
- Panic disorder with agoraphobia
- Agoraphobia without history of panic disorder
- Specific phobia
- Social phobia
- Obsessive-compulsive disorder
- Posttraumatic stress disorder
- Generalized anxiety disorder
- Secondary anxiety disorder caused by a nonpsychiatric medical condition
- Substance-induced (intoxication/withdrawal) anxiety disorder

---

Adapted from American Psychiatric Association: DSM-IV Options Book, 1991, p. B:7.

TABLE 14.40. Symptoms of Panic Attack

- Shortness of breath (hyperventilation)
- Dizziness, unsteady feelings, or faintness
- Palpitations or accelerated heart rate
- Trembling or shaking
- Sweating (clammy hands)
- Choking
- Nausea or abdominal stress
- Numbness or tingling sensations
- Flushes (hot flashes) or chills
- Chest pain or discomfort
- Fear of dying
- Fear of going crazy or doing something uncontrolled

Adapted from American Psychiatric Association: DSM-IV Options Book, 1991, pp. H:1–H:2.

TABLE 14.41.   Characteristics of Anorexia Nervosa

- Refusal to maintain body weight over a minimally normal weight for age and height
- Intense fear of gaining weight or becoming fat, even though underweight
- Disturbance in the way in which one's body weight or shape is experienced

  Places undue importance on body weight or shape in self-evaluation

  Denies the seriousness of the current low body weight
- In females, absence of menstrual cycles when otherwise expected to occur
- Types

  Bulimic type: during the episode of anorexia nervosa, the person engages in recurrent episodes of binge eating

  Nonbulimic type: during the episode of anorexia nervosa, the person does not engage in recurrent episodes of binge eating

Adapted from American Psychiatric Association: DSM-IV Options Book, 1991, p. N:1.

TABLE 14.42. Characteristics of Bulimia Nervosa

- Recurrent episodes of binge eating. An episode of binge eating is characterized by both of the following:

  Eating, within any 2-hour period, an amount of food that is definitely larger than most people would eat in a similar period of time.

  A sense of lack of control over eating during the episode; for example, a feeling that one cannot stop eating or control what or how much one is eating.

- Regularly engages in either self-induced vomiting, use of laxatives or diuretics, strict dieting or fasting, or vigorous exercise to prevent weight gain.

  Purging type: regularly engages in self-induced vomiting or the use of laxatives or diuretics.

  Nonpurging type: use of strict dieting, fasting, or vigorous exercise, but does not regularly engage in purging.

- A minimum average of two binge-eating episodes a week for atleast 3 months.

- Self-evaluation is unduly influenced by body shape and weight.

- The disturbance does not occur exclusively during episodes of anorexia nervosa.

Adapted from American Psychiatric Association: DSM-IV Options Book, 1991, p. N:2.

TABLE 14.43. Alcoholism and Dental Hygiene Treatment

Health effects (150)	Diminished immune response, suppression of immune system defense, increased risk for infection (particularly pulmonary diseases, viral infections), depressed responsiveness to vaccines (especially hepatitis B vaccine [151])
	Alters stomach mucosa, stimulates acid secretion, affects gastric function
	Possible nutritional deficiencies, problems with malabsorption, maldigestion
	Liver damage: cirrhosis, alcoholic hepatitis
	Heavy alcohol consumption increases death rate from cardiovascular disease, increases blood pressure
	Blood disorders: leukopenia, megaloblastic anemia, abnormal iron storage
	Increased risk of neoplasms (150)
	Brain damage (152): dementia associated with alcoholism, alcohol amnestic disorder (Korsakoff's syndrome)
	Reproduction (150):
	Female: menstrual disturbances, secondary sex characteristic loss, infertility, early menopause
	Male: testicular tubule atrophy, testosterone suppression, mature sperm cell loss, feminization, gonadal function failure
	Pregnancy: fetal alcohol syndrome, increased incidence of spontaneous abortion and stillbirth, developmental or behavior problems (153, 154)

continued

TABLE 14.43. Alcoholism and Dental Hygiene Treatment

Dental hygiene care	Possible polysubstance abusers
	Affects all age groups (adolescent, elderly) (155, 156)
	Health/medical history may not reveal alcohol problems; careful presentation of questions is needed
	CAGE questions: four questions; one positive reply can lead to further inquiry (157)
	Have you ever felt you ought to Cut down on your drinking?
	Have people Annoyed you by criticizing your drinking?
	Have you ever felt bad or Guilty about your drinking?
	Have you ever had a drink first thing in the morning to steady your nerves or to get rid of a
	hangover (Eyeopener)?
	Increased risk of oral cancer with heavy alcohol consumers; no other specific oral findings directly
	attributed to alcohol
	Frequently observed characteristics (158):
	Extraoral: alcohol, tobacco breath, body odor; signs of withdrawl; redness of forehead, cheeks,
	nose; acne rosacea; jaundice; evidences of trauma; angular cheilitis
	Intraoral: dry mucosa, lips, tongue; xerostomia; tongue coated, glossitis;; periodontal infection;
	generalized poor oral hygiene; chipped, fractured teeth; tobacco stain; attrition (bruxism);
	caries incidence no greater than usual population's

continued

Gathering of information may serve as a basis for further inquiry/consultation with patient's physician

Monitor vital signs

Check medications: disulfram (Antabuse) (159, 160)

Use nonalcoholic rinses: minute amounts of ingested alcohol can cause an emergency if patient is on disulfram or cause problems with recovering alcoholics

Usual tissue responses post scaling and root planing may be limited

Use caution with power-driven instruments that may cause inhalation of oral microorganisms

Instruction in bacterial plaque control, nutrition, and diet

TABLE 14.44. Cardiovascular Disease and Dental Hygiene Treatment

Classification	Anatomic: diseases of the pericardium, myocardium, endocardium, heart valves, blood vessels
	Etiologic
	Diseases by cause
	Principal causes: infectious agents, atherosclerosis, hypertension, immunologic mechanisms, congenital anomalies
Major cardiovascular diseases	Congenital heart disease
	Anomalies of the anatomic structure of the heart or major blood vessels from developmental irregularities during first 9 weeks *in utero*
	General clinical factors
	Easy fatigue
	Exertional dyspnea, fainting
	Cyanosis of lips, nailbeds
	Poor growth and development
	Chest deformity
	Heart murmurs
	Dental hygiene treatment factors
	Prevention of infective endocarditis
	Elimination of oral disease

continued

Rheumatic heart disease (161, 162)

Complication following rheumatic fever; high percentage have permanent heart valve damage (mitral valve most commonly affected, then aortic valve)

General clinical factors

Stenosis or incompetence of valves

Amount of scarring to valves and mycardium influence heart murmur

Cardiac arrhythmias

Late symptoms: shortness of breath, murmur, angina pectoris, epistaxis, elevated diastolic blood pressure, enlarged left ventricle, increased signs of congestive cardiac failure

Dental hygiene treatment factors

Prevention of infective endocarditis

Maintenance of high level of oral health

Infective endocarditis (161, 163)

Microbial infection of the heart valves or endocardium occuring in proximity to congenital or acquired defects

Subacute infective endocarditis, often referred to as subacute bacterial endocarditis or SBE

Caused by bacteremia that can be created during dental hygiene treatment, surgical procedures (upper respiratory, genitourinary, lower gastrointestinal tracts), or self-induced (any activity that forces bacteria through wall of diseased sulcus or pocket)

continued

TABLE 14.44. Cardiovascular Disease and Dental Hygiene Treatment

Predisposing factors: heart valve damage, infection at portals of entry

Clinical course: symptoms appear within 2 wks (severe fever; appetite and weight loss; weakness; arthralgia; heart murmurs—require hospitalization)

Dental hygiene treatment factors

Patient history must have specific questions related to rheumatic fever, congenital heart defects, cardiac surgery, prosthetic valves, pacemaker, or previous infective endocarditis episode

Prophylactic antibiotic premedication (164); see Tables 5.4, 5.5

Maintenance of oral health: instruction while under antibiotic coverage, before instrumentation, to create a healthier oral environment and reduce incidence of bacteremia

Instrumentation

Reduction of microbes: patient to brush, floss, rinse with antiseptic mouth-rinse

Prevent unnecessary trauma

Hypertension (165): see Tables 14.45, 14.46

Abnormal elevation of blood pressure

Symptom, not a disease entity (contributing risk factor in many vascular diseases or effect/result of underlying pathologic changes)

Primary or essential hypertension: in 90% of cases, idiopathic, predisposing factors (heredity, overweight, race, climate, excess salt in diet, sex, age, stress, cigarette smoking [interrelated with risk factors for atherosclerosis], long-term use of oral contraceptives)

continued

Secondary hypertension: 10% of cases; specific cause such as disorders of the kidney or adrenal or pituitary glands

Dental treatment factors

Postural or orthostatic hypotension can occur when sitting up quickly from supine position, predisposing factor: hypertension medication (166)

Vital signs: blood pressure should be taken at each appointment; for children, once a year beginning at age 3 yrs (165)

Medical history: medications; episodes of headache, dizziness, shortness of breath; memory impairment; concentration difficulties

Diet and nutrition counseling: salt, fat

Tobacco cessation counseling

Hypertensive heart disease (167)

Heart enlargement caused by increased heart load from elevated blood pressure

No specific symptoms; may have hypotension symptoms

Undiagnosed and untreated: severity increases; left ventricular congestive failure

Ischemic heart disease

Acute and chronic cardiac disability caused by arrest or reduction of blood supply to myocardium (imbalance of oxygen supply with myocardium demand)

continued

TABLE 14.44. Cardiovascular Disease and Dental Hygiene Treatment

Often referred to as coronary heart disease or coronary artery disease

Principal cause: atherosclerosis of vessel walls (168)

Predisposing factors: elevated blood lipids, blood pressure; cigarette smoking, diabetes, obesity, insufficient physical activity, stress, family history

Components: angina pectoris, myocardial infarction, congestive heart failure, sudden death

Dental hygiene treatment factors

Medical history: medications, surgery/treatment for heart, vessels

Vital signs

Counseling: diet, nutrition, tobacco cessation

Angina pectoris

Symptom complex/syndrome of chest and adjacent area discomfort from transient and reversible myocardial oxygen deficiency

90% of attacks related to coronary artery atherosclerosis

Predisposing factors: exertion, exercise, emotion, heavy meal, stress

Symptoms:

Characteristic pattern of pain, commonly substernal thoracic, radiating down left arm and up to mandible; duration is seconds to minutes

Possible paleness, faintness, sweating, difficult breathing, anxiety, fear

continued

Dental hygiene treatment factors

Medical history: medications (vasodilator, usually nitroglycerin), history of angina episodes

Vital signs

Have patient bring angina medication to appointment; place it in a readily accessible area (bracket table, counter) in operatory

check purchase date, last usage (potency lost after 6 months out of sealed container)

Procedure for attack

terminate treatment; call for assistance and emergency kit or cart

position patient up comfortably; reassure

administer nitroglycerin sublingually (if xerostomia is present, use a few drops of water)

check patient response; administer second tablet if needed

call for medical assistance if no response after second dose; oxygen administration may be needed

record vital signs, use emergency record

observe recovery, allow to rest before dismissal

keep emergency record in patient's permanent record for reference

Myocardial infarction

Most extreme manifestation of ischemic heart disease: sudden reduction or arrest of coronary blood flow

Also called heart attack, coronary occlusion, coronary thrombosis

continued

TABLE 14.44. Cardiovascular Disease and Dental Hygiene Treatment

Dental hygiene treatment factors

Attack management

sit patient up for comfortable breathing; reassure

administer nitroglycerin

summon medical assistance: call physician, ambulance with paramedic personnel if pain does not

reduce within 3 min after nitroglycerin is administered

record vital signs—use emergency record

administer oxygen

if indicated, apply cardiopulmonary resuscitation

transport to hospital

Counseling for tobacco cessation, diet

Postpone elective dental and dental hygiene appointments 3 mos to 1 yr after attack, until patient's

physician has given release and consent

Congestive heart failure

Syndrome, abnormality of cardiac function causes the inability or failure of the heart to pump blood at a

rate necessary to meet the body tissue needs

Underlying causes: heart valve damage, myocardial failure (result of heart muscle abnormality or

secondary to ischemia)

continued

Precipitating causes: acute hypertensive crisis, massive pulmonary embolism, arrhythmia

Dental hygiene treatment factors

Emergency care for heart failure and acute pulmonary edema

position patient upright for comfortable breathing

administer oxygen

vital signs, use emergency record

reassure patient

get medical assistance—both physician and ambulance

Sudden death: clinical death that occurs within 24 hrs, after onset of symptoms (death within 30 sec is instantaneous death; biologic death takes place when inadequate oxygen is delivered to the brain for 4 to 6 min)

Nearly all sudden deaths are from cardiovascular cause (predominantly coronary atherosclerosis)

Noncardiac examples: cerebral hemorrhage, drug overdose or toxicity, pulmonary thromboembolism

Clinical signs of death: loss of consciousness; no respiration, pulse, or blood pressure; dilated pupils

Emergency care (169)

Immediate oxygen

Basic life support (ventilation, circulation)

Transport to hospital

continued

TABLE 14.44. Cardiovascular Disease and Dental Hygiene Treatment

Cardiac pacemaker	Electronic stimulator: sends specified electrical current to myocardium to control or maintain a minimum heart rate
	External electromagnetic interferences can stop or alter the function (170, 171)
	Newer models have special shielding to protect against interference
	Consult with patient's physician before treating with power-driven devices
	Dental hygiene treatment factors
	Informed consent (172)
	Patient history
	Consult with patient's physician concerning pacemaker, indications for antibiotics premedication, contraindications to treatment
	Position patient to support breathing, circulation
	Consideration of use of lead apron during treatment with electric devices
	Limit dental radiation
	Use manual instrumentation if pacemaker shield information is not known
	Emergency
	Turn off all suspected sources of interference
	Call for medical assistance
	Position patient for cardiopulmonary resuscitation

continued

	Open airway, check for breathing, begin ventilation if needed
	Observe patient
Anticoagulant therapy	Used to prevent embolus and thrombus formation
	Common drugs: heparin (hospital-administered intravenous), coumarin derivatives
	Dental hygiene treatment factors
	Precautions to prevent hemorrhage
	Consultation with patient's physician concerning prothrombin time, contraindications
	Pretest for prothrombin time: within 24 hours before appointment; the safe level for dental hygiene procedures is 1-½ times the normal
	Quadrant scaling and root planing; treat healthiest quadrant first
	Instruction in daily bacterial plaque control
	Local hemostatic measures
	Minimize tissue trauma; control bleeding; do not dismiss patient until bleeding has stopped
	Apply pressure with gauze sponges
	Sutures may be needed
	Periodontal dressing placement
	Check with patient that postoperative instructions are being followed
	Avoidance of vigorous toothbrushing and rinsing for several hrs or next day
	Extraoral ice pack use
	Soft diet, cool food, moderation of activity

continued

TABLE 14.44. Cardiovascular Disease and Dental Hygiene Treatment

Cardiovascular surgery	Completion of all possible dental treatment prior to cardiac surgery Goal to achieve optimum oral health and maintenance by patient Prophylactic antibiotic premedication for patients with prostheses; special regimen for high-risk patients may be needed: check with patient's physician Implanted vascular autographs generally do not need antibiotic premedication: check with physician (173)

TABLE 14.45. Classification of Blood Pressure for Adults Age 18 Years and Older[a]

Category	Systolic (mm Hg)	Diastolic (mm Hg)
Normal[b]	<130	<85
High normal	130–139	85–89
Hypertension[c]		
Stage 1 (mild)	140–159	90–99
Stage 2 (moderate)	160–179	100–109
Stage 3 (severe)	180–209	110–119
Stage 4 (very severe)	≥210	≥120

[a]Not taking antihypertensive drugs and not acutely ill. When systolic and diastolic pressures fall into different categories, the higher category should be selected to classify the individual's blood pressure status. For instance, 160/92 mm Hg should be classified as stage 2, and 180/120 mm Hg should be classified as stage 4. Isolated systolic hypertension (ISH) is defined as SBP ≥140 mm Hg and DBP <90 mm Hg and staged appropriately (for example, 170/85 mm Hg is defined as stage 2 ISH).

[b]Optimal blood pressure with respect to cardiovascular risk is SBP <120 mm Hg and DBP <80 mm Hg. Unusually low readings, however, should be evaluated for clinical significance.

[c]Based on the average of two or more readings taken at each of two or more visits following an initial screening.

Reprinted with permission from *The Fifth Report of the Joint National Committee on Detection, Evaluation, and Treatment of High Blood Pressure.* National High Blood Pressure Education Program, NIH National Heart, Lung, and Blood Institute, NIH Publication No. 93-1088, January, 1993.

TABLE 14.46. Life-Style Modifications for Hypertension Control and/or Overall Cardiovascular Risk

- Lose weight if overweight
- Limit alcohol intake to no more than 1 oz. of ethanol per day (24 oz. beer, 8 oz. wine, or 2 oz. 100-proof whiskey)
- Exercise (aerobic) regularly
- Reduce sodium intake to less than 100 mmol/day (<2.3 g of sodium or <6 g of sodium chloride)
- Maintain adequate dietary potassium, calcium, and magnesium intake
- Stop smoking and reduce dietary saturated fat and cholesterol intake for overall cardiovascular health; reducing fat intake also helps to reduce caloric intake—important for control of weight and type II diabetes

From *The Fifth Report of the Joint National Committee on Detection, Evaluation, and Treatment of High Blood Pressure.* National High Blood Pressure Education Program, NIH National Heart, Lung, and Blood Institute, NIH Publication No. 93-1088, January, 1993.

TABLE 14.47.   Blood Disorders and Dental Hygiene Treatment (see Tables 14.48, 14.49)

General oral factors	Oral manifestations generally exaggerated in presence of bacterial plaque and local predisposing factors
	Oral changes in patients with blood diseases are not necessarily exclusive to systemic blood disorders
	Findings that may suggest blood disorder
	Gingival bleeding: spontaneous or upon gentle probing
	History of problems controlling bleeding
	History of easy bruising, large ecchymoses
	Numerous petechiae
	Marked pallor of mucous membranes
	Tongue papillae atrophy
	Glossodynia
	Acute or chronic infections not responsive to usual treatment
	Severe ulcerations associated nonresponsiveness to treatment
	Exaggerated gingival response to local irritants; NUG characteristics
Anemias classification	Classified into three groups by cause
	Blood loss
	Acute (trauma or disease)
	Chronic (constant slow bleeding from internal lesion)

continued

TABLE 14.47. Blood Disorders and Dental Hygiene Treatment (see Tables 14.48, 14.49)

	Increased hemolysis
	Hereditary hemolytic disorders (e.g., sickle cell anemia)
	Acquired hemolytic disorders (e.g., erythroblastosis fetalis)
	Diminished production of red blood cells
	Nutritional deficiency: inadequate intake, diet; defective absorption (e.g., pernicious anemia); increased nutrient demand (e.g., iron deficiency anemia during pregnancy)
	Bone marrow failure (e.g., aplastic anemia)
Iron deficiency anemia	Oral factors
	Pallor of mucosa and gingiva
	Tongue: atrophic glossitis with filiform papillae loss; when hemoglobin is 10 or below
	Smooth and shiny; glossodynia; secondary irritations from smoking; mechanical trauma; hot or spicy foods
	Treatment with oral ferrous iron in liquid form may stain the teeth
Megaloblastic anemias	Two principal types: pernicious anemia, folate deficiency anemia
	Oral factors
	Tongue
	Atrophic glossitis; burning; pain; inflammation; appearance is flabby, red, smooth, shiny; loss of filiform papillae, sensitive to hot or spicy foods, other irritants; painful swallowing
	Soft tissues may be pale and atrophic; similar appearance to general vitamin B deficiency

continued

Sickle cell anemia (174)	Occurs primarily in the black population and in white populations of Mediterranean origin
	Tests available for screening and diagnosis of sickle cell trait
	Oral factors
	Radiographic (175, 176)
	Decreased radiodensity, increased osteoporosis
	Coarse trabecular pattern with large marrow spaces
	Significant bone loss in children (indicates periodontitis)
	Soft tissues
	May show typical anemia pallor, jaundiced color, pocketing, infection, bleeding
	Need for strict preventive and treatment program
	Dental hygiene treatment factors (177, 178)
	Provide treatment without precipitating a sickle cell crisis
	During sickle cell crisis, only emergency relief treatment
	Consult with physician: antibiotic prophylactic; hematocrit and hemoglobin determination before
	each treatment appointment
	Comprehensive preventive program for minimization of oral infection and etiologic factor control

continued

TABLE 14.47. Blood Disorders and Dental Hygiene Treatment (see Tables 14.48, 14.49)

	Sickle cell crisis: acute form of the disease
	Precipitating factors: may appear any time with or without stimuli; viral or bacterial infections, other systemic diseases, exertion, trauma, temperature change
	Signs and symptoms: severe pain, infarction in various tissues and organs, seizure, stroke, or coma if central nervous system is involved
	Effects: may be reversible to some degree; result in severe physical conditions or be fatal
Polycythemias	Above normal level increase of number and concentration of red blood cells
	Three categories
	Relative polycythemia
	Loss of plasma without loss of red blood cells (dehydration, diarrhea, repeated vomiting, sweating, loss of fluid from burns)
	Contributing factors: smoking, hypertension, obesity, stress (particularly middle-aged men)
	Polycythemia vera (primary polycythemia (179)): actual increase in number of circulating red blood cells, elevated white cell and platelet counts
	Neoplastic condition resulting from a bone disorder
	Occurs more frequently after age 40, more often in men

continued

Oral factors

 tongue, mucous membranes, gingiva deep purplish-red color; gingiva enlarged; bleeding on slight provocation; professional and personal daily oral maintenance can lessen bleeding tendencies

Secondary polycythemia (179): also called erythrocytosis

Increase in numbers of red blood cells caused by

 hypoxia (occuring in residents of high altitudes)

 increase of the hormone erythropoietin (stimulates red cell development in bone marrow), caused by a variety of diseases and tumors

White blood cells

 Leukopenia: decrease in total number of white blood cells (cell production cannot keep pace with turnover rate or when rate of removal of cells accelerates, as in certain disease states)

 Occurrence

  Specific infections (e.g., typhoid fever, influenza, malaria, rubeola, rubella)

  Disease or intoxification of bone marrow (e.g., chronic drug poisoning, radiation, autoimmune reactions, or drug-induced immune reactions)

 Agranulocytosis (180): (malignant neutropenia)

  Rare, serious disease involving destruction of bone marrow (drugs or an autoimmune process are the usual causes)

continued

TABLE 14.47. Blood Disorders and Dental Hygiene Treatment (see Tables 14.48, 14.49)

Oral factors
   Ulceration in mouth and pharynx
   Gingival bleeding
   Increased salivation
   Fetid odor
   Palliative relief only during severe illness: soft diet, soft toothbrushing, possibly using a suction brush
Leukocytosis
   Increase in numbers of circulating white blood cells
   May be caused by inflammatory and infectious states, trauma, exertion (see Table 14.49); most
      extreme abnormal cause is leukemia
Leukemias: malignant neoplasias of immature white blood cells
   Classification: acute or chronic, subdivided by the maturity and type of predominate white cell
      (lymphocytic, myelocytic, or myelogenous) (181)
   Clinical signs and symptoms differ between acute and chronic forms
   Oral factors (182)
      high percentage have oral complications; acute leukemia patients have more problems than do
         chronic leukemia patients

continued

infiltration oral lesions: more pronounced in monocytic leukemia

grossly enlarged, bluish red gingiva (may cover portion of anatomic crowns of teeth)

blunted papillae

soft, spongy consistency

direct drug toxicity (treatment) lesions: use of chemotherapeutic agents

painful ulcerations

spontaneous gingival bleeding

tongue desquamation

xerostomia

secondary infections

bone marrow depression and lymphoid tissue lesions

hemorrhagic manifestations; petechiae and ecchymoses (lips, soft palate, floor of mouth, facial mucosa), spontaneous gingival bleeding on gentle provocation

increased susceptibility to infection: bacterial, fungal, viral, candidiasis is common

Dental hygiene treatment factors

Consultation with patient's physician, hematologist, or oncologist is mandatory

Prophylactic antibiotic premedication

continued

TABLE 14.47. Blood Disorders and Dental Hygiene Treatment (see Tables 14.48, 14.49)

Blood evaluation tests prior to any treatment (see Table 14.48)

Two-way emphasis on aseptic technique

Thorough oral examination to prevent acute problems during chemotherapy

Acute problems during exacerbation

gingival inflammation: palliative treatment—warm saline rinses, nutritious liquid diet with
    supplements, plaque removal with soft toothbrush

scaling when platelet and white blood cell counts permit

posttreatment: control bleeding

diet: first 24 hours, cold clear liquids, then cool soft foods; avoid use of straws

no smoking or tobacco use

avoidance of medications that suppress platelet function (aspirin)

frequent, close follow-up

healing period two to three times longer than normal

candidiasis and other infections

nystatin for *Candida* infection

mouthrinse containing topical anesthetic for relief of pain from oral mucosal ulcerations
    during eating

Oral care during remission: complete preventive, periodontal, and dental care should be completed;
    all measures to obtain and maintain oral health should be instituted

continued

Hemorrhagic disorders	Common tendencies to spontaneous bleeding; moderate to excessive bleeding following trauma or surgical procedure
	Dental hygiene treatment factors
	Moderate to excessive or prolonged bleeding may occur after dental hygiene therapy
	Medical history with questions pertinent to bleeding, bruising tendencies
	Blood disorders; transfusions, previous abnormal bleeding should be followed up with conversational questions
	Consultation with patient's physician concerning recent testing results, need for same-day testing prior to treatment, contraindications, precautions (183)
Hemophilias (184)	Group of congenital disorders of the blood clotting mechanism
	Common types
	Classic hemophilia A
	Hemophilia B or Christmas disease
	von Willebrand's disease
	Occurrence
	Hemophilias A and B are inherited by males through an X-linked recessive trait carried by females (females are rarely affected by hemophilias A or B)
	von Willebrand's disease transmitted by an autosomal codominant trait; occurs in both males and females

continued

TABLE 14.47. Blood Disorders and Dental Hygiene Treatment (see Tables 14.48, 14.49)

Oral factors
  When periodontal infection is more severe, gingival bleeding is common and more extensive
  Personal oral hygiene may be neglected because of fear of bleeding
  Trauma to oral area can result in severe bleeding
Dental hygiene treatment factors
  Prevention and control of bleeding
  May be multihandicapped as a result of internal hemorrhages
  Preliminary evaluation: medical history including hemophilic information; consultation with patient's
      hematologist
  Factor replacement (183) prior to procedures in accord with medical consultation
  Prophylactic antibiotic premedication usually indicated (185)
  Preventive program
    Complete instruction as with any patient
    Proper floss instruction to prevent cutting gingiva
    Aids as needed
    Elimination of oral infections can partially control spontaneous bleeding problems

continued

Instrumentation

Work carefully and thoroughly to minimize tissue trauma and prevent bleeding

Tissue conditioning program—series of appointments

Scaling of small segments one at a time; as tissue heals, root planing can be completed

Probing and periodontal treatment planning may need to be postponed until tissue conditioning is completed

Coordination with medical team; hospitalization for treatment may be indicated

Treatment suggestions

Rubber dam use: thin rather than heavy; Young's frame may eliminate pressure; check clamps for sharp corners; place carefully

Use care in film placement

Bead rims of impression trays

Use caution with high-vacuum suction tips; prevent pulling tissues into tip

Use of periodontal dressing after subgingival scaling and root planing

Never suggest use of aspirin

Frequent maintenance appointments

TABLE 14.48. Tests Used for Blood Evaluation

Test	Normal Range[a]	Causes of Deviations
Hemoglobin	Males: 14–18 g/100 mL Females: 12–16 g/100 mL	Increased in polycythemia, dehydration Decreased in anemias, hemorrhage, leukemias
Hematocrit (volume of packed red cells)	Males: 40–54% Females: 37–47%	Increased in polycythemia, dehydration Decreased in anemias, hemorrhage, leukemias
Bleeding time	Duke: 1–3½ min Ivy: less than 5 min Modified Ivy: 2½–10 min (Mielke template)	Prolonged in disorders of platelet function, thrombocytopenia, von Willebrand's disease, leukemias, aspirin and certain other drug use
Clotting time	Glass tube: 4–8 min	Prolonged in vitamin K deficiency, severe hemophilia, anticoagulant therapy, liver diseases
Prothrombin time (P.T.)	11–15 sec	Prolonged in polycythemia vera, prothrombin deficiency, anticoagulant therapy, vitamin K deficiency, liver diseases, aspirin use
Partial thromboplastin time (P.T.T.)	68–82 sec	Prolonged in hemophilia A and B, von Willebrand's disease, anticoagulant therapy

[a]The normal range varies with the specificity of the technique used. There is also a range variation, depending on the health facility and the laboratory.

TABLE 14.49.   Blood Cells Reference Values

Cell Type	Normal Value	Causes of Increase	Causes of Decrease
Red blood cells	Male 4.5–6.0 Female 4.3–5.5 million/mm^3	Polycythemia Dehydration	Anemias Leukemias Hemorrhage
Platelets	150,000–400,000/mm^3 Wintrobe method 140,000–440,000/mm^3	Polycythemia vera Chronic myelocytic leukemia Sickle cell anemia Rheumatic fever Hemolytic anemias Bone fractures	Acute severe infections Cirrhosis of the liver Thrombocytopenic purpura Acute leukemias Aplastic anemias Pernicious anemia
White blood cells	5,000–10,000/mm^3	Inflammation Overexertion Polycythemia vera	Aplastic anemia Granulocytopenia Drug poisoning Thrombocytopenia Radiation Severe infections

continued

TABLE 14.49. Blood Cells Reference Values

Cell Type	Normal Value	Causes of Increase	Causes of Decrease
Differential White cell count Granulocytes Neutrophils (PMNs)	60–70%	Acute infections Myelogenous leukemia Poisoning Erythroblastosis	Aplastic anemia Granulocytopenia
Eosinophils	1–3%	Allergic diseases Dermatitis Hodgkin's disease Scarlet fever	Aplastic anemia Typhoid fever
Basophils	1%		
Agranulocytes Lymphocytes	20–35%	Certain chronic infections Lymphocytic leukemia Chronic infections Viral diseases	Aplastic anemia Aplastic anemia Myelogenous leukemia Radiation
Monocytes	2–6%	Monocytic leukemias Tuberculosis Infective endocarditis Hodgkin's disease	Aplastic anemia

TABLE 14.50. Diabetes Mellitus and Oral Health (see Tables 14.51, 14.52)

Classification (186, 187)	Diabetes mellitus (DM)
	Type I: insulin-dependent diabetes mellitus (IDDM)
	Type II: noninsulin-dependent diabetes mellitus (NIDDM)
	Nonobese NIDDM
	Obese NIDDM
	Type III: associated with other conditions/syndromes, pancreatic disease, hormonal disease, drug or chemically induced
	Impaired glucose tolerance (IGT)
	Nonobese
	Obese
	Associated with other conditions/syndromes, pancreatic disease, hormonal disease, drug or chemically induced
	Gestational diabetes (GDM)
	Begins or is recognized during pregnancy (previously diagnosed diabetics are not included in this category)
	May be transitory
	Previous abnormality of glucose tolerance (PREVAGT)
	Return to normal glucose tolerance (e.g., after parturition, weight loss)

continued

TABLE 14.50. Diabetes Mellitus and Oral Health (see Tables 14.51, 14.52)

	Potential abnormality of glucose tolerance (POTAGT)
	Increased risk factors: family history or obesity, in mother of neonate weighing more than 9 lbs, in identical twin of diabetic
Periodontal factors (188–190)	Significant risk factor for periodontal infections (lowered resistance, delayed healing)
	Periodontal disease onset may appear at early ages, particularly with insulin-dependent patients
	Findings may include alveolar bone resorption, attachment loss, increased probing depth, increased tooth mobility, possibly with pathologic tooth migration, other signs of occlusal trauma
	Increased susceptibility to periodontal abscess formation
	Severity of tissue response related to bacterial plaque control
	Uncontrolled diabetes
Dental caries	Consistent with age group
	May be slightly higher if decreased saliva/dry mouth or high carbohydrate intake in obese
	Controlled diabetes
	Frequently observed reduced dental caries rate with diet regulation
	Primarily found with poorly controlled or uncontrolled diabetes
Other oral findings	Lips: dry, cracking, angular cheilitis
	Xerostomia
	Mucosa: edematous, red, possibly ulcerated; burning sensations, poor tolerance for removable prostheses

continued

Dental hygiene care	Patient history: additional questions as to medication schedule and type; frequency of medical appointments; last glucose test and results, meal patterns, emergencies that may have occurred related to the diabetes
	Consultation
	With patient's physician prior to any instrumentation
	Degree of control/stability, severity of the diabetes
	Susceptibility to emergency reactions
	Other health problems that may influence treatment
	Indication for antibiotic premedication
	Previous instructions given for diet, care, medication adjustment
	Appointments
	Emphasis on stress prevention and reduction—stress increases glycemia and a tendency toward diabetic acidosis and coma
	Premedication—check with physician
	A person with controlled diabetes is no different than a nondiabetic person
	Presence of periodontal disease may indicate need for antibiotic premedication
	Uncontrolled, unstable diabetes mellitus requires prophylactic antibiotic premedication

continued

TABLE 14.50. Diabetes Mellitus and Oral Health (see Tables 14.51, 14.52)

Time: best in morning, 1-½ to 3 hours after normal breakfast and medication (descending portion of glucose level curve)

Be sure to ask patient if food and medication have been taken

If on long-acting medication, adjust schedule accordingly

Precautions

Do not keep patient waiting

Do not interfere with patient's regular meal/medication schedule

Keep appointments short and stressless as possible

Take other health-related precautions as indicated by patient history

Be prepared for diabetic emergency: keep sugar cubes, orange juice in emergency supplies

Instrumentation

Limit number of teeth to be completed at each appointment

Review and evaluate personal oral hygiene procedures at each appointment

Evaluate tissue response/healing at each appointment

Keep possibility of periodontal abscess formation at a minimum

Avoid undue trauma

continued

	Fluoride	Postpone topical fluoride application if gingival inflammation is present or extensive scaling has been done until gingival tissue shows improvement
		Recommend home use of fluoride
	Instruction	Interrelate oral care with diabetes control
		Bacterial plaque control
		Diet/nutritional counseling in concert with physician instruction
	Maintenance	Regular 2–3 mo. schedule
		Be constantly alert to gingival bleeding, pocket formation
		Soft tissue assessment; attention to areas of irritation
		Routine scaling and planing
Diabetes detection		Early detection and treatment may minimize, postpone, or prevent complications
		Oral health care team responsibility to discover systemic condition before proceeding with dental/dental hygiene treatment to provide safe, effective care
		Patients in diabetes-risk group
		Have close relatives with diabetes
		Women with abnormal obstetric history (spontaneous abortions, stillbirths, babies over 9 lbs. at birth)

continued

TABLE 14.50. Diabetes Mellitus and Oral Health (see Tables 14.51, 14.52)

Obese, particularly age over 40 yrs.
Eye, kidney, coronary artery disease
Early-onset arteriosclerosis
  Postmenopausal women with myocardial infarction
  Men having myocardial infarctions before age 40
Frequent or chronic infections
Symptoms suggestive of diabetes
  Weight changes; weight loss with increased appetite
  Thirst; frequent urination
  Slow-healing cuts, bruises, skin infections
  Pain in extremities (fingers and toes)
  Fatigue and drowsiness
  Recent blood test—test made for blood glucose
  Medical history review at each appointment

TABLE 14.51. Comparison of Characteristics of Insulin-dependent and Noninsulin-dependent Diabetes Mellitus

Characteristics	Insulin-dependent Diabetes Mellitus	Noninsulin-dependent Diabetes Mellitus
Age of onset	Usually less than 25 years; may appear later	Adulthood, particularly older than 40 years; may appear at younger ages
Body weight	Normal or thin	High percentage obese at the time of diagnosis
Onset of clinical symptoms	Rapid/abrupt	Slow/insidious
Severity	Severe	Mild
Diabetic emergency (ketoacidosis)	Common	Rare
Stability	Unstable	Stable
Insulin treatment required	Almost all	Less than 25%
Chronic manifestations	Uncommon before 20 years; prevalent and severe by age 30	Develops slowly with age

TABLE 14.52. Comparison of Insulin Reaction and Diabetic Coma

	Insulin Reaction (Hypoglycemia)	Diabetic Coma (Ketoacidosis)
History (predisposing factors)	Too much insulin Too little food: delayed or omitted Loss of food by vomiting or diarrhea Excessive exercise	Too little insulin: omission of medication or failure to increase dose when requirements increased Too much food Infection Stress Illness of any sort
Cause	Lowered blood glucose with excess insulin in proportion	Decreased glucose utilization when insufficient insulin leads to prolonged increasing acidosis
Occurrence	In insulin-dependent diabetics, particularly the unstable, severe type	Insulin-dependent person who is poorly controlled, unstable, who omits or reduces insulin for emotional or other reasons
Onset	Sudden Slower when long-acting insulin is used	Gradual, over many hours, even days

continued

Physical findings	Skin: moist, increased perspiration Hunger Headache Tremor Pallor Dilated pupils Dizziness, staggering gait Weakness	Skin: flushed and dry Nausea, vomiting Lack of appetite Dry mouth, thirst Soft, sunken eyeballs Increased urination Abdominal pain
Vital signs		
Temperature	Normal or below	Elevated when infection is present
Respirations	Normal	Hyperpnea; acetone breath odor
Pulse	Fast; irregular	Weak; rapid
Blood pressure	Normal or slightly elevated	Lowered; person may be in shock

continued

TABLE 14.52. Comparison of Insulin Reaction and Diabetic Coma

	Insulin Reaction (Hypoglycemia)	Diabetic Coma (Ketoacidosis)
Behavior	Drowsiness	Progressive drowsiness
	Restlessness, anxiety, irritability	Confusion
	Incoordination	Lethargy
	Stupor, confusion	Weakness
	Eventual coma, with or without convulsion	Eventual coma
Treatment	Give sugar to raise the blood glucose level (orange juice, candy, sugar cubes)	Immediate professional care, hospitalization
	Revival: prompt	Keep patient warm
	Unconscious or unresponsive: treated by injection of glucagon[a] or may require intravenous glucose	Fluids for the conscious patient
		Insulin injection
Prevention	Smooth regulation of diabetes with steady diet, insulin, exercise	Early diagnosis of diabetes
		Well-indoctrinated, regulated patient

[a]*Glucagon*, a hormone produced by the alpha cells of the pancreas, increases blood glucose.

REFERENCES

1. **Shrout,** M.K., Comer, R.W., Powell, B.J., and McCoy, B.P: Treating the Pregnant Dental Patient: Four Basic Rules Addressed, *J. Am. Dent. Assoc., 123,* 75, May, 1992.

2. **Hupp,** J.R., Williams, T.P., and Vallerand, W.P.: *The 5-Minute Clinical Consult for Dental Professionals,* Philadelphia, Williams & Wilkins, 1996, p. 439.

3. **Fiese,** R. and Herzog, S.: Issues in Dental and Surgical Management of the Pregnant Patient, *Oral Surg. Oral Med. Oral Pathol., 65,* 292, March, 1988.

4. **Gier,** R.E. and Janes, D.R.: Dental Management of the Pregnant Patient, *Dent. Clin. North Am., 27,* 419, April, 1983.

5. **National Research Council,** Committee on Dietary Allowances, Food and Nutrition Board: *Recommended Dietary Allowances,* 10th ed. Washington, D.C., National Academy of Sciences, Office of Publications, 1989.

6. **Worthington-Roberts,** B.S.: Nutrition During Pregnancy and Lactation, in Mahan, L.K. and Arlin, M.T., eds.: *Krauses' Food, Nutrition & Diet Therapy,* 8th ed. Philadelphia, W.B. Saunders Co., 1992, pp. 151–167.

7. **Carranza,** F.A.: *Glickman's Clinical Periodontology,* 7th ed. Philadelphia, W.B. Saunders Co., 1990, pp. 136–138, 364, 452–455, 576.

8. **Rose,** L.F.: Sex Hormonal Imbalances, Oral Manifestations, and Dental Treatment, in Genco, R.J., Goldman, H.M., and Cohen, D.W., eds.: *Contemporary Periodontics,* St. Louis, The C.V. Mosby Co., 1990, pp. 221–224.

9. **Hoag,** P.M. and Pawlak, E.A.: *Essentials of Periodontics,* 4th ed. St. Louis, The C.V. Mosby Co., 1990, pp. 47–49.

10. **Pindborg,** J.J.: *Atlas of Diseases of the Oral Mucosa,* 5th ed. Philadelphia, W.B. Saunders Co., 1992, pp. 286–288.

11. **Shafer,** W.G., Hine, M.K., and Levy, B.M.: *A Textbook*

    of Oral Pathology, 4th ed. Philadelphia, W.B. Saunders Co., 1983, p. 359.

12. **Casamassimo,** P.S., Griffiths, P., and Nowak, A.: Anticipatory Guidance in Dentistry, *Dentalhygienist news, 5,* 19, Fall, 1992.

13. **Cohen,** M.M., Jr. and Bankier, A.: Syndrome Delineation Involving Orofacial Clefting, *Cleft Palate Carniofac. J., 28,* 119, January, 1991.

14. **Bragger,** U., Schurch, E., Gusberti, F.A., and Lang, N.P.: Periodontal Conditions in Adolescents with Cleft Lip, Alveolus and Palate Following Treatment in a Coordinated Team Approach, *J. Clin. Periodontol., 12,* 494, July, 1985.

15. **Bell,** W.T. and Wright, J.T.: The Cleft Lip and Palate Patient, in Thronton, J.B. and Wright, J.T., eds.: *Special and Medically Compromised Patients in Dentistry.* Littleton, MA, PSG Publishing Co., Inc., 1989, pp. 272–293.

16. **Kaufman,** F.L.: Managing the Cleft Lip and Palate Patient, *Pediatr. Clin. North Am., 38,* 1127, October, 1991.

17. **Garn,** S.M.: Physical Growth and Development, in Friedman, S.B., Fisher, M., and Schonberg, S.K., eds.: *Comprehensive Adolescent Health Care.* St. Louis,Quality Medical Publishing, Inc., 1992, pp. 18–23.

18. **Marlow,** D.R. and Redding, B.A.: *Textbook of Pediatric Nursing,* 6th ed. Philadelphia, W.B. Saunders Co., 1988, pp. 1114–1142.

19. **Hoag,** P.M. and Pawlak, E.A.: *Essentials of Periodontics,* 4th ed. St. Louis, The C.V. Mosby Co., 1990, pp. 35, 46–47.

20. **Carranza,** F.A.: *Glickman's Clinical Periodontology,* 7th ed. Philadelphia, W.B. Saunders, Co., 1990, pp. 138, 451–452.

21. **MacGregor,** I.D.M.: Radiographic Survey of Periodontal Disease in 264 Adolescent Schoolboys in Lagos, Nigeria, *Community Dent. Oral Epidemiol., 8,* 56, February, 1980.

22. **Latcham,** N.L., Powell, R.N., Jago, J.D., and Seymour, G.J.: A Radiographic Study of Chronic Periodontitis in

15 Year Old Queensland Children, *J. Clin. Periodontol.,* *10,* 37, January, 1983.

23. **Gjermo,** P., Bellini, H.T., Santos, V.P., Martins, J.G., and Ferracyoli, J.R.,: Prevalence of Bone Loss in a Group of Brazilian Teenagers Assessed on Bite-wing Radiographs, *J. Clin. Periodontol., 11,* 104, February, 1984.

24. **Wolfe,** M.D. and Carlos, J.P.: Periodontal Disease in Adolescents: Epidemiologic Findings in Navajo Indians, *Community Dent. Oral Epidemiol., 15,* 33, February, 1987.

25. **Aass,** A.M., Albandar, J., Aasenden, R., Tollefesen, T., and Gjermo, P.: Variation in Prevalence of Radiographic Alveolar Bone Loss in Subgroups of 14-year-old Schoolchildren in Oslo, *J. Clin. Periodontol., 15,* 130, February, 1988.

26. **American Academy of Periodontology:** Position Paper: *Periodontal Diseases of Children and Adolescents.* Chicago, A.A.P., 737, North Michigan Avenue, Chicago, IL, 60611, 1991.

27. **Machen,** J.B.: Guidelines for Dental Health of the Adolescent—May, 1986, 1985–86 AAPD Clinical Affairs Committee, *Pediatr. Dent., 9,* 247, September, 1987.

28. **Pankhurst,** C.L., Waite, I.M., Hicks, K.A., Allen, Y., and Harkness, R.D.: The Influence of Oral Contraceptive Therapy on the Periodontium—Duration of Drug Therapy, *J. Periodontol., 52,* 617, October, 1981.

29. **Carranza,** F.A.: *Glickman's Clinical Periodontology,* 7th ed. Philadelphia, W.B. Saunders, Co., 1990, p. 455.

30. **Ibsen,** O.A.C. and Phelan, J.A.: *Oral Pathology for the Dental Hygienist.* Philadelphia, W.B. Saunders Co., 1992, pp. 38–39, 193, 196.

31. **Shafer,** W.G., Hine, M.K., and Levy, B.M.: *A Textbook of Oral Pathology,* 4th ed. Philadelphia, W.B. Saunders Co., 1983, pp. 556–557.

32. **Baum,** B.J.: Current Research on Aging and Oral Health, *Spec. Dentist., 1,* 105, May/June, 1981.

33. **Baum,** B.J.: Age Changes in Salivary Glands and

Salivary Secretion, in Holm-Pedersen, P. and Loe, H., eds.: *Geriatric Dentistry.* St. Louis, The C.V. Mosby Co., 1986, pp. 114–122.

34. **Hix,** J.O. and O'Leary, T.J.: The Relationship Between Cemental Caries, Oral Hygiene Status and Fermentable Carbohydrate Intake, *J. Periodontol., 47,* 398, July, 1976.

35. **Chase,** R.H.: The Management of "Retirement Caries," *J. Mich. Dent. Assoc., 57,* 178, April, 1975.

36. **Seltzer,** S. and Bender, I.B.: *The Dental Pulp. Biologic Considerations in Dental Procedures,* 3rd ed. St. Louis, Ishiyali EuroAmerica, 1990, pp. 324–348.

37. **Zander,** H.A. and Hurzeler, B.: Continuous Cementum Apposition, *J. Dent. Res., 37,* 1035, November–December, 1958.

38. **Tallgren,** A.: The Continuing Reduction of the Residual Alveolar Ridges in Complete Denture Wearers: A Mixed-longitudinal Study Covering 25 years, *J. Prosthet. Dent., 27,* 120, February, 1972.

39. **Gallagher,** J.B.: Insertion and Postinsertion Care, in Clark, J.W., ed.: *Clinical Dentistry,* Volume 5, Revised Edition—1984. Philadelphia, J.B. Lippincott Co., Chapter 14, pp. 1–27.

40. **Atwood,** D.A.: Bone Loss of Edentulous Alveolar Ridges, *J. Periodontol., 50,* 11, Special Issue, 1979.

41. **Welker,** W.A.: Prosthodontic Treatment of Abused Oral Tissues, *J. Prosthet. Dent., 37,* 259, March, 1977.

42. **Iacopino,** A.M. and Wathen, W.F.: Oral Candidal Infection and Denture Stomatitis: A Comprehensive Review, *J. Am. Dent. Assoc., 123,* 46, January, 1992.

43. **American Dental Association,** Council on Prosthetic Services and Dental Laboratory Relations: *Techniques for Denture Identification.* Chicago, American Dental Association, 1984, 12 pp.

44. **Nizel,** A.E.: *Nutrition in Preventive Dentistry: Science and Practice,* 2nd ed. Philadelphia, W.B. Saunders Co., 1980, pp. 507–521.

45. **Atterbury,** R.A.: Preoperative Guidelines for Oral Surgery Patients, *Dent. Surv., 52,* 35, October, 1976.

46. **Chuong,** R.: Perioperative Management of the Surgical

Patient, in Peterson, L.J., ed.: *Oral Maxillofacial Surgery.* Philadelphia, J.B. Lippincott Co., 1992, pp. 63–85.

47. Loe, H., Theilade, E., and Jensen, S.B.: Experimental Gingivitis in Man, *J. Periodontol., 36,* 177, May-June, 1965.

48. Cancer Statistic, 1993, *CA., 43,* 9, January/February, 1993.

49. Silverman, S. and Shillitoe, E.J.: Etiology and Predisposing Factors, in Silverman, S., ed.: *Oral Cancer,* 3rd ed. Atlanta, GA, American Cancer Society, 1990, pp. 7–39.

50. Silverman, S., Gorsky, M., and Greenspan, D.: Tobacco Usage in Patients with Head and Neck Carcinomas: A Follow-up Study on Habit Changes and Second Primary Oral/Oropharyngeal Cancers, *J. Am. Dent. Assoc., 106,* 33, January, 1983.

51. Galante, M., Phillips, T.L., Silverberg, I.J., and Fu, K.: Treatment, in Silverman, S. ed.: *Oral Cancer,* 3rd ed. Atlanta, GA, American Cancer Society, 1990, pp. 65–80.

52. Harrison, L.B. and Fass, D.E.: Radiation Therapy for Oral Cavity Cancer, *Dent. Clin. North Am., 34,* 205, April, 1990.

53. Fleming, T.J.: Oral Tissue Changes of Radiation-oncology and Their Management, *Dent. Clin. North Am., 34,* 223, April, 1990.

54. Jansma, J.: *Oral Sequelae Resulting from Head and Neck Radiotherapy.* Groningen, Drukkerij van Denderen B.V., 1991, pp. 5–50, 117–136.

55. Barker, G.J., Barker, B.F., and Gier, R.E.: *Oral Management of the Cancer Patient. A Guide for the Health Care Profession,* 5th ed. Kansas City, MO, Biomedical Communications, University of Missouri-Kansas City, School of Dentistry, January, 1996. pp. 1–18.

56. Smeltzer, S.C. and Bare, B.G.: *Brunner and Suddarth's Textbook of Medical- Surgical Nursing,* 7th ed. Philadelphia, J.B. Lippincott Co., 1992, pp. 353–358.

57. Peterson, D.E. and Sonis, S.T., eds.: *Oral Complications*

of *Cancer Chemotherapy.* The Hague/Boston/London, Martinus Nijhoff Publishers, 1983, pp. 1–12.

58. **Toth,** B.B., Martin, J.W., and Fleming, T.J.: Oral Complications Associated with Cancer Therapy. An M.D. Anderson Cancer Center Experience, *J. Clin. Periodontol., 17,* 508, August, 1990 (Part II).

59. **Rosenberg,** S.W.: Oral Care of Chemotherapy Patients, *Dent. Clin. North Am., 34,* 239, April, 1990.

60. **Lindquist,** S.F., Hickey, A.J., and Drane, J.B.: Effect of Oral Hygiene on Stomatitis in Patients Receiving Cancer Chemotherapy, *J. Prosthet. Dent., 40,* 312, September, 1978.

61. **Sonis,** S.T., Sonis, A.L., and Lieberman, A.: Oral Complications in Patients Receiving Treatment for Malignancies Other Than of the Head and Neck, *J. Am. Dent. Assoc., 97,* 468, September, 1978.

62. **World Health Organization:** *International Classification of Impairments, Disabilities, and Handicaps.* Geneva, World Health Organization, 1980.

63. **Metal Dynamics Corporation,** 9324 State Road, Philadelphia, PA 19114.

64. **Nowak,** A.J.: Dental Care for the Handicapped Patient—Past, Present, Future, in Nowak, A.J., ed.: *Dentistry for the Handicapped Patient.* St. Louis, The C.V. Mosby Co., 1976, p. 11.

65. **Steinberg,** A.D.: Periodontal Evaluation and Treatment Considerations with the Handicapped Patient, in Nowak, A.J., ed.: *Dentistry for the Handicapped Patient,* St. Louis, The C.V. Mosby Co., 1976, pp. 302–328.

66. **Troutman,** K.C.: Prevention of Dental Disease for the Handicapped, in DePaolo, D.P. and Cheney, H.G., eds.: *Preventive Dentistry.* Preventive Dental Handbook Series, Vol. 2. Littleton, MS, PSG Publishing, 1979, pp. 205–224.

67. **Meador,** H.G.: Toothbrushing: A Sensible Approach for the Mentally Retarded, *Dent. Hyg., 53,* 462, October, 1979.

68. **Nowak,** A.J.: *Dentistry for the Handicapped Patient.* St. Louis, The C.V. Mosby Co., 1976, pp. 167–192.

69. **Pattison,** A.M. and Pattison, G.L.: *Periodontal*

Instrumentation, 2nd ed. Norwalk, CT, Appleton & Lange, 1992, pp. 355–408.

70. **Duncan,** J.L.: Incorporating Oral Hygiene Procedures in Geriatric Nursing Homes, *Dent. Hyg., 53,* 519, November, 1979.

71. **Fred Sammons Inc.,** Box 32, Brookfield, IL 60513.

72. **Albertson,** D.: Prevention and the Handicapped Child, *Dent. Clin. North Am., 18,* 595, July, 1974.

73. **Ettinger,** R.L. and Pinkham, J.R.: Oral Hygiene and the Handicapped Child, *J. Int. Assoc. Dent. Child., 9,* 3, July, 1978.

74. **Williams,** N.J. and Schuman, N.J.: The Curved-bristle Toothbrush: An Aid for the Handicapped Population, *ASDC J. Dent. Child., 55,* 291, July-August, 1988.

75. **Mulligan,** R.A.: Design Characteristics of Electric Toothbrushes Important to Physically Compromised Patients, *J. Dent. Res., 59,* 450, Abstract 731, Special Issue A, March, 1980.

76. **Ettinger,** R.L. and Pinkham, J.R.: Dental Care for the Homebound—Assessment and Hygiene, *Aust. Dent. J., 22,* 77, April, 1977.

77. **Gertenrich,** R.L. and Hart, R.W.: Utilization of the Oral Hygiene Team in a Mental Health Institution, *ASDC J. Dent. Child., 39,* 174, May-June, 1972.

78. **DePaola,** L.G. and Minah, G.E.: Isolation of Pathogenic Microorganisms from Dentures and Denture-soaking Containers of Myelosuppressed Cancer Patients. *J. Prosth. Dent., 49,* 20, January, 1983.

79. **Seto,** B.G., Wolinsky, L.E., Tsutsui, P., and Avera, D.: Comparison of the Plaque-removing Efficacy of Four Nonbrushing Oral Hygiene Devices, *Clin. Prev. Dent., 9,* 9, March-April, 1987.

80. **Capps,** J.S.: New Device for Oral Hygiene, *Am. J. Nurs., 58,* 1532, November, 1958.

81. **Tronquet,** A.A.: Oral Hygiene for Hospital Patients, *J. Am. Dent. Assoc., 63,* 215, August, 1961.

82. **Moi-stir Oral Swabsticks,** Kingswood Laboratories, Inc., 10375 Hague Road, Indianapolis, IN, 46256.

83. **Daeffler,** R.J.: Oral Care, *Hospice J., 2,* 81, Spring, 1986.

84. **Poland,** J.M.: Xerostomia in the Oncologic Patient.

Combating Complications of Treatment, *Am. J. Hospice Care, 4,* 31, May/June, 1987.

85. **Schubert,** M.M., Snow, M., and Stiefel, D.J.: *Dental Treatment of the Spinal Cord Injured Patient.* Disability Dental Instruction, 4919 NE 86th Street, Seattle, WA 98115, 34 pp.

86. **Thornton,** J.B., Sneed, R.C., Tomaselli, C.E., and Boraz, R.A.: Dental Management of Patients with Spinal Cord Injury, *Compendium, 13,* 122, February, 1992.

87. **Wyngaarden,** J.B., Smith, L.H., and Bennett, J.C., eds.: *Cecil Textbook of Medicine,* 19th ed. Philadelphia, W.B. Saunders Co., 1992, pp. 2253–2255.

88. **Keesey,** J.: Myasthenia Gravis, in Rakel, R.E., ed.: *Conn's Current Therapy.* Philadelphia, W.B. Saunders Co., 1993, pp. 902–909.

89. **Wyngaarden,** J.B., Smith, L.H., and Bennett, J.C., eds.: *Cecil Textbook of Medicine,* 19th ed. Philadelphia, W.B. Saunders Co., 1992, pp. 2196–2202.

90. **Burks,** J.S.: Multiple Sclerosis, in Raket, R.E., ed.: *Conn's Current Therapy.* Philadelphia, W.B. Saunders Co., 1993, pp. 892–902.

91. **Sorenson,** H.W.: Physically Handicapped, in Nowak, A.J., ed.: *Dentistry for the Handicapped Patient.* St. Louis, The C.V. Mosby Co., 1976, pp. 23–38.

92. **Danforth,** H.A., Snow, M., and Stiefel, D.J.: *Dental Management of the Cerebral Palsied Patient.* Disability Dental Instruction, 4919 NE 86th Street, Seattle WA 98115, 30 pp.

93. **Regezi,** J.A. and Sciubba, J.: *Oral Pathology. Clinical-Pathologic Correlations,* 2nd ed. Philadelphia, W.B. Saunders Co., 1993, pp. 581–582.

94. **Harris,** E.D.: Rheumatoid Arthritis. Pathophysiology and Implications for Treatment, *N. Engl. J. Med., 322,* 1277, May 3, 1990.

95. **Mulligan,** R.: Late Infections in Patients with Prostheses for Total Replacement of Joints: Implications for the Dental Practitioner, *J. Am. Dent. Assoc., 101,* 44, July, 1980.

96. **Seymour,** R.A., Heasman, P.A., and MacGregor, I.D.M.:

Drugs, Diseases, and the Periodontium. Oxford, Oxford University Press, 1992, pp. 37–38.

97. **National Information Center on Deafness and National Association of the Deaf:** *Deafness: A Fact Sheet.* Washington, D.C., Gallaudet University, 1989.

98. **Riekehof,** L.L.: *The Joy of Signing,* 2nd ed. Springfield, MO, Gospel Publishing House, 1987.

99. **International League Against Epilepsy,** Commission on Classification and Terminology: Proposal for Revised Clinical and Electroencephalographic Classification of Epilepsies and Epileptic Syndromes, *Epilepsia, 22,* 489, August, 1981.

100. **International League Against Epilepsy,** Commission on Classification and Terminology: Proposal for Revised Classification of Epilepsies and Epiletic Syndromes, *Epilepsia, 30,* 389, July/August, 1989.

101. **Malamed,** S.F.: *Handbook of Medical Emergencies in the Dental Office,* 4th ed. St. Louis, The C.V. Mosby Co., 1993, pp. 279–298.

102. **Bredfedt,** G.W.: Phenytoin-induced Hyperplasia Found in Edentulous Patients, *J. Am. Dent. Assoc., 123,* 61, June, 1962.

103. **McCord,** J.F., Sloan, P., and Hussey, D.J.: Phenytoin Hyperplasia Occurring under Complete Dentures: A Clinical Report, *J. Prosthet. Dent., 68, 569,* October, 1992.

104. **Hassell,** T.M., White, G.C., Jewson, L.G., and Peele, L.C.: Valproic Acid: A New Antiepileptic Drug with Potential Side Effect of Dental Concern, *J. Am. Dent. Assoc. 99,* 983, December, 1979.

105. **Hassell,** T.M.: *Epilepsy and the Oral Manifestation of Phenytoin Therapy.* Monographs in Oral Science, Volume 9. London, S. Karger, 1981, pp. 116–127.

106. **Pihlstrom,** B.L.: Prevention and Treatment of Dilantin-associated Gingival Enlargement, *Compendium, 11,* S506, Supplement 14, 1990.

107. **Allen,** S.: The Role of the Dental Hygienist in the Prevention, Control and Treatment of Dilantin Hyperplasia, *Can. Dent. Hyg./Probe, 20,* 139, December, 1986.

108. **Steinberg,** S.C. and Steinberg, A.D.: Phenytoin-induced Gingival Overgrowth Control in Severely Retarded Children, *J. Periodontol., 53,* 429, July, 1982.

109. **O'Neil,** T.C.A. and Figures, K.H.: The Effects of Chlorhexidine and Mechanical Methods of Plaque Control on the Recurrence of Gingival Hyperplasia in Young Patients Taking Phenytoin, *Br. Dent. J., 152,* 130, February 16, 1982.

110. **Tesini,** D.A.: An Annotated Review of the Literature of Dental Caries and Periodontal Disease in Mentally Retarded Individuals, *Spec. Care Dentist., 1,* 75, March-April, 1981.

111. **Pieper,** K., Dirks, B., and Kessler, P.: Caries, Oral Hygiene and Periodontal Disease in Handicapped Adults, *Community Dent. Oral Epidemiol., 14,* 28, February, 1986.

112. **Thornton,** J.B., Al-Zahid, S., Campbell, V.A., Marchetti, A., and Bradley, E.L.: Oral Hygiene Levels and Periodontal Disease Prevalence among Residents with Mental Retardation at Various Residential Settings, *Spec. Care Dentist., 9,* 196, November-December, 1989.

113. **Cooley,** W.C. and Graham, J.M.: Common Syndromes and Management Issues for Primary Care Physicians. Down's Syndrome—An Update and Review for the Primary Pediatrician, *Clin. Pediatr., 30,* 233, April, 1991.

114. **Schendel,** S.A. and Gorlin, R.J.: Frequency of Cleft Uvula and Submucous Cleft Palate in Patients with Down's Syndrome, *J. Dent. Res., 53,* 840, July-August, 1974.

115. **Seymour,** R.A., Heasman, P.A., and Macgregor, I.D.M.: *Drugs, Diseases, and Periodontium.* Oxford, Oxford University Press, 1992, pp. 22–26, and Table 3.3.

116. **Izumi,** Y., Sugiyama, S., Shinozuka, O., Yamazaki, T., Ohyama, T., and Ishikawa, I.: Defective Neutrophil Chemotaxis in Down's Syndrome Patients and Its Relationship to Periodontal Destruction, *J. Periodontol., 60,* 238, May, 1989.

117. **Blumberg,** B.S., Gerstley, B.J.S., Sutnick, A.I., Millman,

I., and London, W.T.: Australian Antigen, Hepatitis Virus and Down's Syndrome, *Ann. N.Y. Acad. Sci., 171,* 486, September 24, 1970.

118. **Dicks,** J.L. and Dennis, E.S.: Down's Syndrome and Hepatitis: An Evaluation of Carrier Status, *J. Am. Dent. Assoc., 114,* 637, May, 1987.

119. **Evenhuis,** H.M.: The Natural History of Dementia in Down's Syndrome, *Arch. Neurol., 47,* 263, March, 1990.

120. **Braff,** M.H. and Nealon, L.: Sedation of the Autistic Patient for Dental Procedures, *ASDC J. Dent Child., 46,* 404, September-October, 1979.

121. **Lowe,** O. and Jedrychowski, J.R.: A Sedation Technique for Autistic Patients Who Require Dental Treatment, *Spec. Care Dentist., 7,* 267, November-December, 1987.

122. **Burkhart,** N.: Understanding and Managing the Autistic Child in the Dental Office, *Dent. Hyg., 58,* 60, February, 1984.

123. **Kamen,** S. and Skier, J.: Dental Management of the Autistic Child, *Spec. Care Dentist., 5,* 20, January-February, 1985.

124. **Felpel,** L.P.: Psychopharmacology, Antipsychotics and Antidepressants, in Neidle, E.A. and Yagiela, J.A., eds.: *Pharmacology and Therapeutics for Dentistry,* 3rd ed. St. Louis, The C.V. Mosby Co., 1989, pp. 162–168.

125. **Barnes,** G.P., Allen, E.H., Parker, W.A., Lyon, T.C., Armentrout, W., and Cole, J.S.: Dental Treatment Needs among Hospitalized Adult Mental Patients, *Spec. Care Dentist., 8,* 173, July-August, 1988.

126. **Friedlander,** A.H. and Liberman, R.P.: Oral Health Care for the Patient with Schizophrenia, *Spec. Care Dentist., 11,* 179, September/October, 1991.

127. **Steifel,** D.J., Truelove, E.L., Menard, T.W., Anderson, V.K., Doyle, P.E., and Mandel, L.S.: A Comparison of the Oral Health of Persons with and without Chronic Mental Illness in Community Settings, *Spec. Care Dentist., 10,* 6, January-February, 1990.

128. **Friedlander,** A.H. and West, L.J.: Dental Management of the Patient With Major Depression, *Oral Surg. Oral Med. Oral Pathol., 71,* 573, May, 1991.

129. **Taylor,** C.M.: *Mereness' Essentials of Psychiatric Nursing,* 13th ed. St. Louis, The C.V. Mosby Co., 1990, pp. 235–243.

130. **Wynn,** R.L.: Pharmacology Today. Antidepressant Medications, *Gen. Dent.,* 40, 192, May-June, 1992.

131. **Friedlander,** A.A. and Brill, N.Q.: The Dental Management of Patients with Bipolar Disorder, *Oral Surg. Oral Med. Oral Pathol,* 61, 579, June, 1986.

132. **Taylor,** C.M.: *Mereness' Essentials of Psychiatric Nursing,* 13th ed. St. Louis, The C.V. Mosby Co., 1990, pp. 249–256.

133. **Inwood,** D.G.: Postpartum Psychotic Disorders, in Kaplan, H.I. and Sadock, B.I., eds.: *Comprehensive Textbook of Psychiatry,* 5th ed. Baltimore, Williams & Wilkins, 1989, pp. 852–856.

134. **Nagy,** L.M. and Charney, D.S.: Panic Disorder with or without Agoraphobia, in Rakel, R.E., ed.: *Conn's Current Therapy.* Philadelphia: W.B. Saunders Co., 1992, pp. 1075–1079.

135. **Felpel,** L.P.: Psychopharmacology, Antipsychotics and Antidepressants, in Neidle, E.A. and Yagiela, J.A., eds.: *Pharmacology and Therapeutics for Dentistry,* 3rd ed. St. Louis, The C.V. Mosby Co., 1989, pp. 178–188.

136. **Snyder,** N.C.: *Dental Hygiene Clinical Applications in Pharmacology.* Philadelphia, Lea & Febiger, 1987, pp. 57–61.

137. **Friedlander,** A.H. and Serafetinides, E.A.: Dental Management of the Patient with Obsessive-Compulsive Disorder, *Spec. Care Dentist.,* 11, 238, November-December, 1991.

138. **King,** L.J.: Treating the Anxious Patient, *Access,* 5, 10, September-October, 1991.

139. **Nadler-Moodie,** M.: *Psychiatric Aspects of General Patient Care.* San Diego, Western School, 1991, pp. 9-3, 9-5.

140. **Gross,** K.B.W., Brough, K.M., and Randolph, P.M.: Eating Disorders. Anorexia and Bulimia Nervosa, *ASDC J. Dent. Child.,* 53, 378, September-October, 1986.

141. **Taylor,** C.M.: *Mereness' Essentials of Psychiatric*

Nursing, 13th ed. St. Louis, The C.V. Mosby Co., 1990, pp. 380–381.

142. **Montgomery, M.T., Ritvo, J., Ritvo, J., and Weiner, K.:** Eating Disorders: Phenomenology, Identification, and Dental Intervention, *Gen. Dent., 36,* 485, November-December, 1988.

143. **Knewitz, J.L. and Drisko, C.L.:** Anorexia Nervosa and Bulimia: A Review, *Compendium, 9,* 244, March, 1988.

144. **Storrie-Lombardi, M.C., Storrie-Lombardi, I.J., Margon, C., and Stiefel, D.J., eds.:** *Dental Treatment of the Patient with a Major Psychiatric Disorder.* A Self-instructional Series in Rehabilitation Dentistry. Seattle, University of Washington School of Dentistry, 1987, p. 36.

145. **American Psychiatric Association,** Task Force on DSM-IV: *DSM-IV Options Book: Work in Progress.* Washington, D.C., American Psychiatric Association, 1991, pp. B-14–B-16.

146. **American Psychiatric Association:** *Diagnostic and Statistical Manual of Mental Disorders,* 3rd ed.—Revised (DSM-III). Washington, D.C., American Psychiatric Association, 1987.

147. **World Health Organization:** International Classification of Diseases (ICD-10). Geneva, World Health Organization, 1993.

148. **Kaplan, H.I. and Sadock, B.J.:** *Pocket Handbook of Clinical Psychiatry.* Baltimore, Williams & Wilkins, 1990, p.1.

149. **Potter, W.Z., Rudorfer, M.V., and Manji, H.:** The Pharmacologic Treatment of Depression, *N. Engl. J. Med., 325,* 633, August 29, 1991.

150. **United States Department of Health and Human Services,** Secretary of Health and Human Services: *Seventh Special Report to the U.S. Congress on Alcohol and Health.* Rockville, MD, National Institute on Alcohol Abuse and Alcoholism, January, 1990, pp. 107–138.

151. **Lybecker, L.A., Mendenhall, C.L., Marshall, L.E., Weesner, R.E., and Myre, S.A.:** Response to Hepatitis B

Vaccine (HBVac) in the Alcoholic, *Hepatology, 3,* 807, Abstract 36, May, 1983.

152. **United States Department of Health and Human Services,** Secretary of Health and Human Services: *Seventh Special Report to the U.S. Congress on Alcohol and Health.* Rockville, MD, National Institute on Alcohol Abuse and Alcoholism, January, 1990, pp. 87–92.

153. **United States Department of Health and Human Services,** Secretary of Health and Human Services: *Seventh Special Report to the U.S. Congress on Alcohol and Health.* Rockville, MD, National Institute on Alcohol Abuse and Alcoholism, January, 1990, pp.139–161.

154. **Gordis,** E. and Alexander, D.: Progress Toward Preventing and Understanding Alcohol-induced Fetal Injury, *JAMA, 268, 3183,* December 9, 1992.

155. **Macdonald,** D.I.: Drugs, Drinking, and Adolescence, *Am. J. Dis. Child, 138,* 117, February, 1984.

156. **Friedlander,** A.H. and Solomon, D.H.: Dental Management of the Geriatric Alcoholic Patient, *Geriodontics, 4,* 23, February, 1988.

157. **Ewing,** J.A.: Detecting alcoholism. The CAGE Questionnaire, *JAMA, 252,* 1905, October, 12, 1984.

158. **Friedlander,** A.H., Mills, M.J., and Gorelick, D.A.: Alcoholism and Dental Management, *Oral Surg. Oral Med. Oral Pathol., 63,* 42, January, 1987.

159. **Aston,** R.: Aliphatic Alcohols, in Neidle, E.A. and Yagiela, J.A., eds.: *Pharmacology and Therapeutics for Dentistry,* 3rd ed. St. Louis, The C.V. Mosby Co., 1989. pp. 594–597.

160. **United States Department of Health and Human Services,** Secretary of Health and Human Services: *Seventh Special Report to the U.S. Congress on Alcohol and Health.* Rockville, MD, National Institute on Alcohol Abuse and Alcoholism, January, 1990, pp. 261–280.

161. **Cotran,** R.S., Kumar, V., and Robbins, S.L.: *Robbins Pathologic Basis of Disease,* 4th ed. Philadelphia, W.B. Saunders Co., 1989, pp. 629–638.

162. **Little,** J.W. and Falace, D.A.: *Dental Management of*

the Medically Compromised Patient, 4th ed. St. Louis, The C.V. Mosby Co., 1993, pp. 128–135.

163. **Little,** J.W. and Falace, D.A.: *Dental Management of the Medically Compromised Patient,* 4th ed. St. Louis, The C.V. Mosby Co., 1993, pp. 98–122.

164. **American Heart Association,** 7320 Greenville Avenue, Dallas, TX 75231, 1997.

165. **United States National Institutes of Health,** National Heart, Lung, and Blood Institute: *The Fifth Report of the Joint National Committee on Detection, Evaluation and Treatment of High Blood Pressure.* Washington, D.C., National Heart, Lung, and Blood Institute, NIH Publication No. 93-1088, January, 1993.

166. **Malamed,** S.F.: *Handbook of Medical Emergencies in the Dental Office,* 4th ed. St. Louis, The C.V. Mosby Co., 1993, pp. 128–135.

167. **Cotran,** R.S., Kumar, V., and Robbins, S.L.: *Robbins Pathologic Basis of Disease,* 4th ed. Philadelphia, W.B. Saunders Co., 1989, pp. 615–617.

168. **Little,** J.W. and Falace, D.A.: *Dental Management of the Medically Compromised Patient,* 4th ed. St. Louis, The C.V. Mosby Co., 1993, pp. 175–195.

169. **Malamed,** S.F.: *Handbook of Medical Emergencies in the Dental Office,* 4th ed. St. Louis, The C.V. Mosby Co., 1993, pp. 424–449.

170. **Escher,** D.J., Parker, B., and Furman, S.: Pacemaker Triggering (Inhibition) by Electric Toothbrush, *Am. J. Cardiol., 38,* 126, July, 1976.

171. **Martinis,** A.J., Jankelson, B., Radke, J., and Adib, F.: Effects of the Myo-monitor on Cardiac Pacemakers, *J. Am. Dent. Assoc., 100,* 203, February, 1980.

172. **Dreifus,** L.S. and Cohen, D.: Implanted Pacemakers: Medicolegal Implications, *Am. J. Cardiol., 36,* 266, August, 1975.

173. **Lindemann,** R.A. and Henson, J.L.: The Dental Management of Patients with Vasculary Grafts Placed in the Treatment of Arterial Occlusive Disease, *J. Am. Dent. Assoc., 104,* 625, May, 1982.

174. **Cotran,** R.S., Kumar, V., and Robbins, S.L.: *Robbins Pathologic Basis of Disease,* 4th ed. Philadelphia, W.B. Saunders Co., 1989, pp. 666–670.

175. **Sanger**, R.G. and Bystrom, E.B.: Radiographic Bone Changes in Sickle Cell Anemia, *J. Oral Med., 32,* 32, April-June, 1977.

176. **Ibsen**, O.A.C., Phelan, J.A., and Vernillo, A.T.: Oral Manifestations of Systemic Diseases, in Ibsen, O.A.C. and Phelan, J.A., eds.: *Oral Pathology for the Dental Hygienist.* Philadelphia, W.B. Saunders Co., 1992, p. 429.

177. **Smith**, H.B., McDonald, D.K., and Miller, R.I.: Dental Management of Patients with Sickle Cell Disorders, *J. Am. Dent. Assoc., 114,* 85, January, 1987.

178. **May**, O.A.: Dental Management of Sickle Cell Anemia Patients, *Gen. Dent., 39,* 182, May-June, 1991.

179. **Cotran**, R.S., Kumar, V., and Robbins, S.L.: *Robbins Pathologic Basis of Disease,* 4th ed. Philadelphia, W.B. Saunders Co., 1989, pp. 691, 735–736.

180. **Shafer**, W.G., Hine, M.D., and Levy, B.M.: *A Textbook of Oral Pathology,* 4th ed. Philadelphia, W.B. Saunders Co., 1983, pp. 732–734.

181. **Cotran**, R.S., Kumar, V., and Robbins, S.L.: *Robbins Pathologic Basis of Disease,* 4th ed. Philadelphia, W.B. Saunders Co., 1989, pp. 722–734.

182. **Little**, J.W. and Falace, D.A.: *Dental Management of the Medically Compromised Patient,* 4th ed. St. Louis, The C.V. Mosby Co., 1993, pp. 445–453.

183. **Little**, J.W. and Falace, D.A.: *Dental Management of the Medically Compromised Patient,* 4th ed. St. Louis, The C.V. Mosby Co., 1993, pp. 423–428.

184. **Mosher**, D.F.: Disorders of Blood Coagulation, in Wyngaarden, J.B., Smith, L.H., and Bennett, J.C., eds.: *Cecil Texbook of Medicine,* 19th ed. Philadelphia, W.B. Saunders Co., 1992, pp. 999–1007.

185. **Mulligan**, R.: Late Infections in Patients with Prostheses for Total Replacement of Joints: Implications for the Dental Practitioner, *J. Am. Dent. Assoc., 101,* 44, July, 1980.

186. **National Diabetes Data Group**, Harris, M. and Cahill, G., Chairmen: Classification and Diagnosis of Diabetes Mellitus and Other Categories of Glucose Intolerance, *Diabetes, 28,* 1039, December, 1979.

187. **Little,** J.W. and Falace, D.A.: *Dental Management of the Medically Compromised Patient,* 4th ed. St. Louis, The C.V. Mosby Co., 1993, pp. 341–360.
188. **Zachariasen,** R.D.: Periodontal Disease and Diabetes Mellitus, *J. Dent. Hyg.,* 66, 259, July-August, 1992.
189. **Seymour,** R.A., Heasman, P.A., and Macgregor, I.D.M.: *Drugs, Disease, and the Periodontium.* Oxford, Oxford University Press, 1992, pp. 20–21, 55–58.
190. **Gottsegen,** R.: Diabetes Mellitus, Cardiovascular Diseases and Alcoholism, in Schulger, S., Yuodelis, R., Page, R.C., and Johnson, R.H., eds.: *Periodontal Diseases,* 2nd ed. Philadelphia, Lea & Febiger, 1990, pp. 273–279.

EMERGENCY CARE

15

Emergency preparedness should be part of a regular orientation of staff, for not only new employees but also long-standing and part-time employees. Location of emergency supplies, routines to follow, and assignment of tasks/personnel during emergency situations should be reviewed on a specified regular basis. Each staff member should have current basic life support certification (some state licensing agencies require CPR certification as a condition for license renewal). Emergency prevention factors are provided in Table 15.1. Basic emergency information is provided in this chapter.

TABLE 15.1. Emergency Prevention

Components	Factors
Patient history	Notation of any medical condition that could cause crisis or emergency during treatment
	Review and update at each appointment
	Notation of allergies or drug reactions
	Illnesses/conditions for which the patient is under the care of a physician
	Medications
Stress minimization (1)	Appointment timing: personal health requirements (both scheduling time and length)
	Minimal waiting time *continued*

TABLE 15.1. Emergency Prevention

Components	Factors
	Previous meal checked
	hunger anxiety
	hypoglycemia
	blood sugar/insulin
Medication	Premedication when indicated
	Pain control during treatment
	Patient's personal prescriptions (asthma inhalers, angina medication, etc.)
Posttreatment care	Instructions for home care, prevention of discomfort
	Follow-up telephone check on patient
Observation/vital signs	General appearance of patient
	Vital signs monitored and recorded
Prevention of accidents to face and eyes (2–4)	Protective eyewear for personnel and patient
	Care in transfer of instruments, medication, materials
	Care in the use of handpieces, ultrasonic scalers, and other power-driven devices that create aerosols, spatter, and ejected debris
	Appropriate working distance from patient's mouth to clinician's eyes
	Use of rubber dam when possible

TABLE 15.2. Emergency Materials and Preparation

Components	Factors
Communication: telephone numbers for medical aid (should be posted at each phone)	Rescue squads with paramedics, 911
	Ambulance service
	Nearest emergency room
	Poison information center
	Physicians: physicians available for emergency calls; patient's personal physician should be listed in the permanent record
Emergency equipment	Every facility should have an emergency cart or kit (5, 6), conveniently located and all personnel should be familiar with the contents
	Contents should be replenished as needed
	Series E portable oxygen tank (low flow regulator, variety of delivery systems including bag-valve mask [Ambu bag], demand valve)
	Airways
	Suction tips (wide diameter, smooth edges)
	Blood pressure equipment
	Magill forceps

continued

TABLE 15.2.   Emergency Materials and Preparation

Components	Factors
	Injectable drugs: antiallergy, antihistamine, disposable syringes and needles[a]
	Tourniquet
	Noninjectable items: oxygen, vasodilator,[a] respiratory stimulant, bronchodilator,[a] antihypoglycemic,[a] antihypertensive,[a] sterile irrigating solution, paper bags for hyperventilation
	Supplementary equipment: pen flashlight, stopwatch, scissors, emesis basin, nonallergenic blanket, board (12 × 24 in.) for CPR in dental chair if patient cannot be moved to floor, commercial cold pack, emergency record form with pen[b] (Fig. 15.1), bandages, sterile dressings, adhesive tape, inflatable splints
Practice and orientation	Regular periodic review of emergency procedures with all staff participating
	Assignment of specific responsibilities for each staff member (each person must be able to assume another member's duties if needed)
	Development of illustrated flow charts for emergencies that show placement of emergency equipment, personnel, and specific assignments; flow charts given to each staff member for memorization

[a]If personnel do not have the proper background/training and experience, drugs should not be kept in the office with the emergency supplies (6).
[b]An emergency form with carbon (one copy to be transported with patient to medical treatment facility; one copy to be filed in patient's record) should be used to document the emergency. The form provides data on the emergency including monitored vital signs for attending medical personnel. It also provides vital data for future oral treatment planning and serves as documentation should legal questions arise (7).

RECORD OF EMERGENCY								
NAME _____					DATE _____		TIME _____	
ADDRESS _____					Onset of Emergency _____			
					CPR Started _____			
					Ambulance Called _____			
Pertinent Medical History _____					Ambulance Arrived _____			
					Hospital Called _____			
					Physician Called _____			
Description of Emergency _____					Patient Left Office _____			
					Attended by: Self _____			
					Relative _____			
					Other _____			

Time								
Blood Pressure								
Pulse								
Respiration								
Pupils								
Skin—color —temperature								
Level of Consciousness								
Medication (specify)								
Other Treatment (specify)								

Comments and Summary	Personnel Attending
	Signature of Team Director:

FIGURE 15.1. Record of emergency. The form is prepared in duplicate. One copy accompanies the patient to the emergency department, and the second copy is retained in the patient's dental record file.

TABLE 15.3. Emergency Care Abbreviations

ACLS:	Advanced cardiac life support
AED:	Automated external defibrillator
AHA:	American Heart Association
ALS:	Advanced life support
BLS:	Basic life support
BCLS:	Basic cardiac life support
CAD:	Coronary artery disease
CPR:	Cardiopulmonary resuscitation
ECC:	Emergency cardiac care
ECG:	Electrocardiogram
EMD:	Emergency medical dispatcher
EMS:	Emergency medical service
EMT:	Emergency medical technician
EMT-D:	Emergency medical technician-defibrillation

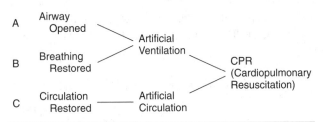

FIGURE 15.2. Basic life support (8).

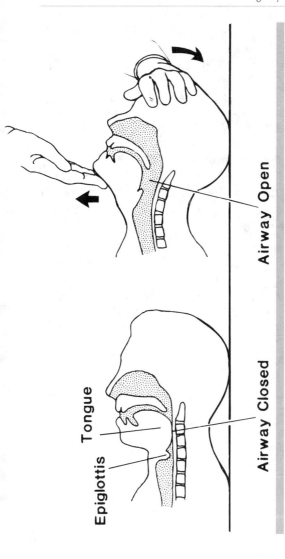

FIGURE 15.3. Chin lift to open airway. **Left,** an unconscious person with the tongue falling back against the posterior wall of the pharynx and obstructing the air passage. **Right,** the head is tilted back and the chin lifted by light pressure under the mandible. When a neck injury is suspected, a jaw thrust is used. See Table 15.5. (Reprinted with permission from Malamed, S.F.: *Handbook of Medical Emergencies in the Dental Office,* 3rd ed. St. Louis, Mosby, 1987, p. 87.)

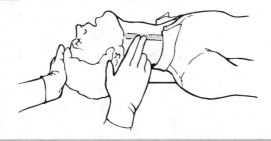

FIGURE 15.4. Carotid pulse. To locate the pulse, two or three fingers are placed on the patient's pharynx. The fingers are then slid down into the groove between the trachea and the neck muscles. With gentle pressure, the pulse can be detected.

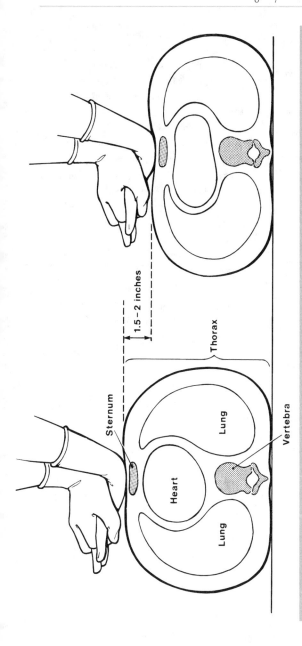

FIGURE 15.5.   External chest compression. **Left,** hands in position on the sternum with the fingers turned up. **Right,** application of firm vertical pressure compresses the heart. The sternum should be compressed 1-½ to 2 inches and then released.

TABLE 15.4. Oxygen Administration

Equipment	*E* cylinder oxygen tank (minimum size recommended), reducing valve, flow meter, tubing, mask, positive pressure bag
Patient breathing: supplemental oxygen	Apply full-face clear mask (fit with good seal) 4–6 L per min
	Monitor breathing, if breathing stops proceed with positive-pressure oxygen
Patient not breathing	Use bag-valve-mask or mouth-to-mask delivery
	Apply full-face clear mask (fit with tight seal)
	Adjust oxygen flow to keep positive-pressure bag inflated
	Compress bag manually
	Adult: 5-sec intervals = 12 respirations/min
	Child: 4-sec intervals
	Watch chest rise and fall; if chest is not moving, recheck airway for obstruction and proceed with airway obstruction management
	Obtain medical assistance

TABLE 15.5. Emergency Reference Chart

Emergency	Signs/Symptoms	Procedure
All cases		Determine consciousness (shake and shout); yell for help
		Place in supine position (if unconscious)
		Identify major problem
		Airway
		Breathing
		Circulation
		Act in accord with findings
		Activate EMS
Respiratory failure	Labored or weak respirations or cessation of breathing	Position
	Cyanosis or ashen-white with blood loss	Supine (not breathing)
	Pupils dilated	Upright (breathing)
	Loss of consciousness	Check for and remove foreign material from mouth
		Establish airway
		Rescue
		Adult: 1 breath every 5 seconds
		Child (1–8): 1 breath every 3 seconds

continued

TABLE 15.5. *(continued)* Emergency Reference Chart

Emergency	Signs/Symptoms	Procedure
		Infant (younger than 1 year): 1 breath every 3 seconds
		Monitor vital signs: blood pressure, pulse, respirations
		Administer oxygen by nonrebreather bag
Airway obstruction	Good air exchange; coughing; wheezing	Sit patient up
		Loosen tight collar, belt
Partial	Poor air exchange; noisy breathing; weak, ineffective cough; difficult respirations; gasping	No treatment; let patient cough
		Reassure patient
	Patient is panicky	Treat for complete obstruction
Complete	Gasping with great effort; no noises	*Conscious patient*
	Patient clutches throat	Perform Heimlich maneuver
	Unable to speak, breathe, cough	Patient becomes unconscious: proceed as for unconscious patient
	Cyanosis	
	Dilated pupils	*Unconscious patient*
		Initiate A-B-C of basic life support

continued

		Unsuccessful breathing attempts: proceed with airway obstruction management
		Perform Heimlich maneuver: 6 to 10 thrusts
		Examine mouth: apply finger sweep
		Open airway: give 2 ventilations
		Repeat manual thrusts and finger sweep until object is expelled
		Try rescue breathing again
		Obtain medical assistance
Hyperventilation syndrome	Lightheadedness, giddiness	Terminate oral procedure
	Anxiety, confusion	Remove rubber dam and objects from mouth
	Dizziness	Position upright or best for comfortable breathing
	Overbreathing (25–30 respiration/min)	Loosen tight collar
	Feelings of suffocation	Reassure patient: explain overbreathing; request that each breath be held to a count of 10
	Deep respirations	Ask patient to breathe deeply (7 to 10/min) into a paper bag adapted closely over nose and mouth; never use a bag for a patient with diabetes
	Palpitations (heart pounds)	Carbon dioxide is indicated, NOT oxygen
	Tingling or numbness in the extremities	

continued

TABLE 15.5. Emergency Reference Chart

Emergency	Signs/Symptoms	Procedure
Hemorrhage	Prolonged bleeding Spurting blood: artery Oozing blood: vein	Compression over bleeding area Apply gauze pack with pressure Bandage pack into place firmly where possible Severe bleeding; digital pressure on pressure point of supplying vessel Watch for shock symptoms
	Bleeding from tooth socket	Pack with folded gauze; do not dab Have patient bite down firmly Do not rinse
	Bleeding of an extremity	Elevate the part: support with pillows or substitute Apply tourniquet only when limb is amputated, mangled, or crushed
	Nosebleed	Tell patient to breath through mouth Apply cold application to nose Press nostril on bleeding side for a few minutes Advise patient not to blow the nose for an hour or more

continued

Syncope (fainting)	Pale gray face, anxiety	Position: Trendelenburg
	Dilated pupils	Loosen tight collar, belt
	Weakness, giddiness, dizziness, faintness, nausea	Place cold, damp towel on forehead
		Crush ammonia vaporole under patient's nose
	Profuse cold perspiration	Keep patient warm (blanket)
	Rapid pulse at first, followed by slow pulse	Monitor vital signs: blood pressure, pulse, respirations
	Shallow breathing	Keep airway open
	Drop in blood pressure	Administer oxygen by nasal cannula
	Loss of consciousness	Keep in supine position 10 minutes after recovery to prevent nausea and dizziness
		Reassure patient, especially during recovery
Shock	Skin: pale, moist, clammy	Position: Trendelenburg
	Rapid, shallow breathing	Keep patient quiet and warm
	Low blood pressure	Monitor vital signs: blood pressure, respirations, pulse
	Weakness and/or restlessness	Keep airway open
	Nausea, vomiting	Administer oxygen by nonrebreather bag
	Thirst, if shock is from bleeding	*Summon medical assistance*
	Eventual unconsciousness if untreated	

continued

TABLE 15.5. Emergency Reference Chart

Emergency	Signs/Symptoms	Procedure
Stroke (cerebrovascular accident)	*Premonitory* Dizziness, vertigo Transient paresthesia or weakness on one side Transient speech defects *Serious* Headache (with cerebral hemorrhage) Breathing labored, deep, slow Chills Paralysis on one side of body Nausea, vomiting Convulsions Loss of consciousness (slow or sudden onset)	*Conscious patient* Turn patient on paralyzed side; semiupright Loosen clothing about the throat Reassure patient; keep calm, quiet Monitor vital signs: blood pressure, pulse, respirations Administer oxygen by nasal cannula Clear airway; suction vomitus because the throat muscles may be paralyzed *Seek medical assistance promptly* *Unconscious patient* Position: supine Basic life support Cardiopulmonary resuscitation if indicated

continued

	Symptoms vary depending on cause	*For all patients* Be calm and reassure patient Keep patient warm and quiet; restrict effort Always administer oxygen when there is chest pain *Call for medical assistance*
Cardiovascular diseases		
Angina pectoris	Sudden crushing, paroxysmal pain in substernal area Pain may radiate to shoulder, neck, arms Pallor, faintness Shallow breathing Anxiety, fear	Position: upright, as patient requests, for comfortable breathing Place nitroglycerin sublingually only when the blood pressure is at or above baseline Administer oxygen by nasal cannula Reassure patient Without prompt relief after a second nitroglycerin, treat as a myocardial infarction
Myocardial infarction (heart attack)	Sudden pain similar to angina pectoris, which also may radiate, but of longer duration Pallor; cold, clammy skin Cyanosis Nausea	Position: with head up for comfortable breathing Symptoms are not relieved with nitroglycerin Monitor vital signs: blood pressure, pulse, respirations Administer oxygen by nonrebreather bag Alleviate anxiety; reassure *Call for medical assistance for transfer to hospital*

continued

TABLE 15.5. Emergency Reference Chart

Emergency	Signs/Symptoms	Procedure
	Breathing difficulty Marked weakness Anxiety, fear Possible loss of consciousness	
Heart failure	Difficult or labored breathing Pulmonary congestion with cough May cough up blood Rapid, weak pulse Dilated pupils May have chest pain	*Urgent medical assistance needed* Place patient in upright position Make patient comfortable: cover with blanket Administer oxygen by nonrebreather bag Reassure patient
Cardiac arrest	Skin: ashen gray, cold, clammy No pulse No heart sounds No respirations Eyes fixed, with dilated pupils; no constriction with light Unconscious	Position: supine Basic life support Check oral cavity for debris or vomitus; leave dentures in place for a seal Begin cardiopulmonary resuscitation; minutes count

continued

Adrenal crisis (cortisol deficiency)	Anxious, stressed Mental confusion Pain in abdomen, back, legs Muscle weakness Extreme fatigue Nausea, vomiting Lowered blood pressure Elevated pulse Loss of consciousness Coma	*Conscious patient* Terminate oral procedure Call for help and emergency kit Place patient in supine position with legs slightly raised Request telephone call for medical assistance Administer oxygen by nonrebreather bag Monitor blood pressure and pulse *Unconscious patient* Place patient in supine position with legs slightly raised Basic life support Try ammonia vaporole when cause is undecided Administer oxygen *Summon medical assistance* Transport to hospital

continued

TABLE 15.5. Emergency Reference Chart

Emergency	Signs/Symptoms	Procedure
Insulin reaction (hyperinsulinism) (hypoglycemia)	Sudden onset	*Conscious patient*
	Skin: moist, cold, pale	Administer oral sugar (cubes, orange juice, candy or frosting)
	Confused, nervous, anxious	Observe patient for 1 hour before dismissal
	Bounding pulse	Determine time since previous meal, and arrange next appointment following food intake
	Salivation	*Unconscious patient*
	Normal to shallow respirations	Basic life support
	Convulsions (late)	Position: supine
		Maintain airway
		Administer oxygen by nonrebreather bag
		Monitor vital signs
		Summon medical assistance
		Administer intravenous glucose

continued

Diabetic coma (ketoacidosis) (hyperglycemia)	Slow onset Skin: flushed and dry Breath: fruity odor Dry mouth, thirst Low blood pressure Weak, rapid pulse Exaggerated respirations Coma	*Conscious patient* Terminate oral procedure Obtain medical care; hospitalization indicated Keep patient warm Administer oxygen by nasal cannula *Unconscious patient* Basic life support *Urgent medical assistance needed*

Allergic reaction
  Delayed
	Skin
	  Erythema (rash)
	  Urticaria (wheals, itching)
	  Angioedema (localized swelling of
	    mucous membranes, lips, larynx,
	    pharynx)
	Respiration
	  Distress, dyspnea
		Skin
		  Administer antihistamine
		Respiration
		  Position: upright
		  Administer oxygen by nasal cannula
		  Epinephrine
		  Airway obstruction
		  Position: supine

continued

TABLE 15.5. Emergency Reference Chart

Emergency	Signs/Symptoms	Procedure
	Wheezing Extension of angioedema to larynx: may have obstruction from swelling of vocal apparatus	Airway maintenance Epinephrine *Summon medical assistance*
Immediate anaphylaxis (anaphylactic shock)	Skin Urticaria (wheals, itching) Flushing Nausea, abdominal cramps, vomiting, diarrhea Angioedema Swelling of lips, membranes, eyelids Laryngeal edema with difficulty swallowing Respiratory distress Cough, wheezing Dyspnea Airway obstruction Cyanosis	Rapid treatment needed (epinephrine) Position: supine (except when dyspnea predominates) Administer oxygen by nonrebreather bag Basic life support Monitor vital signs Cardiopulmonary resuscitation *Summon medical assistance, transfer to hospital*

continued

	Cardiovascular collapse	
	Profound drop in blood pressure	
	Rapid, weak pulse	
	Palpitations	
	Dilation of pupils	
	Loss of consciousness (sudden)	
	Cardiac arrest	
Local anesthesia reactions		
Psychogenic	Reaction to injection, not the anesthetic	See earlier in this table
	Syncope	
	Hyperventilation syndrome	
Allergic (very rare)	Anaphylactic shock	See earlier in this table
	Allergic skin and mucous membrane reactions	
	Allergic bronchial asthma attack	

continued

TABLE 15.5. Emergency Reference Chart

Emergency	Signs/Symptoms	Procedure
Toxic overdose	Effects of intravascular injection rather than increased quantity of drug are more common	Mild reaction
		Stop injection
	Stimulation phase	Position: supine
	Anxious, restless, apprehensive, confused	Loosen tight clothing
		Reassure patient
	Rapid pulse and respirations	Monitor blood pressure, heart rate, respirations
	Elevated blood pressure	Administer oxygen by nasal cannula
	Tremors	*Summon medical assistance*
	Convulsions	Severe reaction
	Depressive phase	Basic life support: maintain airway
	Follows stimulation phase	Administer oxygen by nonrebreather bag
	Drowsiness, lethargy	Continue to monitor vital signs
	Shock-like symptoms: pallor, sweating	Cardiopulmonary resuscitation
	Rapid, weak pulse and respirations	Administration of anticonvulsant
	Drop in blood pressure	
	Respiratory depression or respiratory arrest	
	Unconsciousness	

continued

Epileptic seizure		
Generalized tonic-clonic	Anxiety or depression	Position: supine; do not attempt to move from dental chair
	Pale, may become cyanotic	Make safe by placing movable equipment out of reach
	Muscular contractions	Do not force anything between the teeth; a soft towel or large sponges may be placed while mouth is open
	Loss of consciousness	Open airway; monitor vital signs
		Administer oxygen by nasal cannula
		Allow patient to sleep during postconvulsive stage
		Do not dismiss the patient if unaccompanied
Generalized absence	Brief loss of consciousness	Take objects from patient's hands to prevent their being dropped
	Fixed posture	
	Rhythmic twitching of eyelids, eyebrows, or head	
	May be pale	

continued

TABLE 15.5. Emergency Reference Chart

Emergency	Signs/Symptoms	Procedure
Burns		
First degree	Skin reddened	*First- and Second-degree burns*
Second degree (partial thickness)	Swelling	Do not give food or liquids; anticipate nausea
	Pain	Be alert for signs of shock
	Skin reddened, blisters	Do not apply ointment, grease, or bicarbonate of soda
	Swelling	Immerse in cool water to relieve pain; do not apply ice
	Wet surface	Gently clean with a mild antiseptic
	Pain (more than third degree)	Dress lightly with bandage
	Heightened sensitivity to touch	Elevate burned part
		Obtain medical assistance
Third degree (full thickness)	Leathery look	Request medical assistance and transport system
	Insensitive to touch	Treat for shock
		Basic life support: maintain airway
		Check for other injuries
		Wrap in clean sheet; transport

continued

Chemical burn	Reddened, discolored	Immediate, copious irrigation with water for ½ hour
		Check directions on container from which the chemical came for antidote or other advice
		Burn caused by an acid may be rinsed with bicarbonate of soda, burn caused by alkali may be rinsed in weak acid such as acetic (vinegar)
		Medical assistance needed
Internal poisoning	Signs of corrosive burn around or in oral cavity	Be calm and supportive
		Basic life support: airway maintenance
	Evidence of empty container or information from patient	Artificial ventilation (inhaled poison)
		Record vital signs
	Nausea, vomiting, cramps	*Call Poison Control Center*
		Conscious patient
		Dilute poison in the stomach with 1 or 2 glasses of water or milk
		Induce vomiting by giving 1 tbsp of syrup of ipecac followed by 1 to 2 glasses of water
		Do not induce vomiting if caustic, corrosive, or petroleum products have been ingested

continued

TABLE 15.5. Emergency Reference Chart

Emergency	Signs/Symptoms	Procedure
		Avoid nonspecific and questionably effective antidotes, stimulants, sedatives, or other agents, which may do more harm
		Obtain medical assistance
Foreign body in eye	Tears Blinking	Wash hands
		Ask patient to look down
		Bring upper lid down over lower lid for a moment; move it upward
		Turn down lower lid and examine: if particle is visible, remove with moistened cotton applicator
		Use eye cup: wash out eye with plain water
		When unsuccessful, seek medical attention: prevent patient from rubbing eye by placing gauze pack over eye and stabilizing with adhesive tape
Chemical solution in eye	Tears Stinging	Irrigate promptly with copious amounts of water; turn head so water flows away from inner aspect of the eye; continue for 15 to 20 min

continued

Dislocated jaw	Mouth is open: patient is unable to close	Stand in front of seated patient
		Wrap thumbs in towels and place on occlusal surfaces of mandibular posterior teeth
		Curve fingers and place under body of the mandible
		Press down and back with thumbs, and at same time pull up and forward with fingers (Figure 15.6)
		As joint slips into place, quickly move thumbs outward
		Place bandage around head to support jaw
Facial fracture	Pain, swelling	Place patient on side
	Ecchymoses	Basic life support
	Deformity, limitation of movement	Support with bandage around face, under chin, and tied on the top of the head (Barton)
	Crepitation on manipulation	*Seek prompt transport to emergency care facility*
	Zygoma fracture: depression of cheek	
	Mandibular fracture: abnormal occlusion	
Tooth forcibly displaced (avulsed tooth)	Swelling, bruises, or other signs of trauma, depending on the type of accident	Instruct patient or parent to rinse tooth gently in cool water and place in water or wrap in wet cloth
		Bring to the dental office or clinic *immediately*
		The longer the time lapse between avulsion and replantation, the poorer the prognosis

EMS, emergency medical services

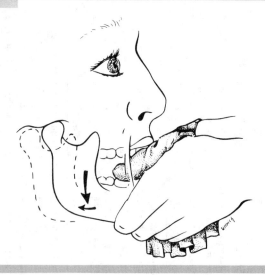

FIGURE 15.6. Treatment for a dislocated mandible. With the thumbs wrapped in toweling and placed on the buccal cusps of the mandibular teeth, the fingers are curved under the body of the mandible. The jaw is pressed down and back with the thumbs while the mandible is pulled up and forward with the fingers to permit the condyle to pass over the articular eminence into its normal position in the glenoid fossa. As the jaw slips into place, the thumbs must be moved quickly aside.

REFERENCES

1. **Malamed,** S.F.: *Handbook of Medical Emergencies in the Dental Office,* 4th ed. St. Louis, The C.V. Mosby Co., 1993, pp. 44–45.
2. **Cooley,** R.L., Cottingham, A.J., Abrams, H., and Barkmeier, W.W.: Ocular Injuries Sustained in the Dental Office: Methods of Detection, Treatment, and Prevention, *J. Am. Dent. Assoc., 97,* 985, December, 1978.
3. **Roberts-Harry,** T.J., Cass, A.E., and Jagger, J.D.: Ocular Injury and Infection in Dental Practice. A Survey and a

Review of the Literature, *Br. Dent. J., 170,* 20, January, 5, 1991.

4. **Wesson,** M.D. and Thornton, J.B.: Eye Protection and Ocular Complications in the Dental Office, *Gen. Dent., 37,* 19, January-February, 1989.

5. **Malamed,** S.F.: *Handbook of Medical Emergencies in the Dental Office,* 4th ed. St. Louis, The C.V. Mosby Co., 1993, pp. 50–89.

6. **Biron,** C.R.: Emergency Drugs, *RDH, 13,* 48, July, 1993.

7. **Robbins,** K.S.: Medicolegal Considerations, in Malamed, S.F., ed.: *Handbook of Medical Emergencies in the Dental Office,* 4th ed. St. Louis, The C.V. Mosby Co., 1993, pp. 91–101.

8. **American Heart Association:** Guidelines for Cardiopulmonary Resuscitation and Emergency Cardiac Care. Recommendations of the 1992 National Conference, *JAMA, 268,* 2171–2302, October 28, 1992.

9. **Malamed,** S.F.: *Handbook of Medical Emergencies in the Dental Office,* 4th ed. St. Louis, The C.V. Mosby Co., 1993, pp. 347–374.

10. **Clark,** W.R.: Burns, in Rakel, R.E., ed.: *Conn's Current Therapy.* Philadelphia, W.B. Saunders Co., 1993, pp. 1131–1136.

11. **Mofenson,** H.C., Caraccio, T.R., and Greensher, J.: Acute Poisonings, in Rakel, R.E., ed.: *Conn's Current Therapy.* Philadelphia, W.B. Saunders Co., 1993, pp. 1148–1192.

CUMULATIVE TRAUMA DISORDERS

16

Practicing clinicians are at risk for a number of problems that affect the hand, wrist, elbow, shoulder, and back (1). Cumulative trauma refers to disorder of the musculo-skeletal, autonomic, and peripheral nervous system caused by repeated stress to tendons, muscles, or nerves. Repeated stresses include awkward positions, forceful grasps, hand/wrist motion, mechanical stresses, vibration, and cold temperature. The most common type of cumulative trauma is carpal tunnel syndrome, also called compression neuropathy. It is a combination of symptoms that result from the compression of the median nerve in the transverse carpal tunnel (1–6).

This chapter discusses the recognition of the risk factors that can lead to a cumulative trauma disorder and strategies to prevent its occurrence. Neutral positions for the hand, wrist, elbow, forearm, and shoulder (7), proper posture, and exercises that strengthen and stretch affected areas are part of prevention.

TABLE 16.1. Symptoms of Carpal Tunnel Syndrome/ Cumulative Trauma

Symptoms (3)	Pain in hand, wrist, shoulder, neck, lower back
	Nocturnal pain in hand(s) and forearm(s)
	Pain in hand(s) while working
	Morning stiffness and numbness
	Daytime numbness and tingling in areas innervated by median nerve
	Loss of strength in hand(s); weakened grip
	Cold fingers
	Increased fatigue
Phelan's test	A test for carpal tunnel syndrome
	Hands are placed back to back with wrists flexed at 90°
	Hold in position for 1 min
	If tingling or numbness occurs, the test is positive
Tinel's sign	Used to diagnose nerve compression in the carpal tunnel
	Tap over the median nerve on ventral side of wrist
	If median nerve is compressed, tingling or electric shooting pain will result

TABLE 16.2. Risk Factors for Cumulative Trauma

Repetition	Constant wrist and forearm flexion, extension, rotation
	Constant tight grasping with thumb and fingers
Force	Firm grasp on instrument handle during scaling and root planing
	Firm grasp on ultrasonic instrument
Awkward posture	Back and shoulders rounded
	Arms elevated
	Elbows bent more than 90°
	Wrist flexed or deviated while fingers grasp
Static posture	Maintaining same position for long period
Vibration	Cumulative use of instruments with vibration (ultrasonic and sonic handpieces)
Mechanical stress	Instruments pressing on nerves or blood vessels in fingers
Cold temperature	Hand washing with cold water
	Cold room temperature
	Cold constricts blood flow

Reprinted with permission from Martha Sanders, Occupational and Sports Medicine Center, Meriden, CT.

TABLE 16.3. Recommendations to Decrease the Incidence of Cumulative Trauma

Hand use	Use proper instrumentation
	Keep wrist in neutral position during forearm rotation
	Minimize extreme wrist flexion and extension
	Vary between intraoral and extraoral fulcrums
	Avoid thumb hypertension
	Wear proper-fitting gloves; avoid glove constriction at thumb joint
Instruments	Select balanced instruments
	Use wide-diameter handles
	Use instruments with handle serrations
	Keep instruments sharp
	Dampen vibration components (ultrasonic, sonic, handpieces)
	Minimize drag on hose; keep hose untangled
Posture	Use alternate work positions
	Keep neutral positions for shoulders, elbow, wrist
	Use properly adjusted clinician's stool with lumbar support
	Use indirect vision (mouth mirror) to avoid awkward, twisted positions
	Stretch forearm, neck, shoulders, and back periodically
Workplace practices	Alternate scheduling of heavy- and light-calculus patients
	Allot adequate time per patient; haste tenses fingers and general posture
	Eliminate wasted motions; minimize reach distances
	Utilize selective polishing to minimize use of handpiece
	Add buffer time to schedule for relaxation and stretching
Body signals	Pay attention to body signals, such as pain and fatigue

Reprinted with permission from Atwood, M.J. and Michalak, C.: The Occurrence of Cumulative Trauma in Dental Hygienists, *WORK, 2*, 17, Summer, 1992.

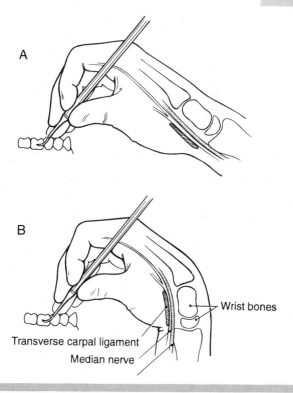

FIGURE 16.1. Effect of wrist position. **A.** The wrist in a neutral position in a straight line with the forearm. **B.** A bent wrist shows cramping of the median nerve in the carpal tunnel of the wrist. Repeated pressure on the median nerve can cause carpal tunnel syndrome.

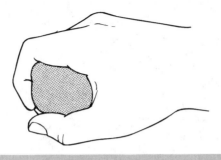

FIGURE 16.2. Exercises with therapy putty. Doing hand exercises with therapy putty develops strength and control and aids in stretching. Putty is available in various resistances and comes with a set of exercises for various muscles of the hands and wrists (5, 6).

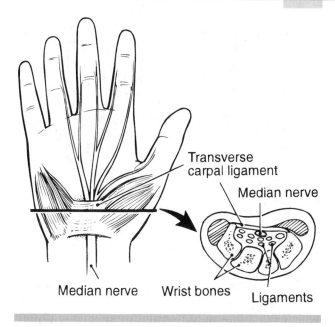

Transverse
carpal ligament

Median nerve

Median nerve   Wrist bones   Ligaments

FIGURE 16.3.   Anatomy of the wrist. **Left,** the median nerve
passes through the transverse carpal tunnel of the wrist and branches
to innervate the thumb, the index and middle fingers, and the medial
aspect of the ring finger. **Right,** a cross section of the wrist shows the
median nerve passing through the carpal tunnel. The tunnel is formed
by the concave arch of the carpal (wrist) bones and roofed over by the
transverse carpal ligament.

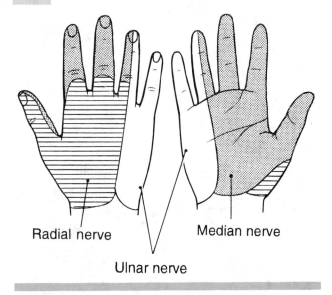

Radial nerve   Median nerve

Ulnar nerve

FIGURE 16.4.   Distribution of the median nerve fibers. The back of the hand on the left and the palm on the right show the distribution of the radial, ulnar, and median nerves.

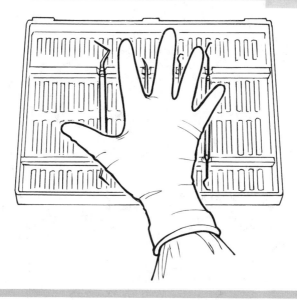

FIGURE 16.5. Stretching fingers prior to instrument retrieval. One of the exercises that can be used during actual clinical practice.

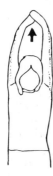

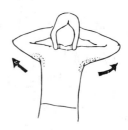

Clasp your fingers over your head and slightly back. Feel a stretch on your arms, shoulders and upper back. Hold for ten seconds.

Lower your hands to behind your neck, keeping your elbows directly out to the side. Hold for ten to fifteen seconds. Feel a stretch in your chest and front shoulders.

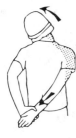

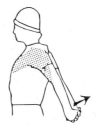

Separate your legs. Tilt your head to your left shoulder, then look at your right arm down, across and behind your back with your left arm. Hold for ten seconds. Repeat on opposite side.

Clasp your hands gently behind your back. Lift your arms backward until you feel a gentle stretch in the arms, shoulders, or chest. Hold for five to fifteen seconds. Keep your chest out and chin in.

FIGURE 16.6. Stretching exercises. Several stretching exercises to benefit the back, neck, shoulders, arms, and hands are recommended to counteract the stress and repetitive body and hand positioning and movements of daily clinical practice. Stretching between patient appointments can be especially beneficial. (Reprinted with permission from Anderson, R.A. and Anderson, J.E.: Stretching. Bolinas, California, Shelter Publications, 1980.)

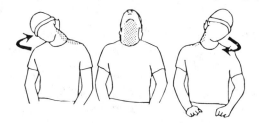

Lean your neck to your right shoulder. Then rotate the neck slowly to the back, left shoulder and down across the chest. Feel a stretch on all sides of the neck. Rotate slowly two to five times.

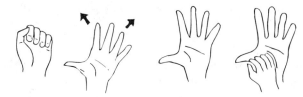

Gently open your hand, then open your fingers wide. Gently close and open them, three to five times periodically and between instrument retrieval.

Open your right hand. Grasp the bulk of your thumb with your opposite hand. Gently move your thumb away from the palm of the hand. Feel a stretch on the base of your thumb, hold for ten seconds. Repeat periodic·ally, especially after forceful or prolonged pinching.

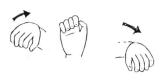

Gently rotate your wrist in small circles clockwise. Perform slowly five times periodically and between procedures and patients.

FIGURE 16.6 *(continued).*

REFERENCES

1. **MacDonald,** G., Robertson, M.M., and Erickson, J.A.: Carpal Tunnel Syndrome among California Dental Hygienists, *Dent. Hyg., 62,* 322, July/August, 1988.

2. **Osborn,** J.B., Newell, K.J., Rudney, J.D., and Stoltenberg, J.L.: Carpal Tunnel Syndrome among Minnesota Dental Hygienists, *J. Dent. Hyg., 64, 79,* February, 1990.

3. **Atwood,** M.J. and Michalak, C.: The Occurrence of Cumulative Trauma in Dental Hygienists, *WORK, 2,* 17, Summer, 1992.

4. **Dobias,** M.T.: Carpal Tunnel Syndrome: Can It Be Prevented?, *Dentalhygienistnews 5,* Winter, 1992.

5. **Gerwatowski,** L.J., McFall, D.B., and Stach, D.J.: Carpal Tunnel Syndrome, Risk Factors and Preventive Strategies for the Dental Hygienist, *J. Dent. Hyg., 66, 89,* February, 1992.

6. **McFall,** D.B., Stach, D.J., and Gerwatowski, L.J.: Carpal Tunnel Syndrome: Treatment and Rehabilitation Therapy for the Dental Hygienist, *J. Dent. Hyg., 67,* 126, March-April, 1993.

7. **Meador,** H.L.: The Biocentric Technique: A Guide to Avoiding Occupational Pain, *J. Dent. Hyg., 67, 38,* January, 1993.

APPENDIX

TABLE A.1. Average Measurements of the Primary Teeth (in Millimeters)

	Tooth	Overall Length	Length of Crown	Length of Root	Width of Crown (Mesial-Distal at Widest Point)
Maxillary	Central incisor	16.0	6.0	10.0	6.5
	Lateral incisor	15.8	5.6	11.4	5.1
	Canine	19.0	6.5	13.5	7.0
	First molar	15.2	5.1	10.0	7.3
	Second molar	17.5	5.7	11.7	8.2
Mandibular	Central incisor	14.0	5.0	9.0	4.2
	Lateral incisor	15.0	5.2	10.0	4.1
	Canine	17.5	6.0	11.5	5.0
	First molar	15.8	6.0	9.8	7.7
	Second molar	18.8	5.5	11.3	9.9

Reprinted with permission from Black, G.V.: *Descriptive Anatomy of the Human Teeth*, 4th ed. Philadelphia. The S.S. White Dental Manufacturing Company, 1897, according to Ash, M.M., ed: *Wheeler's Dental Anatomy, Physiology, and Occlusion*, 7th ed. Philadelphia, W.B. Saunders, Co., 1993, p. 58.

TABLE A.2. Average Measurements of the Permanent Teeth (in Millimeters)

Tooth	Overall Length	Length of Crown	Length of Root	Width of Crown (Mesial-Distal at Widest Point)
Maxillary				
Central incisor	23.5	10.5	13.0	8.5
Lateral incisor	22.0	9.9	13.0	6.5
Canine	27.0	10.0	17.0	7.5
First premolar	22.5	8.5	14.0	7.0
Second premolar	22.5	8.5	14.0	7.0
First molar	B[a] L	7.5	B L	10.0
	19.5 20.5		12 13	
Second molar	B L	7.0	B L	9.0
	17.0 19.0		11 12	
Third molar	17.5	6.5	11.0	8.5

continued

TABLE A.2. Average Measurements of the Permanent Teeth (in Millimeters)

	Tooth	Overall Length	Length of Crown	Length of Root	Width of Crown (Mesial-Distal at Widest Point)
Mandibular	Central incisor	21.5	9.0	12.5	5.0
	Lateral incisor	23.5	9.5	14.0	5.5
	Canine	27.0	11.0	16.0	7.0
	First premolar	22.5	8.5	14.0	7.0
	Second premolar	22.5	8.0	14.5	7.0
	First molar	21.5	7.5	14.0	11.0
	Second molar	20.0	7.0	13.0	10.5
	Third molar	18.0	7.0	11.0	10.0

Reprinted with permission from Ash, M.M.: *Wheeler's Dental Anatomy, Physiology, and Occlusion*, 7th ed. Philadelphia, W.B. Saunders, Co., 1993, p. 15.

[a]B, Buccal measurement; L, Lingual measurement

Related Dental And Professional Organizations

Academy of General Dentistry
211 East Chicago Avenue
Suite 1200
Chicago, IL 60611-2670
(312)440-4300
(312)440-0559 fax

Academy of Dentistry for Persons with Disabilities
(Federation of Special Care Organizations in Dentistry)
211 East Chicago Avenue
17th Floor
Chicago, IL 60611
(312)440-2660
(312)440-2824 fax

American Academy of Periodontology
737 North Michigan Avenue
Suite 800
Chicago, IL 60611-2690
(312)787-5518
(312)787-3670 fax

American Association of Dental Editors
1100 West Lake Street
Suite 240
Oak Park, IL 60301
(708)445-0322
(708)445-0321 fax

American Association of Dental Examiners
211 East Chicago Avenue
Suite 2134
Chicago, IL 60611
(312)440-7464
(312)440-7494 fax

American Association of Dental Schools
1625 Massachusetts Avenue, NW
Washington, DC 20036
(202)667-9433
(202)667-0642 fax

American Association of Hospital Dentists
(Federation of Special Care Organizations in Dentistry)
211 East Chicago Avenue
17th Floor
Chicago, IL 60611
(312)440-2661
(312)440-2824 fax

American Association of Oral & Maxillofacial Surgeons
9700 Bryn Mawr
Rosemont, IL 60018
(708)678-6200
(708)678-6286 fax

American Association of Orthodontists
401 N. Lindberg
St. Louis, MO 63141-7816
(314)993-1700
(314)997-1745 fax

American Association of Public Health Dentistry
AAPHD National Office
10619 Jousting Lane
Richmond, VA 23235-3838
(804)272-8344
(804)272-0802 fax

American Association of Retired Persons
601 E Street, NW
Washington, DC 20049
(202)434-2277

American Cancer Society
1599 Clifton Road N.E.
Atlanta, GA 30333

American Cancer Response Line
(800)227-2345

American Council on Alcoholism
(800)527-5344

American Dental Assistants Association
203 North LaSalle Street
Chicago, IL 60601-1225
(312)541-1550
(312)541-1496 fax

American Dental Association
211 East Chicago Avenue
Chicago, IL 60611
(312)440-2500
(312)440-7494 fax

American Dental Hygienists' Association
444 N. Michigan Avenue
Suite 3400
Chicago, IL 60611
(312)440-8900
(312)440-8929 fax
http://www.adha.org

American Dental Trade Association
4222 King Street
Alexandria, VA 22302
(703)379-7755
(703)931-9429 fax

American Foundation for the Blind
15 East 16th Street
New York, NY 10011

American Heart Association
7320 Greenville Avenue
Dallas,TX 75231

American Public Health Association
1015 15th Street, NW
Washington, DC 20005
(202)789-5600
(202)789-5661 fax

American Society for Geriatric Dentistry
(Federation of Special Care Organizations in Dentistry)
211 East Chicago Avenue
17th Floor
Chicago, IL 60611
(312)440-2600
(312)440-2824 fax

Association of Maternal & Child Health Programs
1350 Connecticut Avenue, NW
Suite 803
Washington, DC 20036
(202)775-0436
(202)775-0061 fax

Association of Schools of Allied Health Professions
1730 M Street, NW
Washington, DC 20036
(202)293-4848
(202)293-4852 fax

American Student Dental Association
211 East Chicago Avenue
Chicago, IL 60611
(312)440-2795
(312)440-2820 fax

Association for Retarded Citizens (of the United States)
500 East Border Street
Suite 300
Arlington, TX 76010-7444
(817)261-6003

Canadian Dental Hygienists' Association
96 Centerpointe Drive
Nepeon, Ontario
Canada K2G-6B1
(613)221-5515
(613)221-7283 fax

Coalition for Oral Health
1625 Massachusetts Avenue, NW
Washington, DC 20036-2212
(202)667-9433 ext. 47
(202)667-0642 fax

Collaborative Family Health Care Coalition
5310 Belt Road, NW
Washington, DC 20015-1961
(202)966-5376
(202)362-0973 fax

Federation of Special Care Organizations in Dentistry
211 East Chicago Avenue
Suite 213
Chicago, IL 60611
(312)440-2660

Group Health Association of America
1129 20th Street, NW
Washington, DC 20036
(202)778-3200
(202)778-8492 fax

Healthy Mothers/Healthy Babies
Center for Preventive Services
Centers for Disease Control and Prevention
1600 Clifton Road
Atlanta, GA 30333

Hispanic Dental Association
188 West Randolph Street
Suite 1811
Chicago, IL 60606
(312)577-4013
(312)577-0052 fax
HDASSOC@AOL.COM e-mail

Institute of Medicine
National Academy of Science
2101 Constitution Avenue NW
Washington, DC 20418
(202)334-3300

International Federation of Dental Hygienists
8802 Higdon Drive
Vienna, VA 22180

**National Academy, Gallaudet University (hearing
    impairment information)**
800 Florida Avenue, N.E.
Washington, DC 20002

National Council on Alcoholism and Drug Dependence
(800)622-2255

National Council on Aging
409 Third Street, SW
Washington, DC 20024
(202)479-1200
(202)479-0735 fax

National Dental Association
National Dental Hygienists' Association
5506 Connecticut Avenue, NW
Suite 24-25
Washington, DC 20015

National High Blood Pressure Education Program
High Blood Pressure Information Center
120/80 National Institutes of Health
Bethesda, MD 20205

National Institute of Dental Research
Building 31 Room 2C35
31 Center Drive MSC-2290
Bethesda, MD 20892-2290
(301)496-4261

National Oral Health Information Clearinghouse
1 NOHIC Way
Bethesda, MD 20892-3500
(301)402-7364, voice
(301)907-8830 fax
(301)656-7581, TTY
nidr@aerie.com e-mail

National Rural Health Association
One West Armour Boulevard
Suite 301
Kansas City, MO 64111
(816)756-3140
(816)756-3144 fax

National Society to Prevent Blindness and Its Affiliates
79 Madison Avenue
New York, NY 10016

Office of Minority Health Resource Center
(800)444-6472

Office Sterilization & Asepsis Procedures
P.O. Box 6297
Annapolis, MD 21401
(410)798-5665
(410)798-6797 fax

Sjögren's Syndrome Foundation, Inc.
382 Main Street
Port Washington, NY 11050
(516)767-2866
(516)767-7156 fax

GLOSSARY

A

Abrasion (ah-bra'shun):

Gingival: a lesion of the gingiva that results from the mechanical removal of the surface epithelium

Tooth: a loss of tooth structure produced by a mechanical cause; abrasion contrasts with erosion, which involves a chemical process

Abscess (ab'ses): a localized collection of pus in a circumscribed or walled-off area formed by the disintegration of tissues

Acute: runs relatively short course; produces pain and local inflammation

Chronic: slow development with little evidence of inflammation; usually an intermittent pus discharge; may follow an acute abscess

Periodontal: localized in the periodontal tissues; also called **lateral** or **parietal**

Absence: a generalized seizure of sudden onset characterized by a brief period of unconsciousness; formerly called **petit mal**

Absorption (ab-sorp'shun): taking up of fluids or other substances by the skin or mucous surfaces; passage of substances to the blood, lymph, and cells from the alimentary canal after digestion

Accessory (ak ses'o re): subordinate, attached or added for convenience

Accessory root canal: a secondary canal extending from the pulp to the surface of the root; frequently found near the apex of a root but may occur higher and provide a connection to a periodontal pocket

Acid (as'id): a chemical substance that undergoes dissociation with the formation of hydrogen ions in aqueous solution; pH less than 7.0

Acid etchant: in sealant placement, the enamel surface is prepared by the application of phosphoric acid, which etches the surface to provide mechanical retention for the sealant

Acidogenic (as'i-do-jen'ik): producing acid or acidity

Acne rosacea (ak'ne ro sa'ce ah): a facial skin condition usually characterized by a flushed appearance; often accompanied by puffiness and a "spider-web" effect of broken capillaries; often associated with alcoholism

Acne vulgaris (ak'ne vul-ga'ris): a chronic inflammatory disease of the sebaceous glands that appears on the face, back, and chest in the form of eruption

Acquired characteristics: those obtained after birth, as a result of environment

Acuity (a-ku i te): sharpness or clearness, especially of the special senses

Acute (a kut'): having rapid onset, a short, severe course, and pronounced symptoms; the opposite of chronic

ADD: attention deficit disorder

Adenopathy (ad e-nop'ah-the): swelling or enlargement of lymph nodes

Adsorption (ad-sorp'shun): the attachment of one substance to the surface of another; the action of a substance in attracting and holding other materials or particles on its surface

Aerobe (a'er-ob): a heterotrophic microorganism that can live and grow in the presence of free oxygen; some are obligate, others facultative; *adj.* aerobic

Aerosol (a'er-o-sol'): an artificially generated collection of particles suspended in air

   Microbial aerosol: a suspension of particles in the air that consists partially or wholly of microorganisms; may be capable of causing an airborne infection

Agar (ah'gar): a gelatin extracted from seaweed, used as a nutrient solidifying agent in bacteriologic culture media; constituent of a reversible hydrocolloid impression material

Agglutination (a-glu' ti-na'shun): the state of being united; adhesion of parts; clumping, as of bacteria or other cells

Akinesia (ah'ki-ne'ze-ah): an abnormal absence of movements

Alkali (al'kah-li): a strong water-soluble base; see **Base Allergen** (al' er-jen): an antigenic substance that produces hypersensitivity; may be inhaled, ingested, or injected or may produce a reaction upon contact with the skin

Allergy (al'er je): a hypersensitive state gained from exposure to a specific substance or allergen; reexposure to the allergen causes a heightened capacity to react

Alloplast (al'lo-plast): a graft of an inert metal or plastic material

Alloy (al'loi): a substance composed of a mixture of two or more metals

Alopecia (al'o-pe'shi-ah): a loss of hair

Alzheimer's disease (altz'hi-merz): a presenile dementia of unknown cause beginning at middle age, affecting nerve cells of the frontal and temporal lobes of the cerebrum and leading to speech defects and progressive loss of mental faculties

Amelia (ah-mel' e ah): the congenital absence of a limb or limbs

Ameloblast (ah-mel'-o-blast): an epithelial cell of the enamel organ; functions in the formation of enamel

Amelogenesis (am'e-lo-jen'e-sis): the production and development of enamel

  Amelogenesis imperfecta: imperfect formation of enamel; hereditary condition in which the ameloblasts fail to lay the enamel matrix down properly or at all

Amenorrhea: the absence of spontaneous menstrual periods in a female of reproductive age

Amniocentesis (am'en-o-sen-te'sis): a testing procedure on fluid aspirated from the amniotic sac to detect chromosomal abnormalities and metabolic disorders of a fetus

Amorphous (ah-mor'fus): without definite shape or visible differentiation in structure

Amylase (am' i laze): an enzyme that converts starch into sugar

Anaerobe (an-a'er-ob): heterotrophic microorganisms that live and grow in complete (or almost complete) absence of oxygen; some are obligate, others facultative; *adj.* anaerobic

Analgesia (an'al-je'ze-ah): insensibility to pain without loss of consciousness; usually induced by a drug, although trauma, a disease process, or a low temperature may produce a general or regional analgesia

Anaphylaxis (an-ah-fi lak'sis): an acute, severe, allergic reaction characterized by sudden collapse, shock, or respiratory and circulatory failure following the injection of an allergen; increased susceptibility to an allergen resulting from previous exposure to it

Anaplasia (an'ah-pla'ze-ah): an irreversible alteration in adult cells toward more primitive (embryonic) cell types; characteristic of tumor cells

Anesthesia (an'es-the'ze-ah): the loss of feeling or sensation, especially loss of tactile sensibility, with or without loss of consciousness

  Block anesthesia: induced by injecting the anesthetic close to a nerve trunk

  Infiltration: induced by injecting the anesthetic directly into or around the tissues to be anesthetized

  Local anesthesia: a loss of sensation in a circumscribed area without loss of consciousness; also called regional anesthesia

  Topical anesthesia: a form of local anesthesia whereby free nerve endings in accessible structures are rendered incapable of stimulation by the application of an anesthetic drug directly to the surface of the area

Aneurysm (an'u-rizm): a sac formed by the localized dilation of the wall of an artery, a vein, or the heart

Angina (an-ji'nah): a disease marked by spasmodic suffocative attacks

  Angina pectoris: acute pain in the chest from decreased blood supply to the heart muscle

Angioneurotic edema (an'je-o-nu-rot'ik e-de'mah): a sudden and temporary appearance of large areas of painless swelling in the subcutaneous tissue or submucosa; a symptom related to allergy; also called angioedema

Anhydrous (an-hi'drus): containing no water

Ankylosis (ang'ki-lo'sis): the union or consolidation of two similar or dissimilar hard tissues previously adjacent but not attached

  Dental ankylosis: the rigid fixation of a tooth to the surrounding alveolus as a result of ossification of the periodontal ligament; prevents eruption and orthodontic movement; union of bone with bone or a union with a tooth, resulting in complete immobility; the periodontal ligament of an ankylosed tooth is completely obliterated

Anlage (ahn'lah-gheh): the earliest primary stage in the development of an organ

Anodontia (an'o-don'she-ah): a congenital absence of all teeth, primary and permanent

Anodyne (an'o-dine): any agent that neutralizes or relieves pain

Anomaly (a nom'a-le): deviation from the normal

Anoxia (an-ok'si-ah): oxygen deficiency; a condition in which the cells of the body do not have or cannot utilize sufficient oxygen to perform normal function

Antabuse (an'tah bus): brand name of the generic drug **disulfiram**; used to deter consumption of alcohol by persons being treated for alcohol dependency by inducing vomiting

Antibody (an'ti-bod'e): a soluble protein molecule produced and secreted by body cells in response to an antigen; capable of binding to that specific antigen

Antidote (an ti-dote): a medicine or other remedy for counteracting the effects of a poison

Antigen (an'ti jen): a substance that is capable, under appropriate conditions, of inducing a specific immune response and of reacting with the products of that response, that is, with the specific antibody

Antimicrobial agent (ann'ti-mi-kro'be-al): any agent that kills or suppresses the growth of microorganisms

Antimicrobial therapy: the use of specific chemical or pharmaceutical agents for the control or destruction of microorganisms, either systemically or at specific sites

Antiseptic (an'ti-sep'tik): a substance that prevents or arrests the growth or action of microorganisms by either inhibiting their activity or destroying them; term used especially for preparations applied topically to living tissue

Apatite (ap'ah-tit): a crystalline mineral component of bones and teeth that contains calcium and phosphate

Hydroxyapatite: the principal mineral component of teeth, bones, and calculus

Fluorapatite (floor ap'ah-tit): the form of hydroxyapatite in which fluoride ions have replaced some of the hydroxyl ions; with fluoride, the apatite is less soluble and therefore is more resistant to the acids formed by plaque bacteria from carbohydrate intake

Fluorhydroxyapatite: apatite formed when low concentrations of fluoride react with tooth mineral; at higher concentrations, calcium fluoride is formed

Aphasia (ah-fa'ze-ah): a defect in, or loss of power of, expression by speech, writing, or signs, or of comprehension of spoken or written language

Apnea (ap'ne-ah): the temporary cessation of breathing; absence of spontaneous respirations

Aphthous ulcer (af'thus ul'ser): aphthous stomatitis; canker sore, vesicle that ruptures after 1 or 2 days and forms a depressed, spherical painful ulcer with elevated rim

Aqueous (a'kwe-us): water; prepared with water

Arch wire: a curved wire positioned in the brackets around the dental arch and held in place by elastomeres or ligatures in orthdontic treatment

Arthroplasty (ar'thro-plas'te): plastic repair of a joint

Articulation (ar-tik'u-la'shun): the place where two or more bones of the skeleton join or unite; a bony joint that may or may not be movable

Artifact (ar'ti fact): caused by the technique used, not a natural occurence; in radiography, a structure, blemish, or unintended radiographic image that may result from the faulty manufacture, manipulation, exposure, or processing of an x-ray film

Ascites (a-si'tez): the accumulation of fluid in the abdominal cavity

Asepsis (a-sep'sis): free from contamination with microorganisms; includes sterile conditions in tissues and on materials, as obtained by exclusion, removing, or killing organisms

　Chain of asepsis: a procedure that avoids transfer of infection. The "chain" implies that each step, related to the previous one, continues to be carried out without contamination

Aseptic technique: procedures carried out in the absence of pathogenic microorganisms

Assessment (ah-ses'ment): the critical analysis and valuation or judgement of the status or quality of a particular condition, situation, or other subject of appraisal

Astringent (ah-strin'jent): a substance that causes contraction or shrinkage and arrest discharges

Ataxia (ah-tak'se-ah): a failure of muscular coordination; irregularity of muscle action

Atrophy (at'ro-fe): wasting; decrease in size; occurs when muscle fibers are not used or are deprived of their blood supply or when the nerve connection is interrupted

Attachment: with reference to the clinical attachment level of the gingival and periodontal tissues:

　New attachment: the union of connective tissue or epithelium with a root surface that has been deprived of its original attachment apparatus; the new attachment may be epithelial adhesion and/or connective adaption or attachment and may include new cementum

Reattachment: the reunion of epithelial and connective tissues with root surfaces and bone such as occurs after an incision or injury

Attachment apparatus: the cementum, periodontal ligament, and alveolar bone

Attenuation (ah-ten' u-a'shun): the process by which a beam of radiation is reduced in intensity when passing through some material; the combination of absorption and scattering processes leads to a decrease in flux density of the beam when projected through matter

Attrition (a trish'un): a gradual wearing away of tooth structure, resulting from mastication

Aura (aw'rah): a warning sensation felt by some people immediately preceding a seizure; may be flashes of light, dizziness, peculiar taste, or a sensation of prickling or tingling

Auscultation (aws'kul-ta'shun): listening for sounds produced within the body; may be performed directly or with a stethoscope

Autism (aw'tizm): a syndrome, beginning in infancy, characterized by extreme withdrawl and an obsessive desire to maintain the status quo

Autograft (aw'to-graft): a graft in which the tissue is obtained from the same individual

Autoimmune disease (aw'to-im-mun): a disease caused by immunologic action of an individual's own cells or antibodies on components of the body

Autonomic (aw to-nom'ik): a division of the nervous system that supplies the sensory innervation for the smooth muscles, heart, and glands; divided into the parasympathetic (craniosacral) and sympathetic (thoracolumbar) systems

Autopolymerization (aw'to-pol-i-mer;i-za'shun): self-curing; a reaction in which a high-molecular-weight product is produced by successive additions of a simpler compound; hardening process of pit and fissure sealants

Avulsion (ah-vul'shun): the tearing away or forcible separation of a structure or part

Tooth avulsion: the traumatic separation of a tooth from the alveolus

B

Bacteremia (bak'ter-e'me-ah): the presence of microorganisms in the blood stream

Bactericide (bak'ter i sid): capable of destroying bacteria

Bacteriostatic (bak ter i-o-stat'ik): capable of inhibiting the growth and multiplication of bacteria

Bardontalgia (aerodontalgia) (bar o don tal'ji ah): the sudden acute pain response in a tooth under reduced atmospheric pressure, notable during high-altitude flying

Base (bas): a chemical substance that in solution yields hydroxyl ions and reacts with an acid to form a salt and water. A base turns red litmus paper blue and has a pH higher than 7.0.

Bifid (bi'fid): cleft into two parts or branches

Bibulous (bib'u-lus): absorbent

Bioburden: a microbiologic load, the number of contaminating organisms present on a surface prior to sterilization or on a surface prior to disinfection

Biocompatible (bi'o-kom-pat' i b'l): harmonious with life; no toxic or injurious effects on biologic function

Biofilm: the surface film that contains microorganisms and other biologic substances

Biohazard: a substance that poses a biologic risk because it is contaminated with biomaterial with a potential for transmitting infection

Biologic indicator: a preparation of nonpathogenic microorganisms, carried by an ampule or a specially impregnated paper enclosed within a package during sterilization and subsequently incubated to verify that sterilization has occurred

BIS-GMA: Bisphenol A-glycidly methacrylate; a plastic material used for dental sealants

Bonding (mechanical): the physical adherence of one substance to another

Booster dose: amount of immunogen (vaccine, toxoid, or other antigen preparation), usually smaller than the original amount, injected at an appropriate interval after the primary immunization to sustain the immune response to that immunogen

Border mold: the shaping of the peripheries of a dressing by manual manipulation of the tissue adjacent to the borders (lips, cheeks) to duplicate the contour and size of the vestibule

Bracket: an attachment that is bonded to the enamel for the purpose of holding the arch wire in orthdontic treatment

Bradycardia (brad e-kar'de-ah): unusually slow heart beat, evidenced by slowing of the pulse rate

Brittle diabetes: a term formerly used to describe very unstable juvenile diabetes; characterized by unexplained oscillation between hypoglycemia and diabetic ketoacidosis

Bruxism (bruk'sizm): a neurogenically related habit of grinding, clenching, or clamping the teeth

Buffer (buf'er): any substance in a fluid that tends to lessen the change in hydrogen ion concentration (reaction) that otherwise would be produced by adding acids or alkalis

C

Cachexia (ka kek'si-ah): a lack of nutrition; wasting; may occur in the course of chronic disease

Calibration (Kal'i-bra'shun): determination of the accuracy of an instrument by measurement of its variation from a standard; determination of accuracy and consistency between examiners to standardize procedures and gain reliability of recorded findings

Calcification (kal si-fi-ka'shyn): the process by which organic tissue becomes hardened by a deposit of calcium and other inorganic salts within its substance

Canker sore: see **Aphthous ulcer**

Capnophilic (kap-no-fil'ik): grows best in the presence of carbon dioxide; usually used in reference to bacteria

Carcinogen (kar-sin'o-jen): an agent that may cause cancer

Carcinoma (kar'si-no'mah): a malignant tumor of epithelial origin

Caries: see **Dental caries**

Cariogenic (kar'e-o-jen'ik): conducive to dental caries

Cariostatic (kar-e-o-sta'tik): exerting an inhibitory action on the progress of dental caries

Carrier: a person who harbors a specific infectious agent in the absence of discernible clinical disease and serves as a potential source of infection. The carrier state may be temporary, transient, or chronic.

    Asymptomatic carrier: an individual who harbors pathogenic organisms without clinically recognizable symptoms; as a carrier and distributor, contacts may become infected

Cartilage (kar'ti lij): firm, elastic, flexible connective tissue that is attached to articular bone surfaces and forms certain parts of the skeleton

Caustic (kaws'tik): an agent that burns or corrodes; destroys living tissue; having a burning taste

Cauterize (kaw'ter ize): to burn, corrode, or destroy living tissue by means of a caustic substance, heated metal, or an electric current

CDCP: United States Centers for Disease Control and Prevention, Department of Health and Human Services, Public Health Service, Atlanta, GA 30333

Cementicle (ce men'ti-k'l): a small globular mass of cementum; may lie free within the periodontal ligament or be attached to the cementum of the root surface

Centric occlusion or habitual occlusion (o kloo'shun): the usual maximum intercuspation or contact of the teeth of the opposing arches

Centric relation: the most unstrained, retruded physiologic relation of the mandible to the maxilla from which lateral movements can be made

Cephalometer (sef'ah-lom'e-ter): an orienting device for positioning the head for radiographic examination and measurement

Cephalometric analysis (sef'ah-lo-met'rik): the process of evaluating dental and skeletal relationships by way of measurements obtained directly from the head or from cephalometic radiographs and tracings made from the radiographs

Cephalometry (sef ah-lom'e tre): a measurement of the bony structure of the head using reproducible latero- and anteroposterior radiographs

Cephalostat (sef'ah-lo-stat'): a head-holding instrument used to obtain cephalometric radiographs

Cerebrovascular accident (CVA): a focal neurologic disorder caused by destruction of brain substance as a result of intracerebral hemorrhage, thrombosis, embolism, or vascular insufficiency; also called stroke

Cheilosis (ke lo'sis): a condition marked by fissuring and dry scaling of the surface of the lips and angles of the mouth; characteristic of riboflavin deficiency

Chemical cure: a mode of self-cure or setting of a dressing in which the ingredients unite in a chemical process that starts as soon as the blending is complete; the setting time is influenced by a warm temperature and the addition of an accelerator

Chemotaxis (ke mo tak'sis): the attraction of living protoplasm to chemical stimuli (e.g., neutrophil movement to inflammation area); a host defense mechanism

Chief complaint: the patient's concern as stated during the initial health history preparation; may be the reason for seeking professional care

Chorea (ko-re'ah): a nervous disorder characterized by irregular and involuntary action of the muscles of the extremities and the face

Chromogenic (kro mo-jen'ik): producing color or pigment

Chronic (kron'ik): characterized by a long, slow course; opposite of acute

Cicatrix (sik'ah-triks): a scar; fibrous tissue left after wound healing

Circumpubertal: on or around the age of puberty

Clearance time: the time from the cariogenic exposure until the food is cleared from the oral cavity; influenced by consistency and quantity of saliva, and by the action of the tongue, lips, and cheeks

Cleft lip: a unilateral or bilateral congenital fissure in the upper lip usually lateral to the midline; can extend into the nares and may involve the alveolar process; caused by defect in the fusion of the maxillary and medial nasal processes

Cleft palate: a congenital fissure in the palate caused by failure of the palatal shelves to fuse; may extend to connect with a unilateral or bilateral cleft lip

Climacteric: the phase in the aging of a woman that marks the transition from the reproductive to the nonreproductive stage

Cleidocranial dysotosis (cli'do kra'ni-al dis-os-to'sis): developmental defect characterized by absence of the development of clavicles and an abnormal shape of the skull

Clinical attachment level: the probing depth measured from a fixed point, such as the cementoenamel junction or other fixed point, to the location of the probe tip at the coronal level of attached periodontal tissues

Coagulation (ko-ag-u-la'shun): changing of a soluble into an insoluble protein; process of changing into a clot

Coagulation factor: the factor essential to normal blood clotting contained within the blood plasma; designated by Roman numerals I to V and VII to XIII; their absence, diminution, or excess may lead to abnormality of clotting

Coaptation (ko-ap-ta'shun): the proper adaptation or union of parts to each other (e.g., ends of a fractured bone, edges of a wound without overlap)

Collagen (kol'ah-jen): white fibers of the connective tissue

Collagenase (kol-laj'e-nas): an enzyme that catalyzes the degradation (hydrolysis) of collagen

Commissure (kom;i-shur): the angle or corner of the eye or lip

Communicable (ko-mu'ni-kah b'l): capable of being transmitted from one person to another

Congenital (kon-jen'i tal): present at and existing from the time of birth

Contagious (kon-ta'jus): communicable; transmissible by contact with an infected or sick person

Contracture (kon-trak'chur): shortening or distortion; permanent, as from shrinkage of muscles, or temporary, from sudden stimulus

Controlled release: the local delivery of a chemotherapeutic agent to a site-specific area; may be a patch to be worn on the skin or a polymeric fiber, such as that used to deliver an agent to a periodontal pocket

Coprolalia (kop'ro-lale-ah): an involuntary utterance of vulgar or obscene words

Core temperature: the temperature of the deep tissues of the body, which remains relatively constant; contrasts with body surface temperature, which rises and falls in response to environment

Corticosteroid (kor'ti-ko-ste'roid): a hormone produced by the adrenal cortex and synthetic equivalent; various steroids have different physiologic effects

Cryosurgery (kri o-ser'jere): surgery performed with the use of extremely low temperature

Cryotherapy (kri o-ther'ah pe): the therapeutic application of cold

Cryptogenic (krip to-jen'ik): of obscure, doubtful, or undeterminable origin

Cumulative trauma: disorders of the musculoskeletal, autonomic, and peripheral nervous system caused by repeated, forceful, and awkward movements of the human body, as well as by exposure to mechanical stress, vibration, and cold temperatures

Curettage (ku're-tahzh'): the scraping or cleaning the walls of a cavity or surface using a curet

    Gingival curettage: a process of debriding the soft tissue wall of a gingival or periodontal pocket

    Closed gingival curettage: the removal of the diseased lining of a soft tissue pocket wall, including pocket and junctional epithelium and the underlying inflamed connective tissue; also called soft tissue curettage

    Open gingival curettage: a surgical flap procedure in which the diseased pocket epithelium and the underlying inflamed connective tissue are removed; also call surgical curettage, open-flap curettage, modified Widman flap, and excisional new attachment procedure (ENAP)

Current: the number of electrons per second passing a given point on a conductor

Cuticle, primary (ku'ti k'l): a delicate membrane covering the crown of a newly erupted tooth; produced by the ameloblasts after they produce the enamel rods. Also called Nasmyth's membrane

Cyst (sist): a sac, normal or pathologic, containing fluid or other material

    Dentigerous cyst: formed by a dental follicle, containing one or more well-formed teeth

    Radicular cyst: an epithelial-lined sac, formed at the apex of a pulpless tooth, containing cystic fluid

Cystic fibrosis (sis'tik fi-bro'sis): a generalized hereditary disorder of primarily young children; characterized by signs of chronic pulmonary disease (result of excess mucus production in the respiratory tract) and pancreatic deficiency

D

Debonding: the removal of brackets and residual adhesive after which the tooth surface is returned to its normal contour

Debridement (da-bred'ment): a form of nonsurgical periodontal therapy accomplished by the mechanical removal of tooth surface irritants using manual and/or ultrasonic methods

Decubitus ulcer (de-ku'bi-tus): an ulcer that usually occurs over a bony prominence as a result of prolonged, excessive pressure from body weight; also called pressure sore or bed sore

Defense mechanism: in psychiatry, an unconscious mental process or coping mechanism that lessens the anxiety associated with a situation or internal conflict and protects the person from mental discomfort

Definitive care: complete care; the end point at which all treatment required at that time has been completed

Deglutition (deg'loo tish'un): the act of swallowing

Dehiscence (de-his'ens): an isolated area in which a root is denuded of bone when the denuded area extends to the margin of the bone. Compare with **fenestration**

Dehydration (de hi dra'shun): the removal of water; the condition that results from undue loss of water

Demineralization (de-min'er-al-i-za'shun): an excessive loss of mineral or inorganic salts from body tissues

Dental caries (den'tal kar'ez): a disease of the calcified structures of the teeth, characterized by decalcification of the mineral components and dissolution of the organic matrix

Dental hygiene: the science and practice of the prevention of oral diseases; the profession of dental hygiene

Dental hygiene diagnosis: the actual or potential oral health problems that are amenable to resolution by a dental hygienist's clinical and educational performance; identifies an existing or potential oral health problem that the dental hygienist is qualified and licensed to treat

Dental hygiene treatment plan: after assessment, pertinent interventions are selected to outline a treatment plan; it consists of those services to be performed by the dental hygienist within the total treatment plan for dental care

Dental hygienist (hi-je'nist): an oral health specialist whose primary concern is the maintenance of oral health and the prevention of oral disease; licensed primary healthcare professional, oral health educator, and clinician; provides preventive, educational, and therapeutic services supporting total health for the control of oral diseases and the promotion of oral health

Dental public health: see **Public health**

Denticle (den'ti k'l): a pulp stone; a relatively large body of calcified substance in the pulp chamber of a tooth

Dentin hypersensitivity: pain arising from exposed dentin typically in response to chemical, thermal, mechanical (tactile), or osmotic stimuli; this pain cannot be explained as arising from any other form of dental defect or disorder (1)

Dentinogenesis imperfecta (den'ti-no-jen'e-sis): a hereditary disorder of dentin formation in which the odontoblasts lay down an abnormal matrix; occurs in both primary and permanent dentitions

Dentition (den-tish'un): the natural teeth in the dental arch
  Succedaneous (suk'se-da'ne-us): the permanent teeth that erupt into the positions of exfoliated primary teeth

Denudation (den'u da shun): laying bare; surgical or pathologic removal of epithelial covering

Desensitization (de-sen'si ti za'shun): the process of removing reactivity or sensitivity

Desquamation (des'kwa-ma'shun): the shedding of the outer epithelial layer of the stratified squamous epithelium or skin or mucosa

Detritus (de tri'tus): debris that adheres to tooth, gingival, and mucosal surfaces

Diagnosis (di-ag-no'sis): a scientific evaluation of existing conditions; the process of determining by examination the nature and circumstances of a diseased condition; the decision reached as to the nature of a disease
  Differential diagnosis: the art of distinguishing one disease from another

Diastema (di-ahs'te-mah): a space or abnormal opening; as a dental term, it is a space between two adjacent teeth in the same dental arch

Diastole (di as'to-le): the phase of the cardiac cycle in which the heart relaxes between contractions and the two ventricles are dilated by the blood flowing into them; diastolic pressure is the lowest blood pressure

Disinfectant (dis in-fek'tant): an agent, usually a chemical, but may be a physical agent, such as x-rays or ultraviolet light, that destroys microorganisms but may not kill bacterial spores; refers to substances applied to inanimate objects

Dislocation: see **Luxation**

Diurnal (di-er'nal): pertaining to or occurring during the daytime or period of light

DNA (deoxyribonucleic acid) (de ok'si-ri-bo nu-kle'ik as'id): occurs in nuclei (chromosomes) of all animal and vegetable cells; repository of hereditary characteristics

Donor site (do'nor sit): an area from which tissue is obtained during surgical procedures such as for a graft

Dorsum (dor'sum): the back surface or a part similar to the back in position; opposite of ventral surface

Duct (dukt): a passage with well-defined walls; especially a tube for the passage of excretions or secretions

Droplet (drop'let): a diminutive drop, such as the particles of moisture expelled while coughing, sneezing, or speaking that may carry infectious agents

Dyspnea (disp'ne-ah): labored or difficult breathing

Dysarthria (dis-ar'thri-ah): disturbances of articulation as a result of emotional stress or paralysis, incoordination, or spasticity of the muscles used for speaking

Dyslexia (dis-lek'se-ah): inability or difficulty in reading, including word blindness and a tendency to reverse letters and words in reading and writing

Dysmenorrhea: difficult and painful menstruation

Dysmorphism (dis-mor'fizm): abnormality of shape

Dysphagia (dis-fa'je-ah): difficulty in swallowing

Dysplasia (dis-pla'zi-ah): abnormal development or growth; an alteration in adult cells characterized by variations in their size, shape, and organization

Dystrophy (dis'tro-fe): degeneration associated with atrophy and dysfunction

E

Ecchymosis (ek'i-mo'sis): a hemorrhagic spot larger than a petechia in the skin or mucous membrane; nonelevated; blue or purplish

Echocardiography (ek'o-kar'de-og'rah-fe): recording of the position and motion of the heart walls and the internal structures of the heart and neighboring tissue by the echo obtained from beams of ultrasonic waves directed through the chest wall; used to show valvular and other structural deformities; the record produced is called an **echocardiogram**

Ectopic (ek-top'ik): out of place; arising or produced at an abnormal site or in a tissue where it is not normally found
   Ectopic oral calcification: pulp stones, denticles, salivary calculi

Edema (e-de'mah): collection of abnormally large amounts of fluid in the intercellular spaces, causing swelling

Pitting edema: pressure on edematous area causes pits, which remain for a prolonged period after pressure is released

Edentulous (e-den'tu-lus): without teeth

Elastomere: an elastoplastic ring or latex elastic used to hold an arch wire in a bracket wing in orthodontic treatment

Electrocardiography (e-lek'tro-kar'de-og'rah-fe): the graphic recording from the body surface of the potential of electric currents generated by the heart as a means of studying the action of the heart muscle; the record produced is called an **electrocardiogram (EKG)**

Electrolyte (e-lek'tro-lit): a conductor; a substance that, in solution, dissociates into electrically charged particles (ions) and thus is capable of conducting an electric current

ELISA or EIA: an enzyme-linked immunoabsorbent assay; a laboratory test to detect antibody in the blood serum

> **Western blot (WB):** a laboratory test for antibody that is more specific than EIA and is used to validate seropositive reactions to the EIA

Emaciation (e-me se-a'shun): the condition of excessive leanness or wasted body tissues

Embolism (em'bol-lizm): the sudden blocking of an artery by a clot of foreign material, an embolus, which has been brought to its site of lodgment by the blood stream; the embolus may be a blood clot (most frequent), or an air bubble, a clump of bacteria, or a fat globule

Emesis basin (em'e-sis): a basin, usually kidney shaped, used for receiving material expectorated or vomited

Emollient (e-mol'yent): softening or soothing; an agent used to soften the skin or other body surface

Endemic (en dem'ik): present in a community or among a group of people; the continuing prevalence of a disease as distinguished from an epidemic

Endodontics (en'do-don'tiks): that branch of dentistry concerned with the etiology, diagnosis, and treatment of diseases of the dental pulp and their sequelae

Endogenous (en'doj'e-nus): produced within or caused by factors within

Endotoxin (en'do-tok'sin): lipopolysaccharide (LPS complex found in the cell wall of many gram-negative microorganisms); contained superficially within periodontally involved cementum

Enolase (e'no las): the enzyme involved in glycolysis and sugar transport

Enzyme (en'zim): an organic compound, frequently protein in nature, that can accelerate or produce by catalytic action some change in a specific substance

EPA: United States Environmental Protection Agency, Washington, DC.

  EPA registered: number on a label indicating that the product has the acceptance of the EPA

Ephebodontics (e-fe bo don'tiks): dentistry for the individual undergoing the transition from childhood to adulthood (adolescence)

Epidemic (ep'i-dem'ik): the occurrence in a community or region of a group of illnesses of similar nature, clearly in excess of normal expectancy and derived from a common source

Epidemiology (ep'i-de'me-ol'o-je): the study of the relationships of various factors that determine the frequency and distribution of diseases in the human community; study of health and disease in populations

Epinephrine (ep'i-nef'rin): a hormone secreted by the adrenal medulla that, among other functions, causes vasodilation of blood vessels of skeletal muscles, vasoconstriction of arterioles of the skin and mucous membranes, and stimulation of heart action; used in local anesthetics for its vasoconstrictive action

Epistaxis (ep'i stak'sis): hemorrhage from the nose

Epithelialization (ep i the le al i za'shun): growth of epithelium over a denuded surface

Epulis: nonspecific term referring to a growth on the gingiva

Ergonomics (er go-nom'iks): a branch of ecology dealing with human factors in the design and operation of machines and the physical environment; in dentistry, the science encompassing all factors that relate to quality and quantity of dental care delivered in comparison to the physical and mental fatigue generated

Erosion (e-ro'zhun): soft tissue, slightly depressed lesion in which the epithelium above the basal layer is denuded

Erythema (er'i-the'mah): red area of variable size and shape; reaction to irritation, radiation, or injury

Erythrocyte (e rith'ro site): red blood cell; specialized cell for the transportation of oxygen

Erythroplakia (e-rith ro pla'ke ah): lesions of the oral mucosa that appear as bright red patches or plaques that cannot be characterized clinically or pathologically as any other disease

Erythropoiesis (e-rith ro-poy e'sis): the formation of red blood cells

Escharotic (es ka rot'ik): corrosive; capable of producing sloughing

Ethics (eth'iks): the science of right conduct; a system of rules or principles governing the conduct of a professional group, planned by them for the common good of man; principles or morality

Etiology (e ti ol'o-je): the science or study of the cause of disease; that which is known about the causes of a disease

Eugenol (u'jen-ol): a constituent of clove oil; used in early periodontal dressings with zinc oxide for its alleged antiseptic and anodyne properties; more recently found to be toxic, to elicit allergic reaction, and to hinder, more than promote, healing

Exfoliate (eks fo'le ate): to fall off in scales or layers; in dentistry, to shed primary teeth

Exodontics (eks'o-don'tiks): a branch of dentistry dealing with the surgical removal of teeth

Exogenous (eks-oj'e-nus): originating outside or caused by factors outside

Exophytic (ek' so-fit'ik): growing inward

Exostosis (ek' sos-to'sis): a benign bony growth projecting from the surface of bone

Exposure incident: a specific eye, mouth, mucous membrane, nonintact skin, or parenteral contact with blood or other potentially infectious material that results from the performance of one's usual professional duties

Extirpation (eks-tir-pa'shun): the complete removal or eradication of a part; in dentistry, the removal of the dental pulp from the pulp chamber and root canal

Extrinsic (eks-trin'sik): derived from or situated on the outside; external

Exudate (eks'u-dat): material, such as fluid, cells, and cellular debris, that has escaped from blood vessels and is deposited in tissues or on tissue surfaces, usually as a result of inflammation

F

Facet (fa-set'): a small flattened surface on a hard body, such as a tooth; a wear facet can result from attrition or repeated parafunctional contact

Facultative (fak'ul-ta'tiv): able to live under more than one specific set of environmental conditions; contrast with **obligate**

Febrile (fe'bril): pertaining to fever; feverish

Fenestration (fen es-tra'shun): an isolated area in which a root is denuded of bone when the marginal bone is intact. Compare with **Dehiscence**

Fermentable (fer men'ta b'l): a term applied to a substance that is capable of undergoing chemical change as a result of the influence of an enzyme; usually applied to substances that break down to an acid or an alcohol; applied to carbohydrate breakdown that forms acid in bacterial plaque

Fetal alcohol syndrome (FAS): an abnormal pattern of growth and development in some children born to chronically alcoholic mothers

Fetor oris (fe'tor o'ris): a foul, offensive odor from the mouth; halitosis

Fibroblast (fi'bro-blast): fiber-producing cell of the connective tissue

Fibrosis (fi-bro'sis): a fibrous change of the mucous membrane, especially the gingiva, as a result of chronic inflammation

Filament (fil'ah-ment): individual synthetic fiber; a single element of a **tuft** fixed into a toothbrush head

Fistula (fis'tu-lah): a commonly used term for a narrow passage or duct leading from one cavity to another, as from a periapical abscess to the oral cavity; see **Sinus tract**

Fluoride (floo'o-rid): a salt of hydrofluoric acid; occurs in many tissues and is stored primarily in bones and teeth

Fluorosis (floo'o-ro'sis): hypocalcification that results from excessive fluoride intake (over 2 ppm) during the development and mineralization of the teeth; depending on the length of exposure and the parts per million (ppm) of the fluoride, the fluorosed area may appear as a small white spot or as severe brown staining with pitting

Focal infection: an infection caused by bacteria or toxins carried in the blood from a distant lesion or focus

Follicle (dental) (fol'i k'l): the sac that encloses the developing tooth before its eruption

Fomite (fo'mit) or **fomes** (fo'mez): an inanimate object or material on which disease-producing agents (microorganisms) may be conveyed

Forensic dentistry (fo ren'sik): the aspect of dental science that relates and applies dental facts to legal problems; encompasses dental identification, malpractice litigation, legislation, peer review, and dental licensure

Fremitus (frem'i-tus): a vibration perceptible by palpation

Frenectomy (fre-nek'o-me): complete removal of a frenum

Frenotomy (fre-not'o-me): partial removal of a frenum

Frenum, *pl.* frena (fre'num) (fre'na): a narrow fold of mucous membrane passing from a more fixed to a movable part, serving in a measure to check undue movement of the part

Friable (fri'a b'l): easily broken or crumbled

Furcation invation: pathologic resorption of bone within a furcation

G

Geriatrics (jer'e-at'riks): the branch of medicine that deals with the problems of aging and diseases of the elderly

Germicide (jer'mi sid): anything that destroys bacteria; applied especially to chemical agents that kill disease germs but not necessarily bacterial spores; applied to both living tissue and inanimate objects

Gerodontics (jer o-don'tiks): that branch of dentistry that treats all problems peculiar to the oral cavity in old age and the aging population; also called geriatric dentistry

Gerontology: study of the aging process; includes the biologic, psychologic, and sociologic sciences

Gestation (jes-ta'shun): pregnancy

Gingivectomy (jin'ji-vek'to-me): the surgical removal of diseased gingiva to eliminate periodontal pockets

Gingivitis (jin'ji-vi'tis): inflammation of the gingival tissues

Gingivoplasty (jin'ji-vo-plas'te): the surgical contouring of the gingival tissue to produce the physiologic architectural form necessary for the maintenance of tissue health and integrity

Glass ionomer (i'on'o-mer): dental material used for restorations and for bases under composite or amalgam restorations;

ionomers adhere to dentin and enamel, release fluoride, reduce microleakage, and prevent secondary (recurrent) dental caries

Glaucoma (glaw-ko'mah): a group of diseases of the eye characterized by intraocular pressure from pathologic changes in the optic disc; person has visual-field defects

Glossitis (glaw si'tis): inflammation of the tongue

Glossodynia (glos'o-din'e-ah): pain in the tongue

Glycerin (glis'er-in): a clear, colorless, syrupy fluid used as a vehicle and sweetening agent for drugs and as a solvent and vehicle for abrasive agents

Glycolysis (gli-kol'i-sis): a process by which sugar is metabolized by bacteria to produce acid

Gnathodynamometer (nath'o-di nah-mom'e ter): an instrument for measuring the force exerted in closing the jaws

Graft (graft): tissues transferred from one site to replace damaged structures in another site
Free graft: the tissue for grafting is completely removed from its donor site
Pedicle graft: the graft remains attached to its donor site
See also **Autograft; Heterograft, Homograft**

Grand mal (grahn mahl): former name for a generalized or major siezure

Granuloma: a nonspecific term applied to a nodular inflammatory lesion containing macrophages and surrounded by lymphocytes
"Pyogenic" granuloma: a misnomer because it does not contain pus but contains blood vessels and inflammatory cells

Grit: with reference to abrasive agents, grit is the particle size

H

Habilitation (ha-bili-ta'shun): the application of measures that will assist a person in obtaining a state of health, efficiency, and independent action

Halitosis (hal-i to'sis): offensive or bad breath; may be related to systemic disease or uncleanliness of the oral cavity

Hawley retainer: a removable plastic and wire appliance used to stabilize teeth; may be modified for special applications during or after orthodontic therapy

HCW: health-care worker; **DHCW:** dental health-care worker

Health (helth): a state of complete physical, mental, and social well-being—not merely the absence of disease

Hemangioma (he-man'ji-o mah): a benign tumor composed of newly formed capillaries filled with blood

Hemorrhage (hem'o rij): bleeding; an escape of blood from the blood vessels

Hemostat (he'mo-stat): an instrument or other agent used to arrest the escape or flow of blood

Heredity (he-red'i-te): the genetic transmission of traits from parents to offspring

Heterograft (het'er-o-graft): a heterologous graft in which the tissue is obtained from another species

Heterotrophic (het'er-o-trof'ik): not self-sustaining; feeding on others

Homeostasis (ho'me-o-sta'sis): the tendency of biologic systems to maintain stability while continually adjusting to conditions that are optimal for survival

Homograft (ho'mo-graft): a homologous graft in which the tissue is obtained from a different individual of the same species

Hormone replacement therapy (HRT): the prescription of a purified or synthetic hormone to correct or prevent undesirable symptoms resulting from the surgical removal or degeneration of the hormone-producing organ

Humectant (hu-mek'tant): a substance contained in a product (such as a dentifrice) to retain moisture and prevent hardening upon exposure to air

Hydrodynamic mechanism: stimuli applied to dentinal tubules cause movement of dentinal fluid, which then stimulates nerve processes in the more pulpal areas of the dentin and/or nerves in the pulp itself; pain-impulse transmission results

Hydrokinetic activity (hi'dro-ki-net'ik): activity relating to motions of fluids or the forces that produce or affect such motions; opposite of hydrostatic

Hydrophilic (hi dro-fil'ik): having a strong affinity for water; as opposed to hydrophobic (repelling water)

Hydrostatic (hi'dro-stat'ik): relating to the equilibrium of a liquid and the pressure exerted by the liquid at rest

Hydrotherapy (hi'dor-ther'ah-pe): the use of a forced intermittent or steady stream of water for cleansing or therapeutic purposes

Hydroxyapatite ceramic: a composition of calcium and phosphate to provide a dense, nonresorbable, biocompatible ceramic used for dental implants; metal implants may be coated with tricalcium phosphate or hydroxyapatite

Hygiene (hi'jen): the science that deals with the preservation of health

Hygroscopic (hi gro-sco'pik): capable of readily absorbing and retaining moisture

Hyperactivity (hi'per-ak-tiv'i-te): abnormally increased activity
   Developmental hyperactivity (hyperkinesia): characterized by constant motion, fidgeting, excitability, impulsiveness, and a short attention span

Hyperglycemia (hi'per-gli-se'me-ah): an abnormally high level of glucose in the blood

Hyperkeratosis (hi'per-ker u to'sis): an abnormal increase in the thickness of the keratin layer (stratum corneum) of the epithelium.
   Benign hyperkeratosis is one of the most common white lesions of the oral mucous membrane.

Hyperkinesis (hi per-ki ne'sis): excessive motility; excessive muscular activity

Hyperplasia (hi'per-pla'zhe): an abnormal increase in volume of a tissue or organ caused by formation and growth of new normal cells

Hyperpnea (hi'perp-ne'ah): an abnormal increase in depth and rate of respiration

Hyperthermia (hi per ther'mia): therapeutically induced hyperpyrexia (high fever)
   Malignant hyperthermia: the rapid onset of extremely high fever with muscle rigidity

Hypertonic (hi per-ton'ik): having excessive tone, tonicity, or activity
   Hypertonic solution: one that has a higher molecular concentration than another with which it is compared; of greater concentration than isotonic

Hypertrophy (hi-per'tro-fe): an increase in the size of tissue or an organ caused by an increase in the size of its constituent cells

Hyperventilation (hi per ven'til a'shun): increased alveolar ventilation with carbon dioxide pressure below normal

Hypnotic (hip-not'ik): inducing sleep

Hypocalcification (hi'po-kal si-fi-ka'shun): a deficiency in the mineral content of a calcified tissue, for example in enamel; results from disturbance in the maturation phase during development; may be caused by systemic, local, or hereditary factors

Hypodontia (hi po-don'shi-ah): a condition of congenitally missing teeth; partial anodontia

Hypoglycemia (hi'po-gli-se'me-ah): an abnormally low level of glucose in the blood; opposite of hyperglycemia

Hypoplasia (hi po-pla'zi-ah): defective or incomplete development; enamel hypoplasia results when the enamel matrix formation is disturbed

    Enamel hypoplasia: incomplete or defective formation of the enamel of either primary or permanent teeth. The result may be an irregularity of tooth form, color, or surface

Hypothermia (hi'po-ther'me-ah): a lower-than-normal body temperature

Hypotonic (hi-po-ton'ik): having diminished tone, tonicity, or activity

    Hypotonic solution: one that has a lesser molecular concentration than another to which it is compared; of less concentration than isotonic

I

Iatrogenic (i-at'ro-jen ik): caused by inadvertent or erroneous diagnosis and/or treatment by a professional

Ictal (ik'tal): pertaining to or resulting from a stroke or an acute epileptic seizure

IDDM: insulin-dependent diabetes mellitus

Idiopathic (id'e-opath'ik): self-originated; of unknown cause

Idiosyncrasy (id e-o-sin'krah-se): any tendency, characteristic, or the like peculiar to an individual

Immunity (i mu'ni-te): an inherited, congenital, or naturally or artificially acquired ability to resist the occurrence and effects of a specific disease

    Acquired immunity: that possessed as a result of having and recovering from a disease or from building up resistance against vaccines, toxins, or toxoids

    Natural immunity: that inherited by the child from the mother or from the race

Passive immunity: that possessed as a result of injection of antibodies or antitoxins of serum from an immune individual or from an animal

Immunocompromised (im'u-no-kom'pro-mizd): when the immune response is attenuated by administration of immunosuppressive drugs, or by irradiation, malnutrition, or certain disease processes

Implant (im'plant): a material or body part that is grafted or inserted within body tissue; an alloplastic inert metal or plastic material or devices grafted or inserted surgically into intact tissues for diagnostic, prosthetic, therapeutic or experimental purposes

Implantation (im plan-ta'shun): the placement within body tissues of a foreign substance in dentistry; a foreign material placed into or on the jawbone to support a crown or partial or complete denture

Impulse: the burst of radiation generated during a half cycle of alternating current; film exposure time is measured in impulses

Incidence (in'si-dens): the rate at which a certain event occurs, such as the number of new cases of a specific disease occuring during a certain period of time

Incipient (in-sip'e-ent): beginning to exist; coming into existence

Incubation (in ku-ba'shun): the keeping of a microbial or tissue culture in an incubator to facilitate development

Index (in'deks): a graduated, numeric scale with upper and lower limits; scores on the scale correspond to a specific criterion for individuals or populations; *pl.* indices (in'di ces) or indexes (in dek'ses)

Indurated (in'du-rat'ed): hardened; abnormally hard

Inert (in-ert'): without intrinsic active properties; no inherent power of action, motion, or resistance

Infection (in-fek'shun): invasion of the body by pathogenic microorganisms and the body's response to the microorganisms and their toxic production; transfer of disease from one part of the body to another or from one person to another

Primary infection: first time; no preexisting antibodies

Latent infection: persistent infection following a primary infection in which the causative agent remains inactive within certain cells

Recurrent infection: symptomatic reactivation of a latent infection

Infectious (in-fek'shus): capable of being transmitted; producing an infection

Infectious waste: contaminated with blood, saliva, or other substances; potentially or actually infected with pathogenic material; officially called "regulated" waste

Infiltration (inn'fil-tra'shun): the diffusion or accumulation in a tissue or cells of substances not normal to it or in amounts in excess of normal

Inflammation (in flah-ma'shun): the reaction of living tissue to injury; a defense reaction of the body characterized by heat, redness, swelling, pain, and loss of function

Informed consent: a medicolegal document that holds providers responsible for ensuring that patients understand the risks and benefits of a procedure or medication before it is administered

Inhibitor (in-hib'i-tor): a substance that arrests or restrains physiologic, chemical, or enzymatic action or the growth of microorganisms

Inlay: a fixed restoration placed within the tooth structure, prepared outside the mouth, and subsequently cemented into the tooth to restore intracoronal tooth structure; may be made of procelain, composite resin, or cast gold

Innoculation (i-nok u la'shun): the introduction of microorganisms or some substance into living tissues or culture media: introduction of a disease agent into a healthy individual to induce immunity

Inorganic (in or-gan'ik): not characterized by organization of living bodies or vital processes; also, pertaining to compounds not containing carbon, except cyanides and carbonates

Insidious (in-sid'e-us): coming on gradually or almost imperceptibly—as in a disease, the onset of which is gradual, with a more serious effect than is apparent

Interdisciplinary team: consists of specialists of many fields; combines expertise and resources to contribute knowledge and resources to provide insight into all aspects of a given special area

Intermaxillary (in ter-mak'si-lar e): between the maxilla and the mandible

Intermaxillary fixation (in'ter-mak'si-lar'e): fixation of the maxilla in occlusion with the mandible held in place by means of wires and elastic bands; the healing parts are stabilized following fracture or surgery

Interocclusal record: a registration of the positional relationship of the opposing teeth or dental arches made in a plastic material; also called the **maxillomandibular relationship record** or "wax bite"

Intervention: to happen or take place between other events; to intervene, as with a specific treatment

Intrapartum: occurring during childbirth

Intrinsic (in-trin'sik): situated entirely within

In vitro (in ve'tro): outside the living body: in a test tube or other artificial environment

In vivo (in ve'vo): in the living body of a plant or animal

Ion (i'on): an electrically charged atom or group of atoms

    Anion (an'i-on): a negatively charged ion, which passes to the positive pole in electrolysis

    Cation (kat'i-on): a positively charged ion, which passes to the negative pole in electrolysis

Iontophoresis (i-on'to-fo-re'sis): the introduction of ions of soluble salts into the body by an electric current; a means of applying medications with the assistance of a small electric current

I.Q.: Intelligence Quotient; the relationship between intelligence and chronologic age

Ischemia (is-ke'me-ah): deficiency of blood caused by functional construction or actual obstruction of a blood vessel

Isoniazid (i'so-ni'ah-zid): antibacterial compound used in the treatment of tuberculosis

Isotonic (i so-ton'ik): having a uniform tonicity or tension; denoting solutions with the same osmotic pressure. See also **hypertonic, hypotonic**

    Isotonic solution: one that has the same molecular concentration as another with which it is compared

Isotope (i'so top): any of two or more forms of a chemical element that have different mass numbers because their nuclei contain different numbers of neutrons. Radioactive isotopes are widely used as tracers in research.

J

Jaundice (jawn'dis): a condition in which there are bile pigments in the blood and deposition of bile pigments in the skin and mucous membranes, with a resulting yellowish appearance

Jurisprudence (joor is-proo'dens): the science of law, its interpretation and application

K

Kaolin (ka'o-lin): a fine white clay; used in pharmacy in ointments and for coating pills

Keratin (ker'ah-tin): a protein material formed as a transformation product of the cellular proteins of the flat cells on the surface of the epithelium; a form of protective adaptation to function

Keratinization (ker ah-tin i-za'shun): the process of formation of a horny protective layer on the surface of stratified squamous epithelium of certain body surfaces, including the epidermis and masticatory oral mucosa

Korotkoff sounds (ko-rot'kof): the sounds heard during the determination of blood pressure; sounds originating within the blood passing through the vessel or produced by vibratory motion of the arterial wall

L

Laceration (las er-a'shun): a wound produced by tearing or irregular cutting

Latent (la'tent): concealed, not apparent; potential

Lavage (lah-vahzh'): a flushing action using large quantities of water or other liquid; also called irrigation

Learning: acquired knowledge or skills through study, instruction, or experience; true learning means that knowledge acquired is applied in everyday living

    Affective domain: the domain of learning concerned with attitudes, interests, and appreciations

    Cognitive domain: the domain of learning concerned with knowledge outcomes and intellectual abilities

    Psychomotor domain: the domain of learning concerned with levels of motor skills

Learning disorders: disorders of academic skills; developmental arithmetic disorder (dyscalculia); writing disorder (dysgraphia); and reading disorder (dyslexia)

Lesion (le'shun): any pathologic or traumatic discontinuity of tissue or loss of function of a part; a broad term that includes wounds, sores, ulcers, tumors, and any other tissue damage

Lethargy (leth'ar-je): condition of drowsiness or sleepiness

Leukocyte (loo'ko sit): white blood corpuscle capable of ameboid movement; it functions to protect the body against infection and disease

Leukoplakia (lu-ko-pla'ke-ah): a white patch or plaque that cannot be characterized clinically or pathologically as any other disease and is not associated with any physical or chemical causative agent except the use of tobacco

License by credential: acceptance for licensure by a regulatory body (state, province) on the evidence from a license obtained in another state where equivalent standards and requirements are required; also called reciprocity, a mutual or cooperative exchange

Ligature: a cord, thread, or stainless steel wire used to secure the arch wire to the bracket in orthodontic treatment

Luxation (luk - sa'shun): a dislocation (e.g., dislocation of the temporomandibular joint, when the head of the condyle moves anteriorly over the articular eminence and cannot be returned voluntarily)

Lymphadenopathy (lim-fad e nop'ah the): disease process affecting a lymph node or lymph nodes

M

Macrocephaly (ma'kro-sef'ah-le): a head that is large in relation to the rest of the body

Malaise (mahl' az'): any vague feeling of illness, uneasiness, or discomfort

Malnutrition (mal'nu-trish'un): poor nourishment resulting from improper diet or some defect of metabolism that prevents the body from utilizing intake of food properly

Manifestation (man'i fe-sta'shun): that which is made evident, especially to the sight and understanding

    Oral manifestation: a symptom or sign of a disease in the oral cavity

Marker: identifier; symptoms or signs by which a particular condition can be recognized; (e.g., clinical and microbiologic markers are used to identify gingival and periodontal infections)

Mastalgia: fullness, soreness, or pain in the breast

Mastication (mas ti-ka'shun): a series of highly coordinated functions that involve the teeth, tongue, muscles of mastication, lips, cheeks, and saliva, in the preparation of food for swallowing and digestion

Matrix (ma'triks): the form or substance within which something originates, takes form, or develops; intercellular substance of a tissue

> **Amalgam matrix:** a thin metal form, usually stainless steel, adapted to a prepared cavity to supply the missing wall so that the amalgam will be confined when condensed into the cavity preparation

Maxillofacial (mak-sil'-o-fa'shal): pertaining to the jaws and the face

Maxillofacial prosthetics: the branch of prosthodontics concerned with the restoration of the mouth and jaws and associated facial structures that have been affected by disease, injury, surgery, or a congenital defect

Menarche: the onset of menstruation, which may occur from ages 9 to 17 years

Menopause (men'o-pawz): the cessation of menstruation; clinically a period of 6 to 12 months of amenorrhea in a female older than 45 years

Metabolism (me-tab'o lizm): the sum total of the chemical changes occurring in the body; a chemical process of transforming foods into complex tissue elements and of transforming complex body substances into simple ones, along with the production of heat and energy

> **Anabolism** (ah-nab'o-lizm): the building up of tissue; maintenance and repair of the body
>
> **Catabolism** (kah-tab o-lizm): the breaking down of tissue into simpler constituents for energy production and excretion

Metaplasia (met'ah-pla'ze-ah): the change of one mature cell type to another form abnormal for that tissue

Metastasis (me-tas'tah-sis): transfer of disease from one organ or body part to another; may be transfer of pathogenic microorganisms or transfer of cells such as malignant tumor cells

Microcephaly (mi'kro-sef'ah-le): a head that is small in relation to the rest of the body

Micron (mi'kron): a unit of linear measurement; one-thousandth of a millimeter

Milliliter (mil i-le'er): one-thousandth part of a liter, usually abbreviated **mL**. Approximately equal to 1 cubic centimeter (cc)

Mineralization (min-er-al-a-za'shun): addition of mineral elements such as calcium and phosphorus to the body or part thereof, resulting in hardening of the tissue

Miniplate osteosynthesis: a method of internal fixation of mandibular fractures utilizing miniaturized metal plates and screws made of titanium or stainless steel

Miscible (mis'i-b'l): capable of being mixed

Monitoring (mon'i tor ing): the overall surveillance of a patient by methods employing the senses of touch, sight, hearing, or smell or by means of devices that operate chemically, physically, or electronically to measure the adequacy of the various physiologic functions

Morbidity (mor-bid'i te): the morbidity rate is the ratio to the total population of individuals who are ill or disabled

Mortality (mor-tal'i te): the mortality rate is the death rate; the ratio of the number of deaths to the total population

Morphology (mor-fol'o-je): the science that deals with form and structure without reference to function

Mucin (mu'cin): secretion of the mucous or goblet cell; a polysaccharide protein that, when combined with water, forms a lubricating solution call mucous; contained in saliva

Murmur (mur'mur): the irregularity of the heartbeat sound caused by a turbulent flow of blood through a valve that has failed to close

Mycoplasma (mi'ko-plaz'mah): pleomorphic, gram-negative bacteria that lack cell walls; many are regular oral cavity residents; some are pathogenic

Myopathy (mi-op'ah-the): any disease of muscle

Myotonia (mi'o-to'ne-ah): a disorder involving the tonic (continuous tension) spasm of a muscle cell

N

Nasmyth's membrane: see **Cuticle, primary**

Necrosis (ne-kro'sis): cell or tissue death within the living body

Necrotizing ulcerative periodontitis (NUP): a severe and rapidly progressive disease that has a distinctive erythema of the free gingiva, attached gingiva, and the alveolar mucosa; extensive soft tissue necrosis that usually starts with the interdental papillae; a marked loss of periodontal attachment; deep probing depths may not be evident because of marked recession

Neonate (ne'o-nat): newborn

> **Neonatal:** refers to the period immediately following birth and continuing through the first month of life

Neoplasm (ne'o-plazm): a new growth comprised of an abnormal collection of cells, the growth of which exceeds and is uncoordinated with that of the normal tissues; see **Precancerous lesion**

Neurosis (nu-ro'sis): a mental disorder that usually involves the use of unconscious defense mechanisms as a means of coping; the individual is not out of touch with reality

NIDD: noninsulin-dependent diabetes mellitus

Nidus (ni'dus): the point of origin or focus of a process

Nonkeratinized mucosa: lining mucosa in which the stratified squamous epithelial cells retain their nuclei and cytoplasm

Nonsurgical periodontal therapy: therapy that includes bacterial plaque removal and plaque control (patient and clinician), supragingival and subgingival scaling, root planing, and the adjunctive use of chemotherapeutic agents; for the control of bacterial infection, desensitization of hypersensitive exposed rooth surfaces and dental hypersensitive exposed root surfaces, and the prevention of dental caries as related to the health of the periodontium

Normotensive (nor'mo-ten'siv): the normal tension or tone; of or pertaining to having normal blood pressure

Nosocomial (nos o-ko'mi-al): denotes a disorder associated with being treated in a hospital that is unrelated to the primary reason for being in the hospital

Nostrum (nos'trum): a quack, patent, or secret remedy

Nutrient (nu'tre-ent): a chemical substance in foods that is needed by the body for building and repair; the six classes of nutrients are proteins and amino acids, fats and fatty acids, carbohydrates (monosaccharides, disaccharides, and polysaccharides), minerals, vitamins, and water

Nystagmus (nis-tag'mus): involuntary, rapid, rhythmic movement of the eyeball

Obligate (ob'li-gat): the ability to survive only in a particular environment; opposite of facultative

Obtundent (ob-tun'dent): having the power to dull sensibility or soothe pain; a soothing or partially anesthetic medicine

Obturator (ob'tu-ra tor): a prosthesis used to close a congenital or acquired opening, such as for a cleft palate, an area lost because of trauma or after surgery for the removal of a diseased area

Occlusal adjustment: a treatment in which the occluding surfaces of teeth are reshaped by grinding to create harmonious contact relationships between the maxillary and mandibular teeth; also known as occlusal equilibration or selective grinding

Occlusal guard: a removable dental appliance usually made of plastic that covers a dental arch and is designed to minimize the damaging effects of bruxism and other oral habits; also called bite guard, mouth guard, or night guard

Occlusal prematurity: any contact of opposing teeth that occurs before the desirable intercuspation

Occupational exposure: reasonably anticipated skin, eye, mucous membrane, or parenteral contact with blood or other potentially infectious materials that may result from the perfomance of one's usual duties

Odontalgia (o-don-tal'je-ah): toothache; pain in a tooth

Odontoblast (o-don'to-blast): connective tissue cell that functions in the formation of dentin

Odontoplasty (o-don'to-plas'te): the reshaping of a portion of a tooth; may be performed for therapeutic or esthetic purposes

Odontolysis (o don tol'i-sis): dissolution or resorption of tooth structure

Oligomenorrhea: menstrual intervals of greater than 45 days

Oncology (ong-kol'o-je): the study or science of neoplastic growth

Onlay: a fixed restoration that is prepared outside the mouth and is subsequently cemented on to the tooth; restores the occlusal surface, the mesial or distal or lingual-facial margins, and covers or replaces one or more cusps

Oral and maxillofacial surgery: that part of dental practice that deals with the diagnosis and surgical and adjunctive treatment of the diseases, injuries, and defects of the oral and maxillofacial region

Orthodontic and dentofacial orthopedics: the specialty area of dentistry concerned with the diagnosis, supervision, guidance, and treatment of the growing and mature dentofacial structure; includes conditions that require movement of teeth and the treatment of malrelationships and malformations of the craniofacial complex

Orthognathics (or'thog-na'thiks): science dealing with the causes and treatment of malposition of the bones of the jaw

Orthopedics (or'tho-pe'diks): the correction of abnormal form or relationship of bone structures; may be accomplished surgically or by application of appliances to stimulated changes in the bone structure through natural physiologic response; orthodontic therapy is orthopedic therapy

Orthopnea (or'thop-ne'ah): the condition of being able to breathe easily only in the upright position

Orthosis (or-tho'sis): an orthopedic appliance or apparatus used to support, align, prevent, or correct deformities or to improve the function of a movable part of the body

Osmosis (oz mo'sis): the passage of a solvent through a semipermeable membrane into a solution of higher molecular concentration, thus equalizing the concentrations on either side of the membrane

Osseous (os'e-us) integration: the apparent direct attachment or connection of osseous tissue to an inert, alloplastic material without intervening connective tissue. Also called **osseointegration**

Osteoclast (os'te-o-klast): cell whose activity initiates the formation of new bone

Osteoectomy, ostectomy (os-te-o-ek'to-mi), (os-tek'to-mi): the removal of tooth-supporting bone for the correction of pockets and onophysiologic bony contours

Osteomyelitis (os'te-o-mi-e-li'tis): acute or chronic inflammation of the bone marrow or of the bone and marrow

Osteoplasty (os'te-plas'te): reshaping of bone: alveoloplasty; plastic contouring of the alveolar process to achieve physiologic contours in the bone and gingival tissues

Osteopenia (os'te-o-pe'ne-ah): reduced bone mass caused by a decrease in the rate of osteoid (new young bone) synthesis to a level insufficient to compensate normal bone destruction

Osteoporosis (os'te-o-po-ro'sis): abnormal rarefaction of bone related to lifetime calcium deficiency and lack of exercise

OTC: over the counter; nonprescription drug; pertains to distribution of drugs directly to the public without a prescription

Otolaryngologist (o to-lar-in-gol'o jist): a medical specialist who treats the ears, throat, pharynx, larynx, nasopharynx, and tracheobronchial tree

Overdenture: a removable denture that covers and is partially supported by one or more remaining natural teeth, roots, and/or dental implants and the soft tissue of the residual alveolar ridge; also called **overlay denture**

P

Palliative (pal'e-a'tiv): affording relief but not a cure

Palpation (pal-pa'shun): perceiving by sense of touch

Palpitation (pal-pi-ta'shun): rapid beating of the heart with or without irregularity in rhythm

Pandemic (pan-dem'ik): widespread epidemic, usually affecting the population of an extensive region, several countries, or sometimes the entire globe

Parafunctional: abnormal or deviated function

Parasite (par'ah-sit): a plant or animal that lives upon or within another living organism and draws its nourishment therefrom; may be obligate or facultative; *adj.* parasitic

Parasympathetic (par ah-sim pah-thet'ik): the craniosacral division of the autonomic nervous system

Parenteral (pah-ren'ter-all): injection by a route other than the alimentary tract, such as subcutaneous, intramuscular, or intravenous

Paresis (pah-re'sis): slight or imcomplete paralysis

Paresthesia (par'es-the'ze-ah): an abnormal sensation, such as burning, prickling, or tingling

Patch: a circumscribed flat lesion larger than a macule; differentiated from the surrounding epidermis by color and/or texture

Pathogenesis (path o-jen'e sis): the course of development of disease, including the sequence of processes or events from inception to the characteristic lesion or disease

Pathogenic (path o-jen'ik): causing disease; disease-producing

Pathognomonic (path og-no-mon'ik): a sign or symptom significantly unique to a disease that distinguishes the disease from other diseases

Pathologic migration: the movement of a tooth out of its natural position as a result of periodontal infection; contrasts with **mesial migration**, which is the physiologic process maintained by tooth proximal contacts in the normal dental arches

Pathosis (path-o'sis): a disease entity

Pediatric dentistry (pe de-at'rik): the practice and teaching of, and research in, comprehensive preventive and therapeutic oral health care of children from birth through adolescence; includes care for special patients beyond the age of adolescence who demonstrate mental, physical, and/or emotional problems

Pedodontics: see **Pediatric dentistry**

Penumbra (pe num'brah): the secondary shadow that surrounds the periphery of the primary shadow; in radiography, it is the blurred margin of an image detail (geometric unsharpness)

Periapical (per e ap'i-kal): around the apex of a tooth

    Periapical tissues: the tissues surrounding the apex of a tooth, including the periodontal ligament and the alveolar bone

Pericoronitis (per i kor-o-ni'tis): inflammation of the soft tissues surrounding the crown of an erupting tooth; frequently seen in association with erupting mandibular third molars and usually accompanied by infection

Peri-implantitis (im-plan-ti'tis): inflammation of the tissue around a dental implant and/or its abutment

Perimylolysis (per i my lol'e sis): erosion of enamel and dentin as a result of chemical and mechanical effects

Periodontics (per e o-don'tiks): the branch of dentistry that deals with the diagnosis and treatment of diseases and conditions of the supporting and surrounding tissues of the teeth or their implanted substitutes

Periodontitis (per'e-o-don-ti'tis): inflammation in the periodontium affecting gingival tissues, periodontal ligament, cementum, and supporting bone

Periodontium (per'e-o-don'she-um): tissues surrounding and supporting the teeth; the two sections are the **gingival unit**, composed of the free and attached gingiva and alveolar mucosa, and the **attachment apparatus**, which includes the cementum, periodontal ligament, and the alveolar process

Periodontology (per e o-don tol'o je): the scientific study of the periodontium in health and disease

Periodontometer (per e-o-don-tom'e ter): an instrument used to measure mobility

Periodontopathic (per e o-don to path'ik): refers to an agent able to induce and/or initiate periodontal pathosis

Periradicular (per i rah-dik'u-lar): around or surrounding the root of a tooth

Permeable (per'me-ah-b'l): permitting passage of a fluid

Petechia (pe-te'ke-ah): a minute hemorrhagic spot of pinpoint to pinhead size

pH: the symbol commonly used to express hydrogen ion concentration, the measure of alkalinity and acidity. Normal (neutral) pH is 7.0. Above 7.0 the solution is alkaline; below, the solution is acidic

  Critical pH: the pH at which demineralization occurs; for enamel, pH 4.5 to 5.5; for cementum, pH 6.0 to 6.7.

Phosphorescence (fos-fo-res'ens): the emission of radiation by a substance as a result of previous absorption of radiation of shorter wave length; contrasts with fluorescence in that the emission may continue for a time after cessation of the ionizing radiation

Physiologic saline solution: a 0.9% sodium chloride solution, which exerts an osmotic pressure equal to that exerted by the blood, and this is compatible with blood

Pica (pi'kah): persistent craving/eating of nonnutritive substances or unnatural articles of food

Placebo effect (plah-se'bo): a positive response to a pain-relieving technique that is enhanced through the power of suggestion

Pleomorphism (ple'o-mor'fism): assumption of various distinct forms by a single organism or within a species; *adj.* pleomorphic

Polyphagia (pol'e-fa'je-ah): excessive ingestion of food

Polymer (pol'i mer): a compound of high molecular weight formed by a combination of a chain of simpler molecules (monomers)

Polyp (pol'ip): any growth or mass protruding from a mucous membrane

  Pedunculated (pe-dung'ku-lat ed): a polyp attached by a thin stalk

Sessile (ses'il): a polyp with a broad base

Postural hypotension (pos'chu-ral hi po-ten'shun): also called **orthostatic** (or tho-stat'ik) **hypotension**: a fall in blood pressure associated with dizziness, syncope, and blurred vision that occurs upon standing or when standing motionless in a fixed position

Potentiation (po-ten'she-a'shun): enhancement of one agent by another so that the combined effect is greater than the sum of the effects of each agent alone

ppm: parts per million; a measure used to designate the amount of fluoride used for optimum level in fluoridated water, dentifrice, and other fluoride-containing preparations

Precancerous lesion: a morphologically altered tissue in which cancer is more likely to occur than in its apparently normal counterpart. A precancerous condition is a generalized state associated with a significantly increased risk of cancer

Precipitate (pre-sip' i tate): to cause a substance in solution to separate out in solid particles *(verb)*; that which is separated out is called the precipitate

Precision attachment: a type of connector that consists of a metal receptacle and a close-fitting part; the metal receptacle usually is included within the restoration of an abutment tooth, and the close-fitting part is attached to a pontic or removable partial denture framework

Predisposition (pre-dis-po-zish'un): a concealed but present susceptibility to disease, which may be activated under certain conditions

Premedication (pre med-i-ka'shun): preliminary treatment, usually with a drug, to prevent untoward results that may be caused by the treatment to be performed

Premenstrual syndrome (PMS): a cluster of behavioral, somatic, affective, and cognitive disorders that appears in the premenstrual (luteal) phase of the menstrual cycle and that resolve rapidly with the onset of menses

Prevalence (prev'ah-lens): the total number of cases of a specific disease or condition in existence in a given population at a certain time

Probing depth: the distance from the gingival margin to the location of the periodontal probe tip at the coronal border of attached periodontal tissues

Prodrome (pro'drom): an early or premonitory symptom of a disease

Profession: an occupation or calling that requires specialized knowledge, methods, skills, and preparation, from an institution of higher learning, in the scholarly, scientific, and historic principles underlying such methods and skill; a profession continuously enlarges its body of knowledge, functions autonomously in formulation of policy, and maintains high standards of achievement and conduct. Members of a profession are committed to continuing study, place service above personal gain, and are committed to providing practical services vital to human and social welfare.

Prognosis (prog-no'sis): a forecasting of the probable course and termination of a disease and the response to treatment; the prospect of recovery from a disease as indicated by the nature and symptoms of the case

Proliferation (pro-lif e-ra'shun): reproduction or multiplication of similar forms

Prosthodontics (pros tho-don'tiks): the branch of dentistry pertaining to the restoration and maintenance of oral function, comfort, appearance, and health of the patient by the restoration of natural teeth and/or the replacement of missing teeth and contiguous oral and maxillofacial tissues with artificial substitutes

Proteolytic (pro te-o-lit'ik): effecting the digestion of proteins

Pseudomembrane (soo'do-mem'bran): a loose membranous layer of exudate containing microorganisms, precipated fibrin, necrotic cells, and inflammatory cells produced during an inflammatory reaction on the surface of a tissue

p.s.i.: pounds per square inch

Psychosomatic (si co-so-mat'ik): pertaining to the mind-body relationship; having body symptoms of a psychic, emotional, or mental origin

Ptosis (to'sis): falling or sinking down; drooping of the upper eyelid

Ptyalin (ti'ah-lin): an enzyme occuring in the saliva that converts starch into maltose and dextrose

Pubescence (pu-bes'ens): coming to the age of puberty or sexual maturity

Public health: the science and art of preventing disease, prolonging life, and promoting physical health and efficiency through organized community efforts

Dental public health: the art of preventing and controlling dental diseases and promoting oral health through organized community efforts

Pulp stone: see **Denticle**

Pulpectomy (pul-pek'to me): the removal of the pulp chamber and root canals of a tooth

Pulpotomy (pul-pot'o-me): the removal of a portion of the pulp of a tooth, usually meaning the coronal portion

Pulse pressure (puls): the difference between systolic and diastolic blood pressure; normally 30 to 40 mm Hg

Punctate (punk'tat): marked with points or punctures differentiated from the surrounding surface by color, elevation, or texture

Purpura (pur'pu-rah): a hemorrhage into the tissues, under the skin, and through the mucous membranes; produces petechiae and ecchymoses

Thrombocytic purpura: a hemorrhage in which circulating platelets are decreased

Purulent (pu'rro-lent): containing, forming, or discharging pus

Pyorrhea (pi o-re'ah): a purulent discharge; discharge of pus. Formerly a name for advanced, severe periodontal disease

Pyramidal (pi-ram'i-dal): shaped like a pyramid

Pyramidal tracts: collections of motor nerve fibers arising in the brain and passing down through the spinal cord to motor cells in the anterior horns

Pyrexia (pi-rek'se-ah): an abnormal elevation of the body temperature above 37.0°C (98.6°F)

Pyrophosphate (pi'ro-fos'fat): inhibitor of calcification that occurs in the parotid saliva of humans in variable amounts; anticalculus component of "tartar-control" dentifrices

Q

Quadrant (kwod'rant): any one of the four parts or quarters of the dentition, with the dividing line of the maxillary or mandibular teeth at the midline between the central incisors

R

Radiotherapy: radiation therapy

Raphe (ra'fe): a ridge, furrow, or seam-like union between two parts or halves of an organ or structure

Rarefaction (rar e fak'shun): being or becoming less dense

R.D.A.: Recommended Dietary Allowances: recommendations for the average amounts of nutrients that should be consumed daily by healthy people

Recolonization (re kol'o-ni-za'shun): regrowth or multiplication of a particular bacterium or species; in periodontal therapy, the regrowth of the flora or a particular periodontal pathogen of a periodontal pocket after reduction or apparent elimination during therapy

Rectification: conversion of alternating current (AC) to direct current (DC); a rectifier changes AC to DC

Recurrent (re kur'ent): returning after intermissions

Refractory (re-frak'to-re): not readily responsive to treatment

Rehabilitation (re-ha-bil i-ta'shun): a restoration to the former state of health, efficiency, and independent action; regeneration

Reliability: the ability of an index or test procedure to measure consistently at different times and under a variety of conditions; reproducibility; consistency

Remineralization (re-min'er-al-i-za'shun): the restoration of mineral elements; enhanced by the presence of fluoride; remineralized lesions are more resistant to the initiation of dental caries than is normal tooth structure

Remission (re-mish'un): a decrease or arrest of the symptoms of a disease; also the period during which such decrease occurs

Reparative dentin: a type of secondary dentin formed along the pulpal wall as a protective mechanism; has fewer, less regular dental tubules; may form throughout life in response to extensive wear, erosion, dental caries, or restorative procedures

Replantation (re plan-ta'shun): the replacement into its own alveolar socket of a traumatically or otherwise removed tooth

Resection (re-sek'shun): an operation in which a part of a tissue or an organ is removed

   Root resection: removal of a root from a multirooted tooth

   Hemisection: removal of half of a tooth

Resorption (re-sorp'shun): removal of bone or tooth structure by pressure; gradual destruction of dentin and cementum of the root, as with the primary teeth prior to shedding; in orthodontic tooth movement, bone formation on one side compensates for resorption of bone on the other side

Rest: a rigid stabilizing extension of a fixed or removable partial denture that contacts a remaining tooth or teeth; prevents movement toward the mucosa and transmits functional forces to the teeth

Resuscitation (re-sus i-ta'shun): the restoration of life or consciousness; the restoration of heartbeat and respiration

Retinopathy (ret'i-nop'ah-the): a noninflammatory disease of the retina; identified by the chronic disease of which it is a symptom

Retrovirus (ret'ro-vi'rus): a virus with RNA core genetic material; it requires that the enzyme reverse transcriptase to convert its RNA into proviral DNA

Rh factor: agglutinogens of red blood cells responsible for isoimmune reactions such as occur in erythroblastosis fetalis and in incompatible blood transfusion; erythroblastosis fetalis results when a mother is Rh negative and develops antibodies against the fetus that is Rh positive

Rheumatic (roo-mat'ik): pertaining to or affected with rheumatism, which is a general term pertaining to conditions characterized by inflammation or pain in muscles or joints

RNA (ribonucleic acid) (ri bo-noo-kla'ik as'id): occurs in nuclei and cytoplasm of all cells; stores and transfers genetic information

Root planing: a definitive treatment procedure designed to remove altered cementum or surface dentin that is rough, impregnated with calculus, or contaminated with toxins or microorganisms

r.p.m.: revolutions per minute

Rubefacient (roo'be-fa'shent): reddening of the skin

Ruga (roo'gah): ridge, wrinkle, fold

Palatal rugae (roo'gi): the irregular ridges in the mucouse membrane covering the anterior part of the hard palate

S

Sanitation: the process by which the number of organisms on inanimate objects is reduced to a safe level. It does not imply freedom from microorganisms, and generally refers to a cleaning process

Saprophyte (sap'ro-fit): any organism that lives upon dead or decaying organic matter

Saturated (sach;e-rat'ed): holding all of a solute that can be dissolved in the solution

SBE: subacute bacterial endocarditis

Scaling: instrumentation of the crown or root surfaces to remove bacterial plaque, calculus, and stains

Sclerosis (skle-ro'sis): induration or hardening

Scoliosis (sko le o'sis): curvature of the spine

Screening:

    Population: assessment of many individuals to disclose certain characteristics or a certain disease entity

    Individual: brief assessment for initial evaluation and classification of needs for additional examination and treatment planning

Sealant: organic polymer that bonds to an enamel surface by mechanical retention accommodated by projections of the sealant into micropores created in the enamel by etching; the two types of sealants, filled and unfilled, are composed of BIS-GMA

    Filled sealant: contains, in addition to BIS-GMA, microparticles of glass, quartz, silica, and other fillers used in composite restorations; fillers make the sealant more resistant to abrasion

Sedation (se-da'shun): allaying stress, irritability, or excitement; the act of calming, especially by the administration of a sedative drug by inhalation, oral administration, or parenteral injection (intramuscular or intravenous)

    Conscious sedation: a minimally depressed level of consciousness that retains the patient's ability to maintain an airway independently and continously and to respond to verbal command or physical stimulation; may be produced by pharmacologic or nonpharmacologic methods or a combination of the two

    Deep sedation: a controlled state of depressed consciousness accompanied by the partial loss of reflexes, including inability to respond purposefully to verbal command; produced by a pharmacologic or nonpharmacologic method or a combination of the two

Seizure (se'hur): paroxysmal spell of transitory alteration in consciousness, motor activity, or sensory phenomenon; convulsion

Senescence (se-nes'ens): process or condition of growing old; physiologic aging not necessarily related to chronologic age

Senility (se-nil i-te): old age; feebleness of body and mind occurring with old age

Septum (sep'tum): a dividing wall, partition, or membrane

Sequestrum (se-kwes'trum): a piece of necrosed bone that has become separated from the surrounding bone; usually the necrosed bone is being expelled from the body

Seroconversion (se'ro-kon-ver'shun): after exposure to the etiologic agent of a disease, the blood changes from negative ("seronegative") to positive ("seropositive") serum marker for that disease; the time interval for conversion is specific for each disease

Serologic diagnosis: the identification of a disease by serum markers of that specific condition

Serum (se'rum): the clear, liquid part of blood separated from its more solid elements after clotting; the blood plasma from which fibrinogen has been removed in the process of clotting

Serum marker: a specific finding (such as an antibody or antigen) by laboratory blood analysis that identifies an existing disease state

Sharpey's fibers: penetrating connective tissue fibers by which the tooth is attached to the adjacent alveolar bone; the fiber bundles penetrate cementum on one side and alveolar bone on the other

Shedding (viral): the presence of virus in body secretions, excretions, or body surface lesions with a potential for transmission

Shelf life: the stability of an item after it has been prepared; the length of time a substance or preparation can be kept without changes occurring in its chemical structure or other properties

Sinus tract (si'nus trakt): a pathologic sinus or passage leading from an abscess cavity or hollow organ to the surface or from one cavity to another; formerly known as a fistula

Slough (sluf): a mass of dead tissue in, or cast out of, living tissue

Slurry: thin, semifluid suspension of a solid in a liquid

Smear layer: thin tenacious, amorphous layer of microcrystalline particles that remains on instrumented dentinal surfaces whenever they are cut or root planed; the particles are burnished together and on to the underlying surface in a manner that prevents the layer from being rinsed off or scrubbed away; the layer is removed during acid-etching; the particles may cover the dentinal surface and obturate the tubules

Sordes (sor'dez): foul matter that collects on the lips, teeth, and oral mucosa in low fevers; consists of debris, microorganisms, epithelial elements, and food particles; forms a crust

Space maintainer: prosthetic replacement for prematurely lost primary teeth to prevent closure of the space before eruption of the permanent successors

Speech aid prosthesis: a prosthetic device with a posterior section to assist with palatopharyngeal closure; also called a bulb, speech bulb, or prosthetic speech appliance

Splint: an apparatus, appliance, or device used to prevent motion or displacement of fractured or movable parts

Dental splint: designed to immobilize and stabilize teeth in the same dental arch

Spondylitis (spon'di-li'tis): inflammation of the vertebrae

Sporicide (spo'ri-sid): a substance that kills spores

Stabile (sta'bil): not moving, stationary, resistant; opposite of labile

Heat stabile (thermostabile): resistant to moderate degrees of heat

Status epilepticus (sta'tus ep'e-lep'ti cus): rapid succession of epileptic spasms without intervals of consciousness; life threatening; emergency care is urgent

Sterilization: a process by which all forms of life, including bacterial spores, are destroyed by physical or chemical means

STI: sexually transmitted infection

Stock: the extention of a toothbrush handle where the tufts are attached

Stomatitis (sto ma-ti'tis): inflammation of the oral mucosa because of local or systemic factors

Subclinical (sub-klin'i k'l): without clinical manifestations; said of the early stages of a disease

Subluxation (sub-luk-sa'shun): partial or incomplete dislocation: see **Luxation**

Submerged tooth (sub-merjd'): a tooth that is below the line of occlusion and may be ankylosed; intrusion; infraocclusion

Substantivity: the ability of an agent to be bound to the pellicle and tooth surface and to be released over an extended period of time with the retention of its potency

Subsurface lesion: a demineralized area below the surface of the enamel created by acid that has passed through micropores between enamel rods; is subject of remineralization by the action of fluoride

Subtraction radiography: a photographic or digital method of eliminating background anatomic structures from the final image, thus bringing out the differences between the pre- and postprocedure radiographic images

    Digital subtraction radiography: a radiographic image subtraction method in which the pre- and postprocedure radiographic images are digitized into the computer memory; these images are subtracted from each other within the computer memory, and the resultant subtracted image is displayed on the monitor

Sulcular (sul'ku-lar) **brushing:** a method in which the end-rounded filament tips are activated at and just below the gingival margin for the purpose of loosening and removing bacterial plaque from the gingival sulcus

Supernumerary tooth (su per-nu'mer-ar e): extra tooth; one that is in excess of the normal number

Supersaturated (soo'per-sat'u-rat-ed): a solution containing more of an ingredient than can be held in solution permanently

Supervision: a term applied to the legal relationship between the dentist and the dental hygienist in a practice. Each practice act defines the type of supervision required

Supine (soo'pin): a flat position with the head and feet on the same level

Supportive periodontal treatment: an extension of periodontal therapy; includes procedures performed at selected time intervals to review the general health history, reassess the status of periodontal health, and provide preventive oral hygiene care; also called **periodontal maintenance** or **preventive maintenance**

Suppuration (sup u-ra'shun): the formation of pus

Suture (su'chur): a stitch or series of stitches made to secure apposition of the edges of a surgical or traumatic wound

    Absorbable suture: becomes absorbed in body fluids and disappears

Continuous suture: made with an uninterruped length that connects each stitch with the previous one

Interrupted suture: one in which each stitch is made with a separate piece of material

Swage (swaj): to fuse, as with suture material, to the end of a suture needle

Sympathetic nervous system: that part of the autonomic (involuntary) nervous system that arises in the thoracic and first three lumbar segments of the spinal cord

Syncope (sin'ko-pe): a temporary loss of consciousness caused by a sudden fall in blood pressure, resulting in generalized cerebral ischemia; commonly referred to as fainting

Syndrome (sin'drom): a group of symptoms and signs that, when considered together, characterize a disease or lesion

Synergistic (sin er-jis'tik): acting jointly; enhancing the effect of another drug, force, or agent

Systemic (sis-tem'ik): pertaining to or affecting the whole body

Systole (sis'to-le): the contraction, or period of contraction, of the heart, especially the ventricles, during which blood is forced into the aorta and the pulmonary artery; systolic pressure is the highest, or greatest pressure

T

Tachycardia (tak'e-kar'de-ah): an unusually fast heart beat; at a rate greater than 100 beats per minute

Tactile (tak'til): pertaining to the touch; perceptible to the touch

Tactile discrimination: the ability to distinguish relative degrees of roughness and smoothness; also called tactile sensitivity

Taste bud: a receptor of taste on the tongue and oropharynx; goblet-shaped cells oriented at right angles to the surface of the epithelium

Tardive dyskinesia (tar'div dis-ki-ne'ze-ah): involuntary movements of the mouth, lips, tongue, and jaws; usually associated with long-term use of antipsychotic medication

Temporomandibular disorder (TMD): a collective term that includes a wide range of disorders of the masticatory system that are characterized by one or more of the following: pain in the preauricular area, temporomandibular joint (TMJ), and muscles of mastication, with limitation or deviation in mandibular motion and TMJ sounds during mandibular function

Tensile strength: the maximum stress that a material is capable of sustaining; usually expressed in pounds per square inch (psi)

Tensile: susceptible to extension; capable of being stretched

Tension test: the application of tension at the mucogingival junction by retracting the cheek, lip, and tongue to tighten the alveolar mucosa and test for the presence of attached gingiva; an area of missing attached gingiva is revealed when the alveolar mucosa and the frena are connected directly to the free gingiva

Teratogen (ter'ah-to-jen): nongenetic factors that cause malformation and disease syndromes in utero

Teratoma (ter a to'mah): a neoplasm composed of multiple tissues, including tissues not normally found in the organ in which it arises

Therapeutic (ther ah-pu'tik): pertaining to the treating or curing of disease; curative

Therapy (ther'ah-pe): the treatment of disease

Threshold (thresh'old): that amount of stimulus that just produces a sensation

Pain threshold: that amount of stimulation that just produces a sensation of pain

Thrombus (throm'bus): a blood clot attached to the intima of a blood vessel; may occlude the lumen; contrast with embolus

TIA: transient ischemic attack; a brief episode of cerebral ischemia that results in no permanent neurologic damage; symptoms are warning signals of impending CVA (stroke)

Tic: an involuntary purposeless movement of muscle that usually occurs under emotional stress; a twitching, especially of facial muscles

Tincture (tingk'chur): an alcoholic solution of a drug or other chemical substance

Tinnitus (ti-ni'tus): noise in the ears; ringing, buzzing, or roaring

Titanium: a uniquely biocompatible metal used for implants, either in the commercially pure form or as an alloy

Titanium alloy: the most common titanium alloy (Ti-6AI-4V) used for dental implants contains 6% aluminum to increase strength and decrease weight and 4% vanadium to prevent corrosion

Tomography: a radiographic technique that provides a distinct image of a selected plane through the body; the images of structures that lie above and below that plane are blurred

Tone (ton): the normal degree of vigor and tension; a healthy state of a part

Tonguetie (tung'ti): abnormal shortness of the frenum of the tongue, resulting in limitation of the motion of that organ

Tongue thrust: the infantile pattern of the suckleswallow movement in which the tongue is placed between the incisor teeth or alveolar ridges; may result in an anterior open bite, deformation of the jaws, and abnormal function

Topical (top'i-k'l): on the surface; pertaining to a particular spot; local

Topography (to-pog'rah-fe): the detailed description and analysis of the features of an anatomic region or of a specific part

Torus (to'rus): a bony elevation or prominence usually located on the midline of the hard palate (torus palatinus) and the lingual surface of the mandible in the premolar area (torus mandibularis)

Tourette's syndrome: multiple motor and one or more vocal tics; may involve squatting, twirling, grunts, barks, sniffs, and coprolalia

Toxic (tok'sik): poisonous

Toxicity (toks-is'i-te): the state or quality of being poisonous; the degree of virulence of a toxic microbe or a poison; the capacity of a drug to damage body tissue or seriously impair body functions

Toxin (tok'sin): any poisonous substance of a microbial, vegetable, or animal origin that causes symptoms after a period of incubation; can induce the elaboration of specific antitoxins in suitable animals

Toxoid (tok'soid): a toxin treated by heat or a chemical agent to destroy its deleterious properties without destroying its ability to combine with, or stimulate the formation of, antitoxin (e.g., tetanus, diphtheria)

Tracheotomy (tra ke-ot'o-me): a surgical operation to provide an artificial opening into the trachea

Transdermal medication: a drug delivered by a patch on the skin; a mode for slow release over extended time

Transmissible (trans mis'si b'l): capable of being carried across from one person to another

Transmission (horizontal): the passage of an infectious agent from one individual to another

  Vertical transmission: the passage of an infectious agent from one generation to another by breast milk or across the placenta

Transplant (trans'plant): tissue removed from one part of the body and placed at a different site

Transplantation (trans-plan-ta'shun): implanting a tissue or organ that has been taken from another part of the same body or from another person

  Autotransplantation: transfer of a tissue or organ to another place in the same person

Trauma (traw'mah): an injury; damage; impairment; external violence, producing body injury or degeneration

Trauma from occlusion: injury to the periodontium that results from occlusal forces in excess of the reparative capacity of the attachment apparatus; also called occlusal traumatism

Treatment (tret'ment): the management and care of a patient for the purpose of curing a disease or disorder

Tremor (trem'or): involuntary trembling or quivering

Trendelenburg (tren-del'en-berg): the modified supine position when the head is lower than the heart

Trimester: a period of three months; one third of a pregnancy

Trismus (triz'mus): motor disturbance of the trigeminal nerve, especially spasm of the masticatory muscles with difficulty in opening the mouth

Tuberculin test (Mantoux) (too-ber'ku-lin test) (Mantoo'): a test for the presence of active or inactive tuberculosis

U

Ulceration (ul'se-ra'shun): the formation or development of an ulcer with a loss of epithelial surface and sloughing of necrotic inflammatory tissue

Universal precautions: an approach to infection control in which all human blood and certain human body fluids are treated as if known to be infectious for HIV, HBV, and other blood-borne pathogens

U.S.R.D.A.: United States Recommended Daily Allowance;

used for labeling purposes for protein, five vitamins, and two minerals

Urticaria (ur ti-ka're-ah): hives; nettle rash; an eruption of itching wheals usually of systemic origin. May be caused by a state of hypersensitivity to foods or drugs, foci of infection, physical agents (heat, cold, light, friction), or psychic stimuli

V

Validity: the ability of an index or test procedure to measure what it is intended to measure

Vector (vek'tor): a carrier that transfers an infectious microorganism from one host to another

   Biologic vector: an arthropod vector in whose body the infecting organisms multiply before becoming infective to the recipient

Vehicle (ve'i k'l): a substance possessing little or no medicinal action, used as a medium to confer a suitable consistency or form to a drug

Velopharyngeal insufficiency (vel'-o-fah-rin'je-al): an anatomic or functional deficiency in the soft palate or the muscle affecting closure of the opening between the mouth and nose in speech; results in a nasal speech quality

Velum (ve'lum): a covering structure or veil

   Palatine velum (or velum palatinum): the soft palate

Veneer: a layer of tooth-colored material (composite or porcelain) that is bonded or cemented to a prepared tooth surface

Ventral (ven'tral): anterior, front surface: opposite of dorsal surface

Verruca (ve-roo'kah): a wart-like growth

Vertigo (ver'ti-go): the sensation of rotation or movement of one's self (subjective vertigo) or of one's surroundings (objective vertigo); a subtype of dizziness, but not a synonym

Viron (vi're-on): a complete virus particle made up of the **nucleoid** (genetic material) and **capsid** (the protein shell that protects the necleoid)

Virulence (vir'u-lens): the degree of pathogenicity or the disease-evoking power of an infectious agent

Virulent (vir'u-lent): capable of causing infection or disease

Virus (vi'rus): a subcellular genetic entity capable of gaining entrance into a limited range of living cells and capable of replication only within such cells; a virus contains either DNA or RNA, but not both

Viscosity (vis-kos'i-te): stickiness; ability of a fluid to resist change in shape or arrangement during flow

Visible-light cure: light activation using a photocure system; shorter curing time than sel-cure (chemical cure); does not start setting until the light is activated, thereby allowing longer working time for adapting the material

Volatile (vol'ah-til): tending to evaporate readily

W

Waste:

Infectious: capable of causing an infectious disease

Contaminated: items that have contacted blood or other body secretions

Hazardous: poses a risk to humans or the environment

Toxic: capable of having a poisonous effect

Regulated: contaminated, hazardous, and otherwise useless waste that requires special disposal methods outlined by the OSHA

Wheal (hweel, wel): an acute, circumscribed transitory area of edema of the skin; an urticarial lesion; see **Urticaria**

White spot: a term used to describe a small area on the surface of enamel that contrasts in appearance with the rest of the surface and may be visible only when the tooth is dried; two types of white spots can be differentiated: an area of demineralization and an area of fluorosis (also referred to as an "enamel opacity")

Whitlow (hwit'lo): a purulent infection or abscess involving the end of a finger; also called a felon

Window period: the time between exposure resulting in infection and the presence of detectable serum antibody; the antibody test is negative but the infectious agent is transmissible during the window period

X

Xeroradiography (ze'ro-ra'de-og'rah-fe): a dry process that produces prints of x-ray images by means of a seleniumplate, which records an image through the radiation-induced discharge of a positive electrostatic potential

Xerosis (ze-ro'sis): an abnormal dryness with particular reference to the eye (xerophthalmia), skin (xeroderma), or mouth (xerostomia); it may be a result or sign of certain nutritional deficiencies, drugs, or medical conditions

Xerostomia (ze ro-sto me-ah): dryness of the mouth caused by functional or organic disturbances of the salivary glands

REFERENCE

1. Addy, M.: Etiology and Clinical Implications of Dentine Hypersensitivity, *Dent. Clin. North Am., 34,* 503, July, 1990.

INDEX